MACHINE LEARNING AND DEEP LEARNING TECHNIQUES FOR MEDICAL SCIENCE

Artificial Intelligence (AI): Elementary to Advanced Practices

Series Editors: Vijender Kumar Solanki, Zhongyu (Joan) Lu, and Valentina E Balas

In the emerging smart city technology and industries, the role of artificial intelligence is getting more prominent. This AI book series will aim to cover the latest AI work, which will help the naïve user to get support in solving existing problems and for the experienced AI practitioners it will assist in shedding light on new avenues in the AI domains. The series will cover the recent work carried out in AI and its associated domains; it will cover Logics, Pattern Recognition, NLP, Expert Systems, Machine Learning, Block-Chain, and Big Data. The work domain of AI is quite deep, so it will be covering the latest trends that are evolving with the concepts of AI and it will be helping those new to the field, practitioners, students, as well as researchers, to gain some new insights.

Enabling Technologies for Next Generation Wireless Communications
Edited by Mohammed Usman, Mohd Wajid, and Mohd Dilshad Ansari

Artificial Intelligence (AI)
Recent Trends and Applications
Edited by S. Kanimozhi Suguna, M. Dhivya, and Sara Paiva

Deep Learning for Biomedical Applications
Edited by Utku Kose, Omer Deperlioglu, and D. Jude Hemanth

Cybersecurity
Ambient Technologies, IoT, and Industry 4.0 Implications
Gautam Kumar, Om Prakash Singh, and Hemraj Saini

Industrial Internet of Things
Technologies, Design, and Applications
Edited by Sudan Jha, Usman Tariq, Gyanendra Prasad Joshi, and Vijender Kumar Solanki

Machine Learning And Deep Learning Techniques For Medical Science
Edited by K. Gayathri Devi, Kishore Balasubramanian and Le Anh Ngoc

For more information on this series, please visit: https://www.routledge.com/Artificial-Intelligence-AI-Elementary-to-Advanced-Practices/book-series/CRCAIEAP

MACHINE LEARNING AND DEEP LEARNING TECHNIQUES FOR MEDICAL SCIENCE

Edited by
K. Gayathri Devi, Kishore Balasubramanian, and Le Anh Ngoc

CRC Press
Taylor & Francis Group
Boca Raton London New York

CRC Press is an imprint of the
Taylor & Francis Group, an **informa** business

First edition published 2022
by CRC Press
6000 Broken Sound Parkway NW, Suite 300, Boca Raton, FL 33487-2742

and by CRC Press
4 Park Square, Milton Park, Abingdon, Oxon, OX14 4RN

CRC Press is an imprint of Taylor & Francis Group, LLC

Library of Congress Cataloging-in-Publication Data
Names: Gayathri Devi, K. G., editor.
Title: Machine learning and deep learning techniques for medical science / edited by K. Gayathri Devi, Kishore Balasubramanian, Le Anh Ngoc.
Description: First edition. | Boca Raton : CRC Press, 2022. |
Series: Artificial intelligence (AI): elementary to advanced practices | Includes bibliographical references and index. |
Summary: "This book presents the integration of machine learning and deep learning algorithms that can be applied in the healthcare sector to reduce the time needed by doctors, radiologists, and other medical professionals to analyze, predict, and diagnose conditions with accurate results"-- Provided by publisher.
Identifiers: LCCN 2021059672 (print) | LCCN 2021059673 (ebook) | ISBN 9781032104201 (hardback) | ISBN 9781032108827 (paperback) | ISBN 9781003217497 (ebook)
Subjects: LCSH: Medical informatics. | Machine learning. | Deep learning (Machine learning) | Artificial intelligence--Medical applications. | Medical technology.
Classification: LCC R858 .M316 2022 (print) | LCC R858 (ebook) | DDC 610.285--dc23/eng/20220120
LC record available at https://lccn.loc.gov/2021059672
LC ebook record available at https://lccn.loc.gov/2021059673

ISBN: 978-1-032-10420-1 (hbk)
ISBN: 978-1-032-10882-7 (pbk)
ISBN: 978-1-003-21749-7 (ebk)

DOI: 10.1201/9781003217497

Typeset in Times
by MPS Limited, Dehradun

Contents

Editor Biographies ix
List of Contributors xi

Chapter 1 **A Comprehensive Study on MLP and CNN, and the Implementation of Multi-Class Image Classification using Deep CNN** 1

S. P. Balamurugan

Chapter 2 **An Efficient Technique for Image Compression and Quality Retrieval in Diagnosis of Brain Tumour Hyper Spectral Image** 27

V. V. Teresa, J. Dhanasekar, V. Gurunathan, and T. Sathiyapriya

Chapter 3 **Classification of Breast Thermograms using a Multi-layer Perceptron with Back Propagation Learning** 45

Aayesha Hakim and R. N. Awale

Chapter 4 **Neural Networks for Medical Image Computing** 75

V. A. Pravina, P. K. Poonguzhali, and A. Kishore Kumar

Chapter 5 **Recent Trends in Bio-Medical Waste, Challenges and Opportunities** 97

S. Kannadhasan and R. Nagarajan

Chapter 6 **Teager-Kaiser Boost Clustered Segmentation of Retinal Fundus Images for Glaucoma Detection** 109

P M Siva Raja, R P Sumithra, and K Ramanan

Chapter 7 **IoT-Based Deep Neural Network Approach for Heart Rate and SpO_2 Prediction** 121

Madhusudan G. Lanjewar, Rajesh K. Parate, Rupesh D. Wakodikar, and Anil J. Thusoo

Chapter 8 **An Intelligent System for Diagnosis and Prediction of Breast Cancer Malignant Features using Machine Learning Algorithms** 143

Ritu Aggarwal

Chapter 9 **Medical Image Classification with Artificial and Deep Convolutional Neural Networks: A Comparative Study** 153

Amen Bidani, Mohamed Salah Gouider, and Carlos M Travieso-Gonzalez

Chapter 10 **Convolutional Neural Network for Classification of Skin Cancer Images** 175

Giang Son Tran, Quoc Viet Kieu, and Thi Phuong Nghiem

Chapter 11 **Application of Artificial Intelligence in Medical Imaging** 195

Sampurna Panda and Rakesh Kumar Dhaka

Chapter 12 **Machine Learning Algorithms Used in Medical Field with a Case Study** 203

M. Jayasanthi and R. Kalaivani

Chapter 13 **Dual Customized U-Net-based Based Automated Diagnosis of Glaucoma** 221

C. Thirumarai Selvi, J. Amudha, and R. Sudhakar

Chapter 14 **MuSCF-Net: Multi-scale, Multi-Channel Feature Network using Resnet-Based Attention Mechanism for Breast Histopathological Image Classification** 243

Meenakshi M. Pawer, Suvarna D. Pujari, Swati P. Pawar, and Sanjay N. Talbar

Chapter 15 **Artificial Intelligence is Revolutionizing Cancer Research** 263

B. Sudha, K. Suganya, K. Swathi, and S. Sumathi

Chapter 16 **Deep Learning to Diagnose Diseases and Security in 5G Healthcare Informatics** 279

Partha Ghosh

Chapter 17 New Approaches in Machine-based Image Analysis for Medical Oncology 333

E. Francy Irudaya Rani, T. LurthuPushparaj, E. Fantin Irudaya Raj, and M. Appadurai

Chapter 18 Performance Analysis of Deep Convolutional Neural Networks for Diagnosing COVID-19: Data to Deployment 361

K. Deepti

Chapter 19 Stacked Auto Encoder Deep Neural Network with Principal Components Analysis for Identification of Chronic Kidney Disease 385

Sanat Kumar Sahu and Pratibha Verma

Index 397

Editor Biographies

Dr. K. Gayathri Devi has 21 years of experience working as a Professor in the Department of Electronics and Communication Engineering, Dr. N.G.P Institute of Technology, Tamil Nadu, India. She received her B.E. degree in ECE from Coimbatore Institute of Technology (1998), and M.E degree from Dr Mahalingam College of Engineering and Technology, (2005) and Ph.D. from Medical Image Processing (2016) under the affiliation of Anna University, Chennai. She has published 3 patents, 26 papers, 3 book chapters, and 24 conference publications. She is an editor of the book "Artificial Intelligence Trends for Data Analytics Using Machine Learning and Deep Learning Approaches" published by CRC Press, Taylor & Francis Group. She is also a reviewer of several SCI and Scopus indexed journals. She has completed 21 online certification courses from NPTEL, Coursera, Mathworks and Great Learning and Topper in the NPTEL courses "Digital Image Processing of Remote Sensing Images" and "Outcome based pedagogic principles for effective teaching". Received Grant from Anna University Chennai and ICMR to conduct programmes. She is a life member in ISTE, IETE and IAENG.

Dr. Kishore Balasubramanian has more than 17 years of academic experience in imparting Engineering Education. He received his Bachelor's Degree in Electronics and Instrumentation from Bharathiar University, India, Master's Degree in Applied Electronics from Anna University, India and Ph.D. (Information and Communication Engineering) from Anna University, India. His research interests include Medical Image Processing and Computer Vision. He is an active reviewer in many SCI and Scopus indexed journals, conferences and editor in several scientific international journals. He has authored three books in the field of Analog Electronics and has published papers in international and national journals. He has received grants from CSIR, DRDO (Government Funding agencies) for conducting Faculty Development Programmes, Workshops and Conferences. He is a member of ISTE, IRED and IAENG. Presently he is working as an Assistant Professor (Senior Scale) in the Department of EEE and holds the additional portfolio as Training Officer (Career Planning and Guidance Cell) at Dr. Mahalingam College of Engineering & Technology, India.

Dr. Le Anh Ngoc is a Director of Swinburne Innovation Space, Swinburne University of Technology (Vietnam). He received his B.S in Mathematics and Informatics from Vinh University and VNU University of Science, Master's degree in Information Technology from Hanoi University of Technology, Vietnam, and Ph.D. degree in Communication and Information Engineering from the School of Electrical Engineering and Computer Science, Kyungpook National University, South Korea, in 2009. His general research interests are Embedded and Intelligent Systems, Communication Networks, the Internet of Things, Image/Video Processing, AI & Big Data Analysis. On these topics, he published more than 60 papers in International journals and Conference proceedings. He served as a Keynote Speaker, TPC member, Session chair, Book Editor, and Reviewer of The international conferences and journals (Email: nle@swin.edu.au).

Contributors

Ritu Aggarwal
Maharishi Markandeshwar Institute of Computer Technology and Business Management
Mullana, Ambala, Haryana, India

J. Amudha
Department of EEE
Dr Mahalingam College of Engineering and Technology
Pollachi, Tamil Nadu, India

M. Appadurai
Department of Mechanical Engineering
Dr. Sivanthi Aditanar College of Engineering
Tamil Nadu, India

R. N. Awale
Veermata Jijabai Technological Institute
Mumbai, India

S. P. Balamurugan
Department of Computer and Information Science
Faculty of Science
Annamalai University
Tamil Nadu, India

Amen Bidani
SMART Lab, ISG
University of Tunis
Tunis, Tunisia

Rakesh Kumar Dhaka
School of Nursing Sciences
ITM University
Gwalior, India

J. Dhanasekar
Department of ECE
Sri Eshwar College of Engineering
Coimbatore, Tamil Nadu, India

K. Deepti
Dept of ECE
Vasavi College of Engineering(A)
Osmania University
Hyderabad, India

Partha Ghosh
Department of Computer Science and Engineering
Government College of Engineering and Ceramic Technology
Kolkata, West Bengal, India

Mohamed Salah Gouider
SMART Lab, ISG
University of Tunis
Tunis, Tunisia

V. Gurunathan
Department of ECE
Dr. Mahalingam College of Engineering and Technology
Pollachi, Tamil Nadu, India

Aayesha Hakim
Veermata Jijabai Technological Institute
Mumbai, India

M. Jayasanthi
Department of ECE
PSG Institute of Technology and Applied Research
Coimbatore, Tamil Nadu, India

A. Kishore Kumar
Department of Robotics & Automation
Sri Ramakrishna Engineering College
Coimbatore, Tamil Nadu, India

R. Kalaivani
Department of ECE
Erode Sengunthar Engineering College
Erode, Tamil Nadu, India

S. Kannadhasan
Department of Electronics and Communication Engineering
Cheran College of Engineering
Tamil Nadu, India

Quoc Viet Kieu
ICTLab
University of Science and Technology of Hanoi
Vietnam Academy of Science and Technology
Hanoi, Vietnam

Madhusudan G Lanjewar
School of Physical and Applied Sciences
Goa University
Taleigao Plateau, Goa, India

R. Nagarajan
Department of Electrical and Electronics Engineering
Gnanamani College of Technology
Tamil Nadu, India

Thi Phuong Nghiem
ICTLab
University of Science and Technology of Hanoi
Vietnam Academy of Science and Technology
Hanoi, Vietnam

Sampurna Panda
Department of EC&EE
Institute of Technology & Management
Gwalior, India

Rajesh K. Parate
Department of Electronics
S. K. Porwal College
Kamptee, India

Swati P. Pawar
Department of Electronics and Telecommunication Engineering
SVERIs College of Engineering Pandharpur
University of PAH
Solapur, India

Meenakshi M. Pawer
Department of Electronics and Telecommunication Engineering
SVERIs College of Engineering
Pandharpur
University of PAH
Solapur, India

P. K. Poonguzhali
Department of Electronics and Communication Engineering
Hindusthan College of Engineering and Technology
Tamil Nadu, India

V. A. Pravina
Department of Electronics and Communication Engineering
DMI College of Engineering
Tamil Nadu, India

Suvarna D. Pujari
Department of Electronics and Telecommunication Engineering
SVERIs College of Engineering Pandharpur
University of PAH
Solapur, India

T. Lurthu Pushparaj
Department of Chemistry (PG), TDMNS College
Tamil Nadu, India

E. Fantin Irudaya Raj
Department of Electrical and Electronics Engineering
Dr. Sivanthi Aditanar College of Engineering
Tamil Nadu, India

K Ramanan
Rohini College of Engineering and Technology
Tamil Nadu, India

E. Francy Irudaya Rani
Department of Electronics and Communication Engineering
Francis Xavier Engineering College
Tamil Nadu, India

Sanat Kumar Sahu
Department of Computer Science
Govt. K.P.G. College Jagdalpur (C.G.)
Chhattisgarh, India

T. Sathiyapriya
Department of ECE
Dr. Mahalingam College of Engineering and Technology
Pollachi, Tamil Nadu, India

C. Thirumarai Selvi
Department of ECE, Sri Krishna College of Engineering and Technology
Coimbatore, Tamil Nadu, India

Siva Raja P M
Amrita College of Engineering and Technology
Nagercoil, India

Sudha B
Department of Biochemistry
Biotechnology and Bioinformatics
Avinashilingam Institute for Home Science and Higher Education for Women
Coimbatore, Tamil Nadu, India

R. Sudhakar
Department of ECE
Dr Mahalingam College of Engineering and Technology
Pollachi, Tamil Nadu, India

Suganya K
Department of Biochemistry
Biotechnology and Bioinformatics
Avinashilingam Institute for Home Science and Higher Education for Women
Coimbatore, Tamil Nadu, India

Sumathi S
Department of Biochemistry
Biotechnology and Bioinformatics
Avinashilingam Institute for Home Science and Higher Education for Women
Coimbatore, Tamil Nadu, India

Swathi K
Department of Biochemistry
Biotechnology and Bioinformatics
Avinashilingam Institute for Home Science and Higher Education for Women
Coimbatore, Tamil Nadu, India

Sanjay N. Talbar
Department of Electronics and Telecommunication Engineering
SGGS, Nanded
Maharashtra, India

V. V. Teresa
Department of ECE
Sri Eshwar College of Engineering
Coimbtaore, Tamil Nadu, India

Anil J Thusoo
Govt. Secondary School
Kupwara, India

Giang Son Tran
ICTLab
University of Science and Technology of Hanoi
Vietnam Academy of Science and Technology
Hanoi, Vietnam

Carlos M Travieso-Gonzalez
IDeTIC
Universidad de Las Palmas de Gran Canaria
Las Palmas, Spain

Pratibha Verma
Department of Computer Science
Dr. C.V. Raman University Bialspur (C.G.)
Chhattisgarh, India

Rupesh D Wakodikar
Department of Electronics
N. H. College
Bramhapuri, India

1 A Comprehensive Study on MLP and CNN, and the Implementation of Multi-Class Image Classification using Deep CNN

S.P. Balamurugan
Assistant Professor/Programmer, Department of Computer and Information Science, Faculty of Science, Annamalai University, Tamil Nadu, India

CONTENTS

1.1 Introduction ... 2
1.2 The Processes of the Neural Network ... 2
1.2.1 Basics of Neural Network ... 2
1.2.1.1 Architecture of Neural Network ... 3
1.2.1.2 Working Principles of Neural Network ... 3
1.2.1.3 Learning Methods of Neural Network ... 4
1.2.1.4 Drawbacks of Neural Network ... 4
1.2.2 Convolutional Neural Network (CNN) Algorithm ... 5
1.2.2.1 Merits of CNN over MLP ... 5
1.2.2.2 Contents of CNN ... 5
1.2.2.3 Working of CNN Algorithm ... 5
1.2.2.4 Deep CNN ... 10
1.3 Experimental Procedure ... 11
1.3.1 Preparing the Dataset ... 11
1.3.2 Model Training and Testing ... 11
1.4 Results and Discussion ... 12
1.4.1 MNIST Dataset Image Classifications ... 12
1.4.2 CIFAR-10 Dataset Image Classifications ... 16
1.5 Conclusion ... 22
References ... 24

DOI: 10.1201/9781003217497-1

1.1 INTRODUCTION

Its use in various fields has increased as the efficiency of computer-assisted image processing has improved. Basic image processing techniques include restoration, enhancement, segmentation, and classification, etc. Image classification is critical in image processing. The goal of image classification is to assign images to the same class category automatically [1]. The classification may be carried out in two ways such as supervised and unsupervised. The two processes involved in image classification are training and testing. During training, the visual features are retrieved and combined to generate a unique description for each class. Depending on the type of classification challenge, such as binary or multi-class classification, the preceding method is repeated for all classes. The test images are presented to the trained model to categorize the class during testing. This assigning of classes is done based on the training features. Deep learning, also known as hierarchical learning has been a hot topic in machine learning research since 2006. Deep learning is a class of machine learning algorithms that use multiple layers of non-linear information processing for supervised or unsupervised feature extraction, transformation, pattern analysis, and classification, according to a standard definition [2]. One of the most widely used types of ANN approaches is the MLP approach. It is a member of the ANN's FFNN class structure. An FFNN framework of MLP comprises neuron that is gathered in layers. In the MLP method, the entire input nodes in input and hidden layers are dispersed to several hidden layers [3,4]. The CNN is applied in image prediction and classification, and a minimal rate of error is accomplished that is less than the maximum human error rate [5,6]. Additionally in [6], CNN is utilized for training the maximum number of images and classifying the tomato leaf's diseases. It is one of the interventions in CNN which has accomplished maximum prediction and classification. The DCNN model will convolve more of the input data. It extracts more relevant features and achieves better accuracy for bigger datasets than CNN [7,8]. In [7], DCNN is employed for classifying the interstitial lung infection from CT imaging, and in [8]; it is used to determine whether COVID-19 is present in radiological imaging.

The goal of this study is to show that a Deep Convolutional Neural Network (DCNN) is effective at image classification. The datasets used for testing the algorithm includes handwritten digits and various objects like automobile, deer, horse, ship, etc [9,10]. The residual of the chapter is laid out as follows. The processes of MLP, CNN, and DCNN are explained in Section 1.2. The experimental approach is described in Section 1.3. Finally, Section 1.4 discusses the experimental results achieved with the models offered.

1.2 THE PROCESSES OF THE NEURAL NETWORK

The Neural Network's operation is split into two portions. Section 1.2.1 describes the fundamental concepts of Neural Network and Section 1.2.2 elaborates the working principles of CNN and the function of layers.

1.2.1 Basics of Neural Network

Neural networks are mathematical models that store information using learning techniques inspired by the brain. A neural network's building blocks are perceptrons, which are similar to biological bricks. The output of a network with a single perceptron will be in binary format. A multilayer perceptron (MLP) is created when more than one perceptron is present and connected in a layered fashion to form a neural network. In MLP, the first layer's output is fed into the second, and so on, until the output layer adds up the entire activation. The network's final decision is aided by the entire activation. Because neural networks are employed in machines, they are referred to as 'Artificial Neural Networks'.

1.2.1.1 Architecture of Neural Network

It is composed of three parts:

- Input layer
  Initial data gave through this layer and it represents the dimensions of the input vector.
- Hidden (computation) layers
  This layer serves as a bridge between the input and output layers, performing all computations.
- Output layer

For a given input, generate the ultimate outcome (Figure 1.1).

1.2.1.2 Working Principles of Neural Network

Consider a neural network with two input values, single hidden layer with three nodes, and two output layer nodes at the end (Figure 1.2).

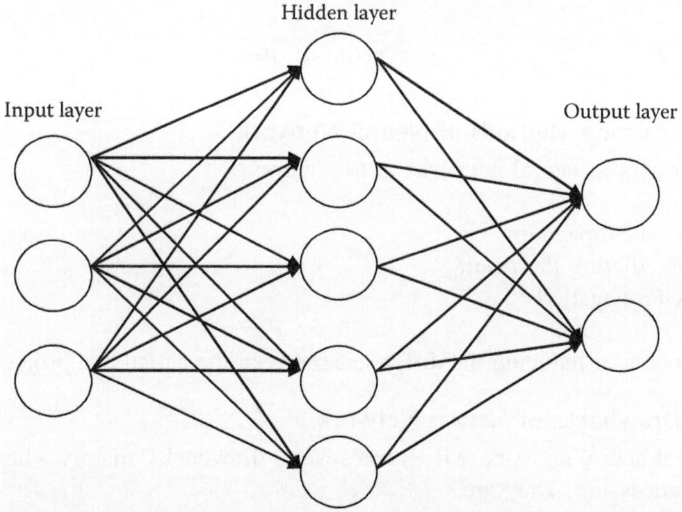

FIGURE 1.1 Neural network architecture.

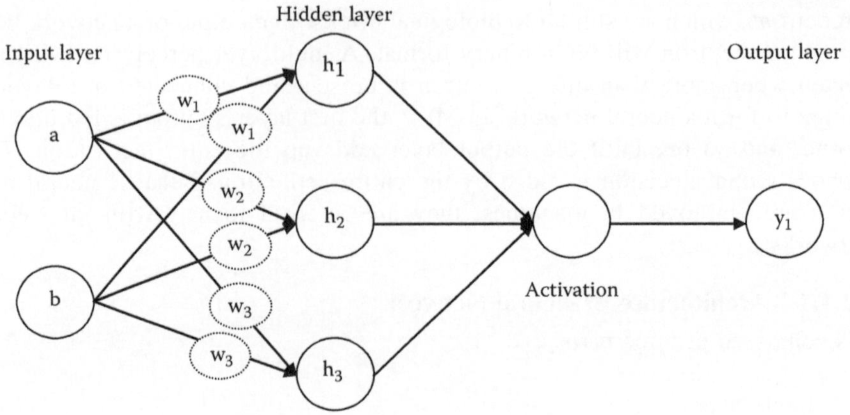

FIGURE 1.2 Neural network with weights and activation.

Step 1 Initialize the weights w1, w2, and w3 at random
Step 2 Data from the input layer is multiplied by corresponding weights and given to the hidden layer

$$h_1 = (a^*w_1) + (b^*w_1)$$
$$h_2 = (a^*w_2) + (b^*w_2)$$
$$h_3 = (a^*w_3) + (b^*w_3)$$

Step 3 The projected outcome is obtained by passing the output of the hidden layer through a non-linear function known as the activation function

$$y\_ = fn\,(h_1, h_2, h_3)$$

1.2.1.3 Learning Methods of Neural Network

Learning occurs in neural networks in two ways:

- Forward-Propagation
  It is predicting the result
- Back-Propagation

It is the process of reducing the difference between the actual and projected results

1.2.1.4 Drawbacks of Neural Network

A traditional neural network (MLP) has several drawbacks, mainly when it comes to image processing. They are,

- The quantity of weights hastily will become unmanageable for huge images

- Cannot handle translations, that is they are not translation invariant
- Loses the spatial information when the image is flattened

1.2.2 Convolutional Neural Network (CNN) Algorithm

The name 'Convolutional Neural Network' refers to the network's use of the mathematical process convolution, which is a type of linear operation. This section explains the merits of CNN, contents of CNN, working principles of CNN algorithm, and Deep CNN briefly.

1.2.2.1 Merits of CNN over MLP

CNN is extensively used for image classification and object detection. It has several advantages over MLP. They are,

- CNN's are capable of working with image data in 2D. So, there is no need to flatten the input images to 1D like MLP. It helps in retaining the spatial properties of images.
- It finds the relevant traits without the need for human intervention
- It converges faster than the MLP model
- It has the highest accuracy than MLP in image prediction
- It is also computationally efficient

1.2.2.2 Contents of CNN

A CNN is made up of layers, each of which uses a differential equation to convert one volume of activations to another. It means that each layer converts data from values and passes it along to the next layers for further generalization. Typically, the CNN is made up of two components. They are,

- Convolution block – It is made up of two layers: a convolution layer and a pooling layer. The feature extraction process would not be complete without this block.
- Fully Connected block – It is made out of a simple neural network design that is fully connected. Based on the convolutional block's input, this block does categorization (Figure 1.3).

1.2.2.3 Working of CNN Algorithm

Convolutional layers, pooling layers, and fully connected layers are the three layers that play a key part in the CNN algorithm's operation. There are two more important parameters to consider: the drop out layer and the activation function, both of which are detailed further below Figure 1.4.

1.2.2.3.1 Convolution Layer

The input images are processed using convolution layers to extract various information. Convolution is conducted between the input image and a filter of a given size, such as M x N, in this case. The dot product is calculated between the filter and

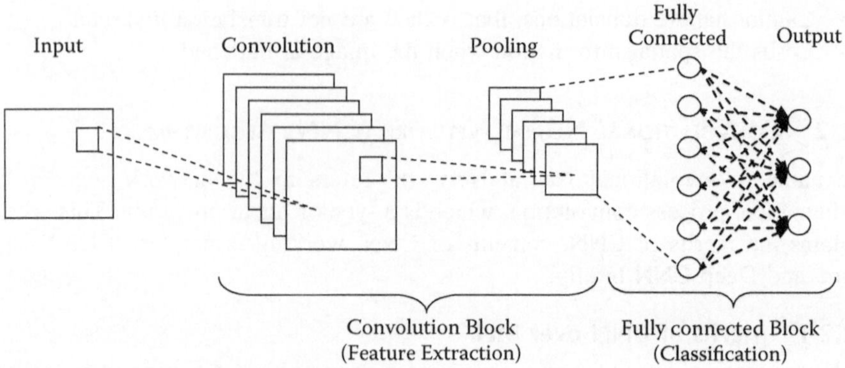

FIGURE 1.3 Basic architecture of CNN.

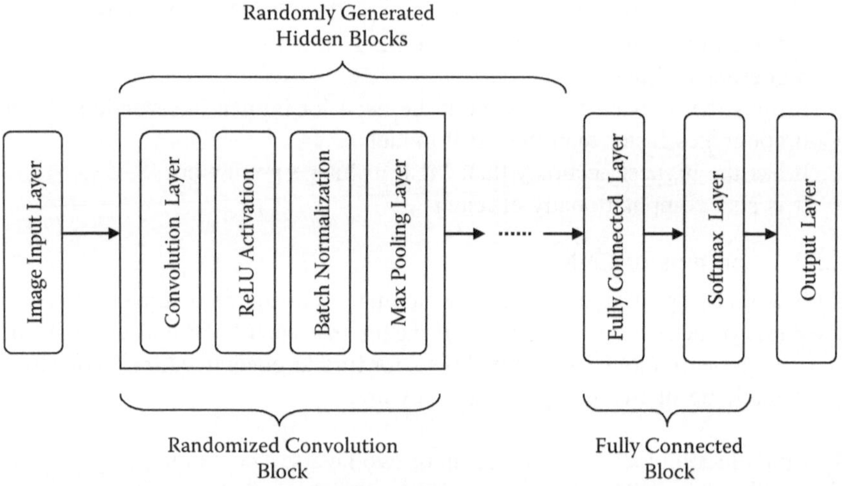

FIGURE 1.4 Different layers of CNN architecture.

the portion of the input image that corresponds to the filter's size by sliding the filter over it.

The feature map is the result, and it contains information about the image such as its corners and edges. This feature map is also provided to additional layers, which use it to learn a variety of different features from the input image.

Figure 1.5 shows the evaluation of convolved features from the input image by applying the filter. For example, let apply the filter on the left top corner of the input image, the corresponding feature is calculated in the following way.

Portion of input image (A) = [2 3 9; 7 0 1; 6 5 3]

Filter/Kernel (B) = [1 0 −1; 2 4 −2; 1 0 1]

A * (convolve) B = 2 * 1 + 3 * 0 + 9 * −1 + 7 * 2 + 0 * 4 + 1 * −2 + 6 * 1 + 5 * 0 + 3 * 1 = 14

Input

2	3	9	0	2	3
7	0	1	3	5	4
6	5	3	1	3	3
5	7	6	5	5	4
1	2	3	4	5	7
8	9	9	5	2	1

*

Filter

1	0	-1
2	4	-2
1	0	1

=

Feature Map

14	7	17	19
46	29	7	16
39	38	30	31
23	24	24	21

FIGURE 1.5 Working of convolution.

0	0	0	0	0	0	0	0
0	2	3	9	0	2	3	0
0	7	0	1	3	5	4	0
0	6	5	3	1	3	3	0
0	5	7	6	5	5	4	0
0	1	2	3	4	5	7	0
0	8	9	9	5	2	1	0
0	0	0	0	0	0	0	0

FIGURE 1.6 Actual matrix is surrounded by a '0' padding.

Padding The pixels on the corners will only be covered once in the above process, but the pixels in the middle will be covered multiple times. It arises two major downsides, they are

- Reduced outputs
- Information is being lost in the image's corners

To get around these limits, padding was introduced. Padding the picture matrix entails adding additional row and column of solely zeros on all sides. In reality, these variables being '0' would not provide any additional information, but they would aid in accounting for the previously unaccounted-for variables to be given greater priority (Figure 1.6).

Striding In convolution, rather than shifting the filter one row or column at a time, shift it two or three rows or columns at a time. It aids in reducing the amount of computations as well as the result matrix's size. This does not result in data loss for large images, but it does reduce the computational cost on a large scale.

For example, let assume, the input image matrix is 5 × 5 and the filter size is 3 × 3, after applying the filter on the image with a stride of 1, then it produces the output feature matrix with the size of 3 × 3.

In the above example, let apply the same filter with the stride of 2, the output feature matrix will be generated with the size of 2 × 2.

After striding, the dimension of the output matrix can be calculated by using the following formula.

$$floor\left(\frac{x + 2p - f}{s} + 1\right) \times floor\left(\frac{x + 2p - f}{s} + 1\right) \quad (1.1)$$

Where,

x – input image size
p – padding of 0's length
f – filter size
s – stride length

Let consider the Figure 1.7(a), where, n = 5, p = 0, f = 3 and s = 1,

Apply the above values in eqn. (1.1), the dimension of output matrix is,

$$floor\left(\frac{5 + 2(0) - 3}{1} + 1\right) \times floor\left(\frac{5 + 2(0) - 3}{1} + 1\right) \quad (1.2)$$

$$floor\,(3) \times floor\,(3) = 9 \quad (1.3)$$

Let consider the Figure 1.7(b), where, n = 5, p = 0, f = 3 and s = 2,

Apply these values in eqn. (1.1), the dimension of output matrix is,

$$floor\left(\frac{5 + 2(0) - 3}{2} + 1\right) \times floor\left(\frac{5 + 2(0) - 3}{2} + 1\right) \quad (1.4)$$

$$floor\,(2) \times floor\,(2) = 4 \quad (1.5)$$

(a)

(b)

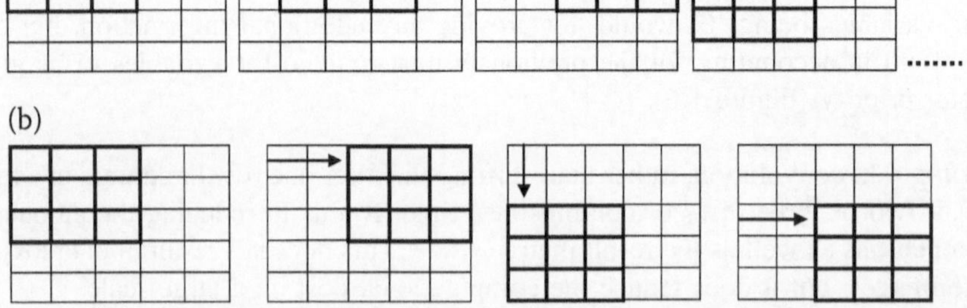

FIGURE 1.7 (a) Convolution with stride = 1, (b) Convolution with stride = 2.

1.2.2.3.2 Pooling Layer

A Pooling layer is frequently added after a Convolutional layer. The ultimate goal of this layer is to lower computational expenses by reducing the size of the convolved feature map. The feature map formed by the convolution layer is summarized by the pooling layer, which summarizes the features discovered in a specific location. As a result, rather than using the complete set of features created by the convolution layer, additional operations are done on these features. It aids in making the model more resistant to changes in the position of features in the input image.

Pooling Layer Types The largest element from the feature map is picked in Max Pooling. After max-pooling, the output would be a feature map with the most prominent features from the preceding feature map.

The average of the items present in the region of the feature map covered by the filter is calculated using Average Pooling.

The dimension of the output matrix can be computed using the following formula after pooling.

$$\left(\frac{n_h - f}{s} + 1\right) \times \left(\frac{n_w - f}{s} + 1\right) \times n_c \tag{1.6}$$

Where,

n_h – feature map's height
n_w – feature map's width
n_c – channel count in the feature map
f – filter size
s – length of stride

Let consider the Figure 1.8(a), where, $n_h = 4$, $n_w = 4$, $n_c = 1$, $f = 2$ and $s = 2$,

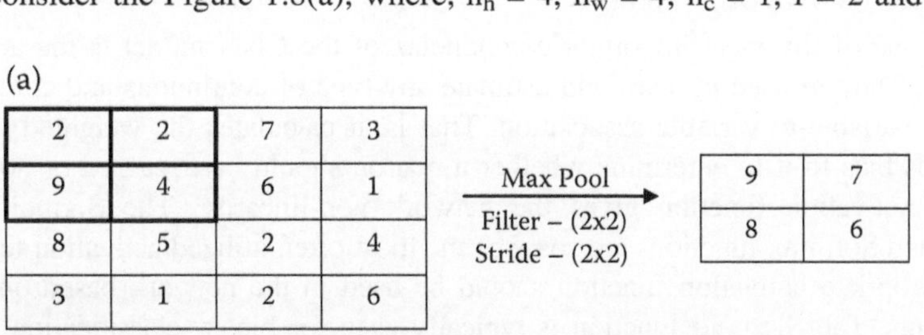

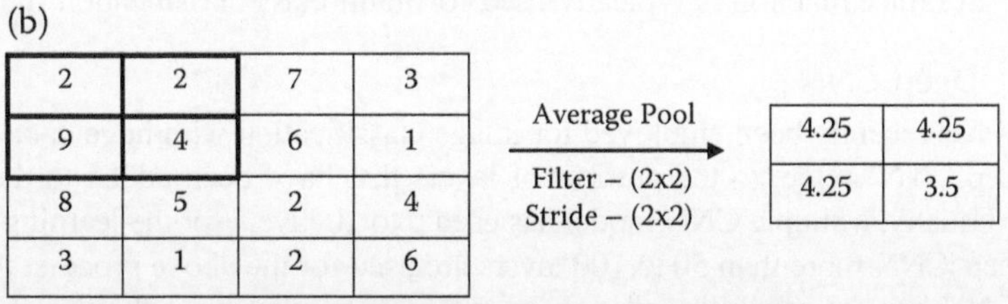

FIGURE 1.8 (a) Max pooling with stride = 2, (b) Average pooling with stride = 2.

Apply these values in eqn. (1.6), the dimension of output matrix is,

$$\left(\frac{4-2}{2}+1\right)\times\left(\frac{4-2}{2}+1\right)\times 1 \quad (1.7)$$

$$(2)\times(2)\times 1 = 4 \quad (1.8)$$

1.2.2.3.3 Fully Connected Layer (FC)

FC is made up of weights and biases, as well as neurons, and is used to connect the neurons between two layers. The output layer is normally placed after the fully connected layers. The input image from the previous layers is flattened and supplied to the fully connected layer in CNN architecture. The flattened vector is then sent through a few additional FC levels, which are where the mathematical operations are normally performed. The classifying procedure begins here.

The convolutional layers' output represents the data's high-level characteristics. While that output could be flattened and connected to the output layer, the best approach to learn nonlinear combinations of these features is to add a fully connected layer.

1.2.2.3.4 Dropout

When all features are connected to the fully connected layer, the training dataset is prone to overfitting. Overfitting occurs when a model performs well on training data but not on new data, resulting in a negative influence on the model's performance.

A dropout layer is utilized to overcome this problem, in which a few neurons are removed from the network during the training process, resulting in a smaller model. When a dropout of 0.2 is reached, 20% of the nodes in the network are dropped at random.

1.2.2.3.5 Activation Functions

Finally, one of the most important components of the CNN model is the activation function. They're used to learn and estimate any type of continuous and complicated network variable-to-variable association. That is, it calculates the weighted sum and then adds bias to it to determine whether a neuron should be triggered or not.

The Activation function gives the network non-linearity. The Sigmoid, tanH, ReLU, and Softmax functions are some of the most often utilized activation functions. The appropriate activation function should be used in the network based on the requirements. The Sigmoid function is typically used for binary classification models, while the Softmax function is typically used for multi-class classification models.

1.2.2.4 Deep CNN

A DCNN has recently been employed for image classification with huge datasets. The term 'Deep CNN' refers to the number of layers that have been added to the neural network. Usually, a simple CNN model has used 5 to 10 layers for the learning process but in Deep lCNN more than 50 to 100 layers are used for the above process. And also a Deep CNN has the capability of learning vital information from the inputs without human intervention and combining them to enable the description of a dormant model

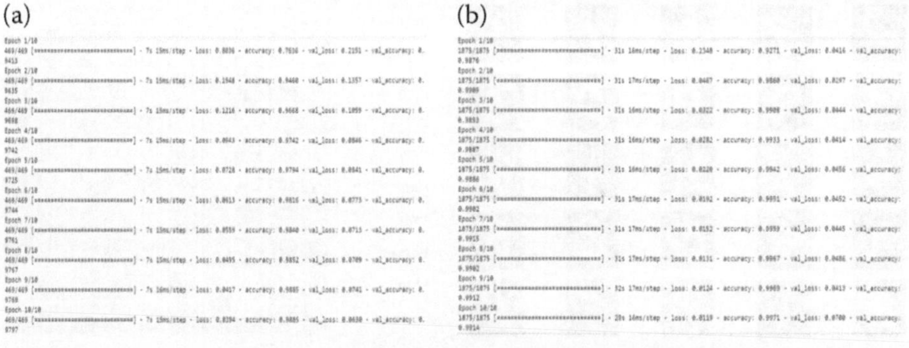

FIGURE 1.9 Evaluation of training and validation using (a) CNN (b) DCNN.

for pattern recognition. So a Deep CNN achieves better accuracy than Simple CNN models. Figure 1.9 shows the evaluation of training and validation history for the same dataset using CNN and DCNN. It clearly illustrates that DCNN achieves better accuracy in both training and validation.

1.3 EXPERIMENTAL PROCEDURE

The experimental procedure was implemented in two divisions. Division 3.1 describes the preparation of the dataset for the experimentation and division 3.2 explains the procedure followed in splitting the dataset for training and testing purposes.

1.3.1 Preparing the Dataset

The accuracy of the model is assessed using two different benchmark datasets: MNIST and CIFAR-10. There are 60000 training images and 10000 test images in the MNIST dataset. The CIFAR-10 dataset contains 60000 images, among them 50000 images are utilized for training purposes and the residual 10000 images are used for testing. Images in both datasets are grouped into 10 classes. Here the images are converted to grayscale before being given to the network because the designed model is not handled colour information. Also, the images are resized to 28 × 28 for easy handling. The pyramid reduction approach is used to reduce the size to 28 × 28 because the images from the datasets are larger. The image pyramid is a technique that uses reduced image representation to facilitate effectively scaled convolution. It consists of a series of duplicates of an original image that are gradually lowered in sample density and resolution (Figure 1.10).

1.3.2 Model Training and Testing

There are two types of image datasets: training datasets and testing datasets. Typically, 80% of photos are used in the training phase, whereas 20% are used in the testing process. The three layers that make up a neural network are the input layer, hidden layer, and output layer. The number of neurons in the input layer is the

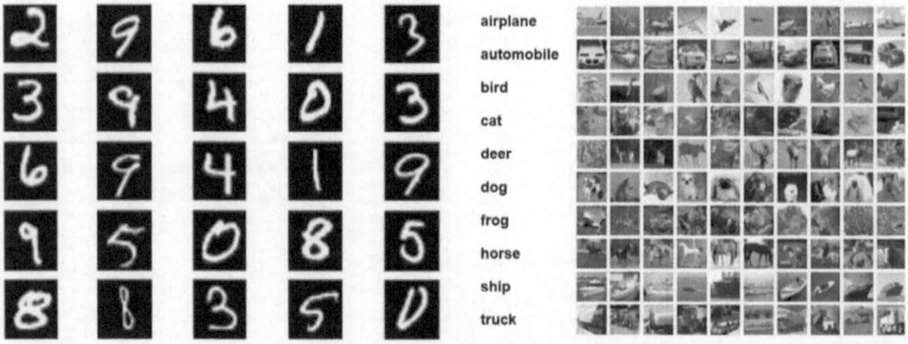

FIGURE 1.10 MNIST and CIFAR-10 dataset – sample images.

same as the number of features chosen in the previous step. The number of neurons in the output layer is proportional to the number of classes in the network. Experiments are used to determine the number of hidden neurons. The weighted sum of the outputs of all the neurons to which it is linked is the relevant neuron's input. A neuron's output is a non-linear function of the input it receives. The ultimate aim of the training is to reduce the error rate between the network output and desired output. The error may be calculated by using the following equation (1.9).

$$\nabla \mathrm{E(t)} = \frac{1}{K \times N} \sum_{k=1}^{K} \sum_{n=1}^{N} \left(\mathrm{d}_n^k - y_n^k \right)^2 \tag{1.9}$$

Where K is the number of the input image, N is the count of training images, d_n^k is the desired output and the network's actual output is y_n^k. The error gradient $\nabla E(t)$ is calculated through the partial derivatives of the error function. Once the error is computed, the optimization algorithm is used to minimize the error and train the network. Here, the 'RMSprop' optimization is utilized. The neural network parameters are modified throughout the training process. The Neural Network settings are set after the training phase, followed by the testing phase.

1.4 RESULTS AND DISCUSSION

The results of image categorization for two different datasets are discussed in this section. The presented method is simulated utilizing Python 3.7.0 tool. The sample images are displayed in Figure 1.9. The findings for the MNIST dataset are shown in section 1.4.1, while the results for the CIFAR-10 dataset are shown in section 1.4.2.

1.4.1 MNIST Dataset Image Classifications

The confusion matrix generated by the MLP technique on the classification of MNIST images is given in Figure 1.11. Besides, the confusion matrix generated by the CNN model is given in Figure 1.12 and the DCNN model is given in Figure 1.13.

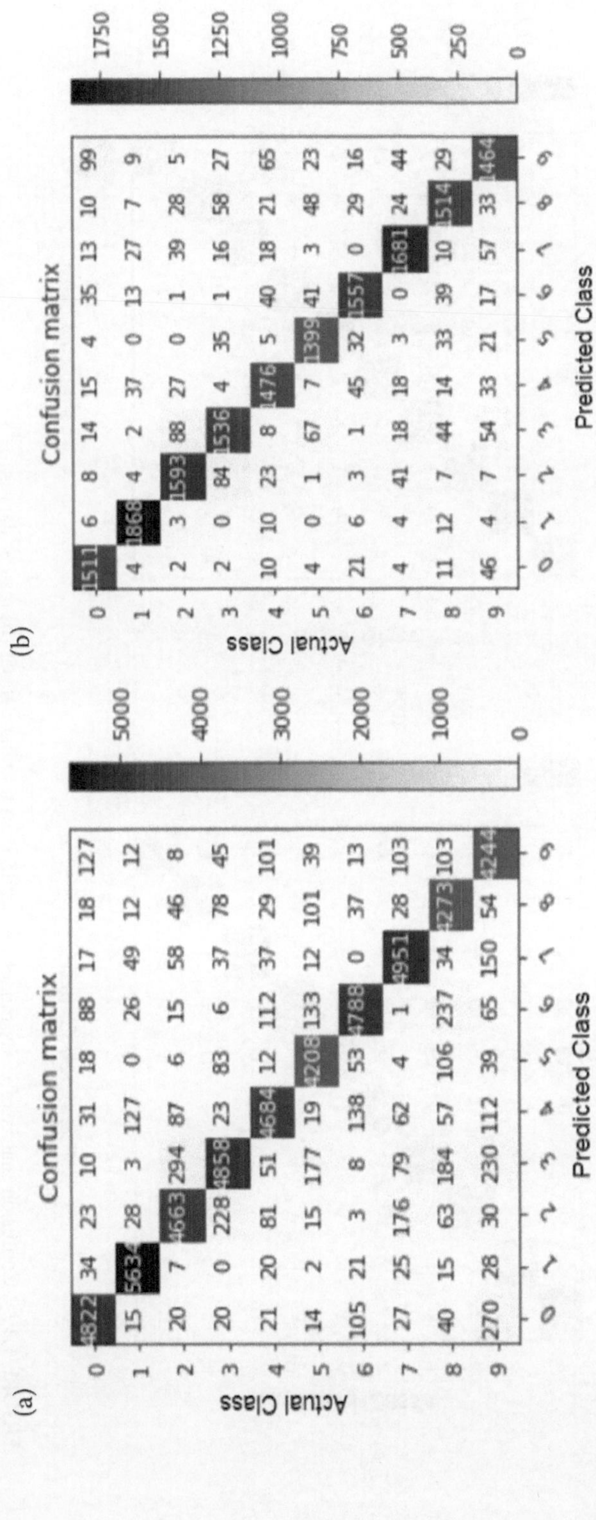

FIGURE 1.11 Confusion matrix of MLP model for MNIST (a) training dataset (b) testing dataset.

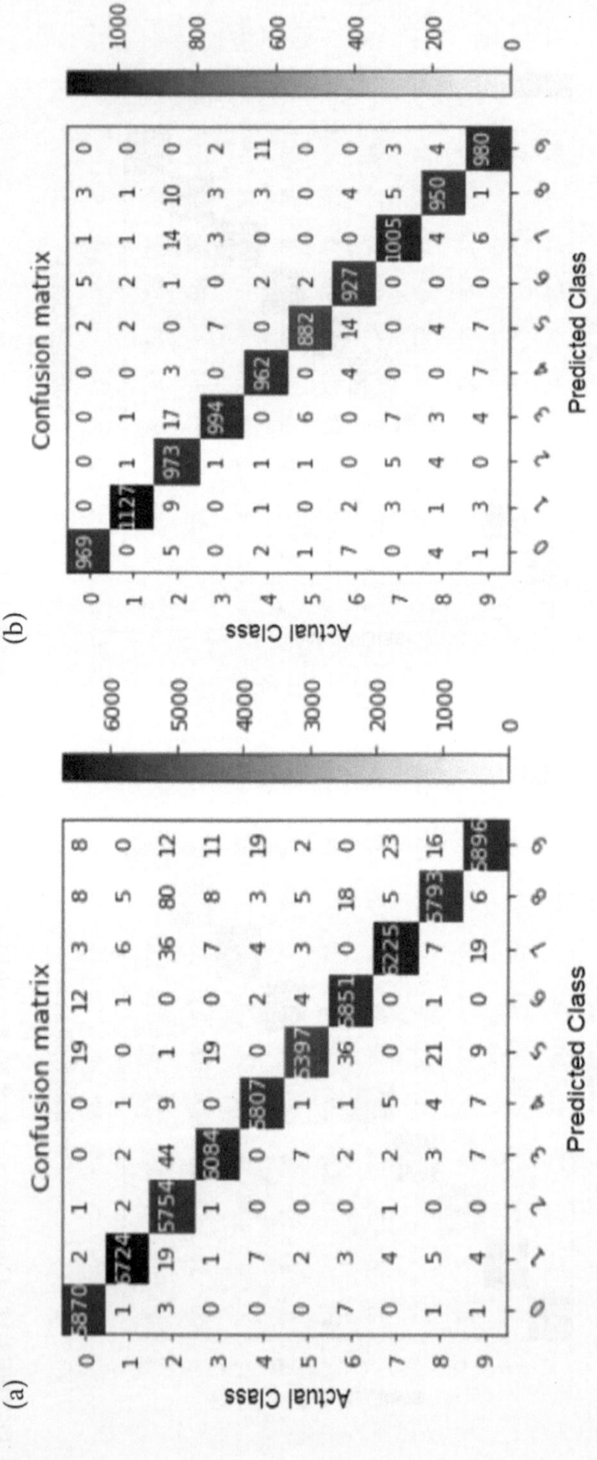

FIGURE 1.12 Confusion matrix of CNN model for MNIST (a) training dataset (b) testing dataset.

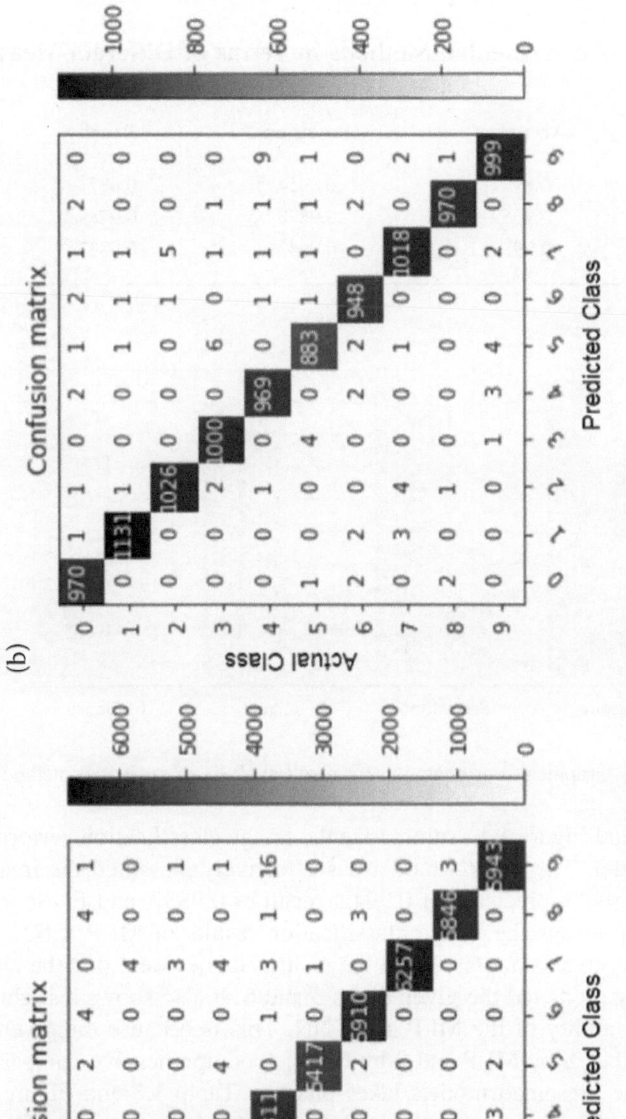

FIGURE 1.13 Confusion matrix of DCNN model for MNIST (a) training dataset (b) testing dataset.

TABLE 1.1
Result Analysis of Presented Methods in Terms of Different Measures for MNIST

Methods	Accuracy	Precision	Recall	F1-Score
MLP	0.8937	0.8954	0.8873	0.8894
CNN	0.9659	0.9878	0.9789	0.9812
DCNN	0.9983	0.9942	0.9837	0.9864

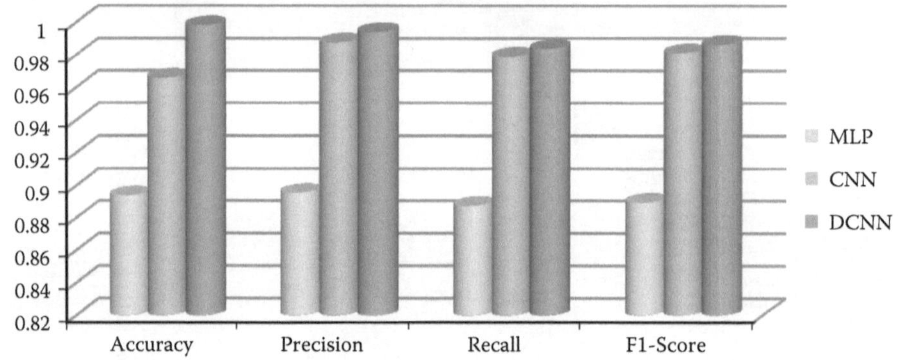

FIGURE 1.14 Graphical representation for result analysis of presented methods for MNIST.

Table 1.1 and Figure 1.14 summarize the image classification performance of the presented model. The DCNN model has effectively classified the images with an accuracy of 0.9983, precision of 0.9942, recall of 0.9837, and F1-Score of 0.9864.

Table 1.2 portrays the image classification results of MLP, CNN, and DCNN models for the given samples. From the results, it is evident that the DCNN model has effectively predicted the given digits 3 and 6. It also shows a slight decrease in the predictive ability of the MLP and CNN. This is because the given digit 3 has been predicted as 8 by MLP and 9 by CNN. A comprehensive comparative results analysis of the presented models takes place in Table 1.3 and Figure 1.15. From these values, it is apparent that the DCNN model is better than the MLP and CNN models.

1.4.2 CIFAR-10 Dataset Image Classifications

The confusion matrix generated by the MLP technique on the classification of CIFAR-10 images is given in Figure 1.16. Besides, the confusion matrix generated by the CNN model is given in Figure 1.17 and the DCNN model is given in Figure 1.18.

TABLE 1.2
Prediction Results Generated by Presented Models for Different Digits

Input image	MLP		CNN		DCNN	
	Prediction Score	**Predicted Digit**	**Prediction Score**	**Predicted Digit**	**Prediction Score**	**Predicted Digit**
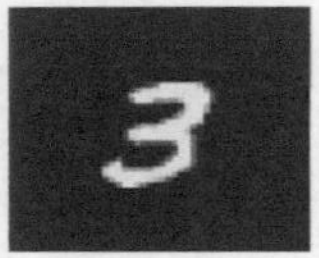	[2.00913968e-04 5.91005997e-04 2.15221417e-02 7.30199461e-03 8.59525304e-03 1.09598162e-02 1.06621664e-04 2.11524617e-02 9.26556384e-01 3.01340677e-03]	Thresholded Score: [0 0 0 0 0 0 0 0 1 0] Digit: 8	[2.2369113e-06 8.0744321e-08 5.7980878e-04 1.8824078e-01 6.1479645e-05 5.8901078e-05 3.5250773e-06 5.9361319e-06 7.0129982e-03 8.0403429e-01]	Thresholded Score: [0 0 0 0 0 0 0 0 0 1] Digit: 9	[4.8647796e-14 1.0964681e-10 9.6834723e-05 9.9280965e-01 8.9020479e-13 4.0718442e-07 1.0084744e-16 9.5953623e-10 7.4570711e-10 7.0932130e-03]	Thresholded Score: [0 0 0 1 0 0 0 0 0 0] Digit: 3
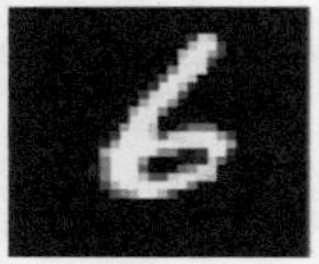	[1.22677295e-03 5.14925733e-04 6.66435637e-03 1.40520261e-04 2.72911708e-02 5.91280587e-03 9.25327899e-01 3.43654171e-05 3.09296476e-02 1.95753599e-03]	Thresholded Score: [0 0 0 0 0 0 1 0 0 0] Digit: 6	[2.5232079e-05 6.3475850e-11 1.0780598e-08 5.0491741e-04 5.4549833e-04 1.8582511e-04 9.9872893e-01 2.6589416e-12 9.0612257e-06 4.5235279e-07]	Thresholded Score: [0 0 0 0 0 0 1 0 0 0] Digit: 6	[4.8783041e-21 8.7868579e-20 1.7532738e-16 3.9073188e-20 8.6013051e-20 1.1510676e-15 1.0000000e+00 8.7845207e-33 5.7963187e-19 2.6382374e-24]	Thresholded Score: [0 0 0 0 0 0 1 0 0 0] Digit: 6

TABLE 1.3
Comparative Analysis of Training and Validation History for MNIST

Methods	Train_Loss	Val_Loss	Train_Acc	Val_Acc
MLP	1.9086	1.2210	0.8801	0.8937
CNN	0.1535	0.0982	0.9357	0.9659
DCNN	0.0436	0.0852	0.9739	0.9983

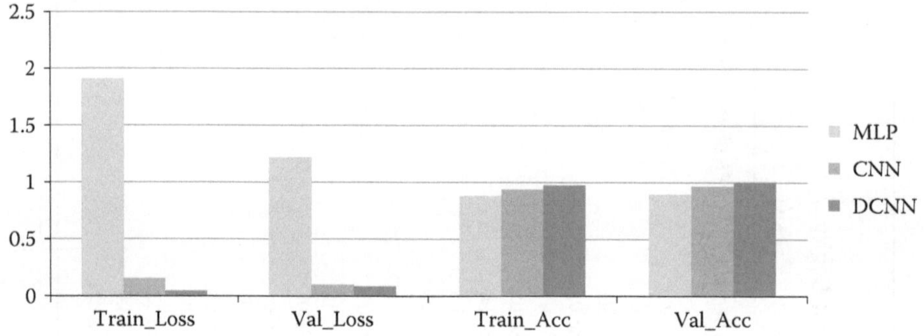

FIGURE 1.15 Graphical illustration for comparative analysis of training and validation history for MNIST.

Table 1.4 and Figure 1.19 summarize the image classification performance of the presented model. The DCNN model has effectively classified the images with an accuracy of 0.9014, precision of 0.8959, recall of 0.8864, and F1-Score of 0.8875.

Table 1.5 summarizes the image classification results of MLP, CNN, and DCNN models for the given samples. The results clearly show that the DCNN model has effectively predicted the given samples automobile and horse. But the MLP has predicted the automobile as a ship and the CNN has predicted it as a truck. A complete comparative results analysis of the presented models takes place in Table 1.6 and Figure 1.20. From these values, the DCNN model is found to be superior and appeared as an effective image classification model.

By looking into the above comparative analysis, it can be confirmed that the DCNN model has accomplished effective image classification performance over the other techniques.

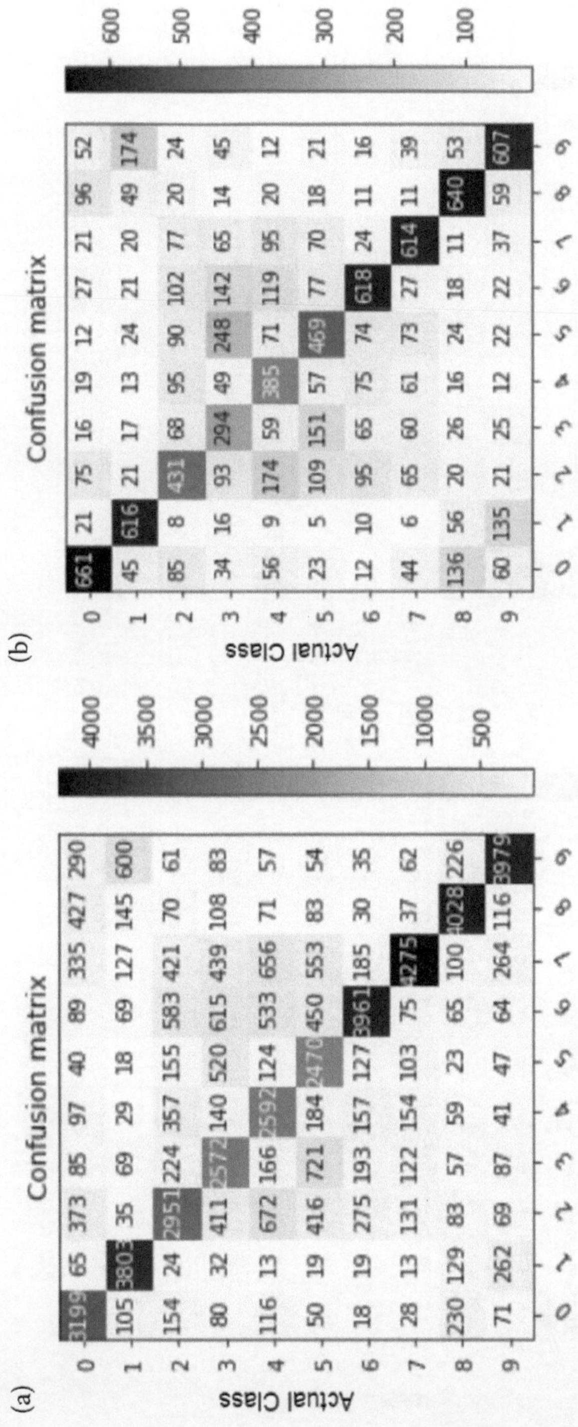

FIGURE 1.16 Confusion matrix of MLP model for CIFAR-10 (a) training dataset (b) testing dataset.

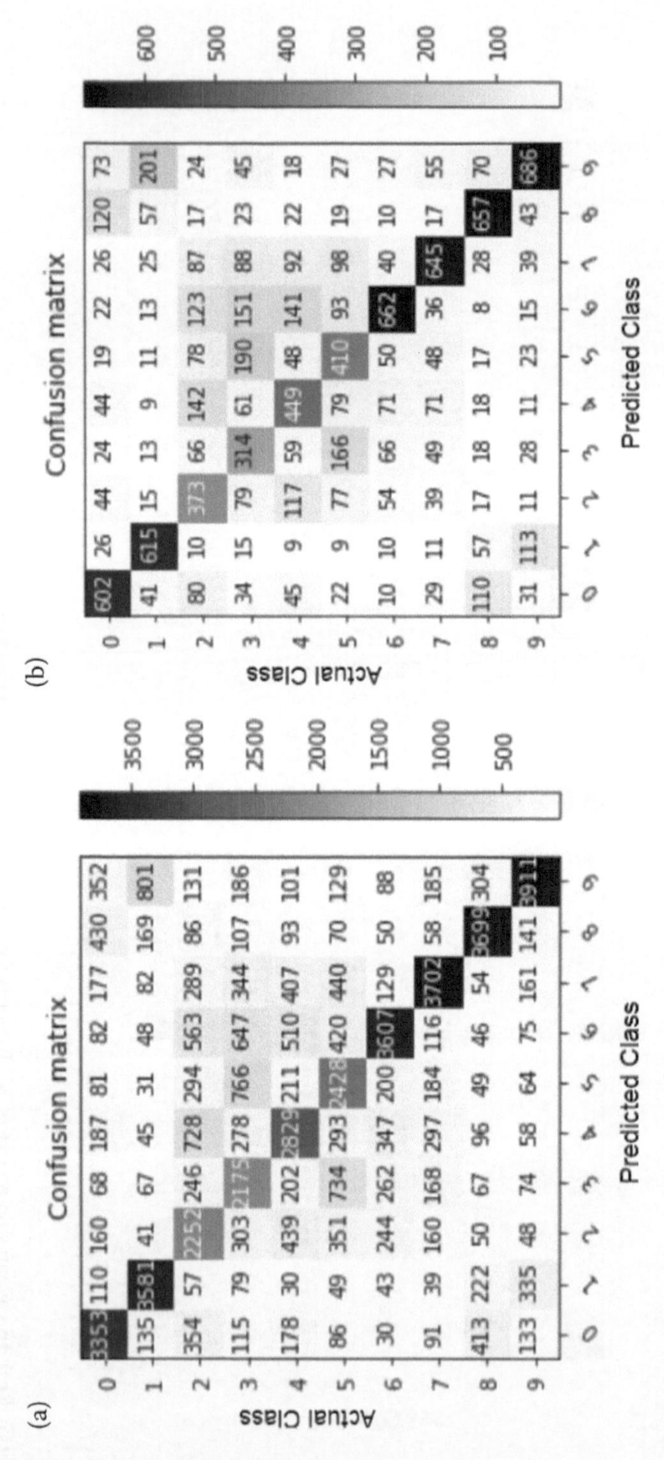

FIGURE 1.17 Confusion matrix of CNN model for CIFAR-10 (a) training dataset (b) testing dataset.

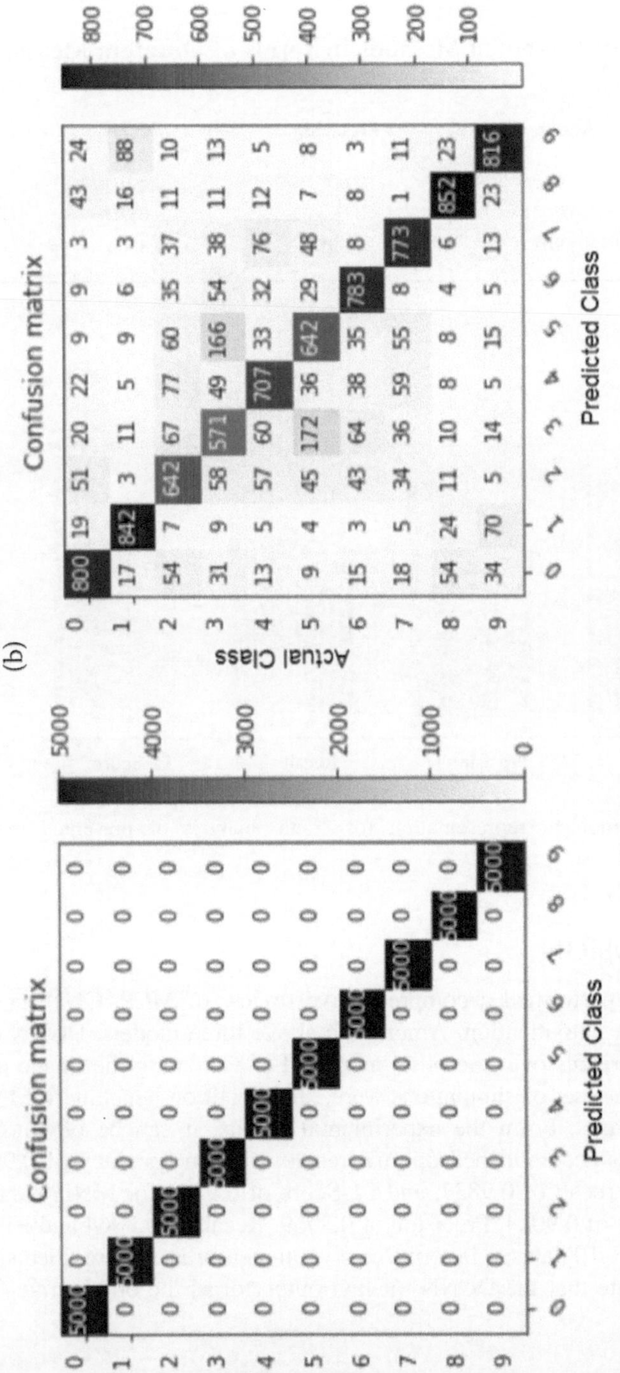

FIGURE 1.18 Confusion matrix of DCNN model for CIFAR-10 (a) training dataset (b) testing dataset.

TABLE 1.4
Result Analysis of Presented Methods in Terms of Different Measures for MNIST

Methods	Accuracy	Precision	Recall	F1-Score
MLP	0.6158	0.6081	0.6010	0.6017
CNN	0.7021	0.6934	0.6852	0.6860
DCNN	0.9014	0.8959	0.8864	0.8875

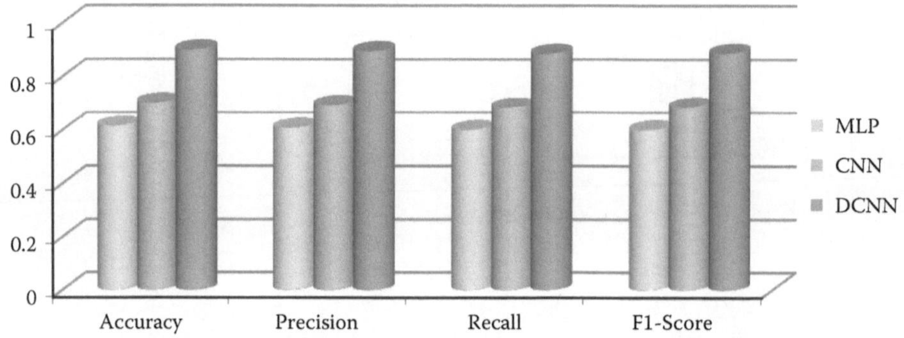

FIGURE 1.19 Graphical representation for result analysis of presented methods for CIFAR-10.

1.5 CONCLUSION

The chapter has performed a comprehensive review of MLP, CNN, and DCNN models for image classification. Among the above three models, DCNN exhibited superior characteristics over the other models. For validating the image classification performance, a set of simulations were carried out on benchmark MNIST and CIFAR-10 databases. From the experimental results, it can be obvious that the DCNN model has accomplished optimal results with an accuracy of 0.9983, precision of 0.9942, recall of 0.9837, and F1-Score of 0.9864 for MNIST dataset and with an Accuracy of 0.9014, Precision of 0.8959, Recall of 0.8864 and F1-Score of 0.8875 for CIFAR-10 dataset. In terms of several measures, the provided simulation results demonstrate that the DCNN method outperforms the other strategies.

TABLE 1.5
Prediction Results Generated by Presented Models for Different Objects

Input image	MLP		CNN		DCNN	
	Prediction Score	Predicted Class	Prediction Score	Predicted Class	Prediction Score	Predicted Class
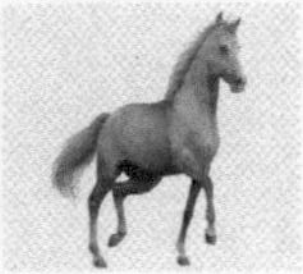	[7.7998244e-08 4.6624723e-07 3.7035336e-06 2.8177901e-06 5.4669528e-13 1.3182037e-01 2.1716358e-02 8.4645605e-01 6.9680251e-14 1.9974350e-07]	Thresholded Score: [0 0 0 0 0 0 0 1 0 0] Class: 7 Label: Horse	[1.5980469e-06 4.8422838e-10 2.6365095e-07 2.2712295e-07 5.2281009e-11 1.5338340e-04 3.8448385e-16 9.1782576e-01 2.2018753e-02 2.6871886e-08]	Thresholded Score: [0 0 0 0 0 0 0 1 0 0] Class: 7 Label: Horse	[1.9946109e-24 2.5004898e-21 1.5775133e-15 3.4273462e-05 4.8722887e-19 2.6060965e-13 1.3107702e-24 9.9990571e-01 2.5270626e-09 1.3508437e-14]	Thresholded Score: [0 0 0 0 0 0 0 1 0 0] Class: 7 Label: Horse
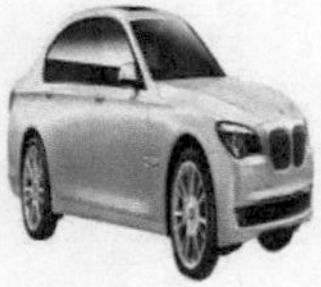	[6.1390233e-11 1.1133318e-05 2.2406834e-05 1.7419775e-04 1.6770286e-08 7.6780608e-03 1.3093304e-13 1.2797749e-05 9.9209189e-01 9.5676724e-06]	Thresholded Score: [0 0 0 0 0 0 0 0 1 0] Class: 8 Label: Ship	[4.6675690e-09 7.3125422e-11 5.4727249e-08 4.2234283e-06 1.2168361e-11 2.1183946e-09 1.8432037e-18 1.0365518e-07 1.1486064e-07 9.9999547e-01]	Thresholded Score: [0 0 0 0 0 0 0 0 0 1] Class: 9 Label: Truck	[2.3716780e-08 9.9993718e-01 1.2674458e-07 2.3581324e-06 1.4572389e-05 3.8353828e-05 2.1381297e-08 3.3912852e-07 5.3096960e-06 1.6103827e-06]	Thresholded Score: [0 1 0 0 0 0 0 0 0 0] Class: 1 Label: Automobile

TABLE 1.6
Comparative Analysis of Training and Validation History for CIFAR-10

Methods	Train_Loss	Val_Loss	Train_Acc	Val_Acc
MLP	0.2683	1.1858	0.8067	0.6158
CNN	0.2015	1.0310	0.9197	0.7021
DCNN	0.0339	0.9199	1.1808	0.9014

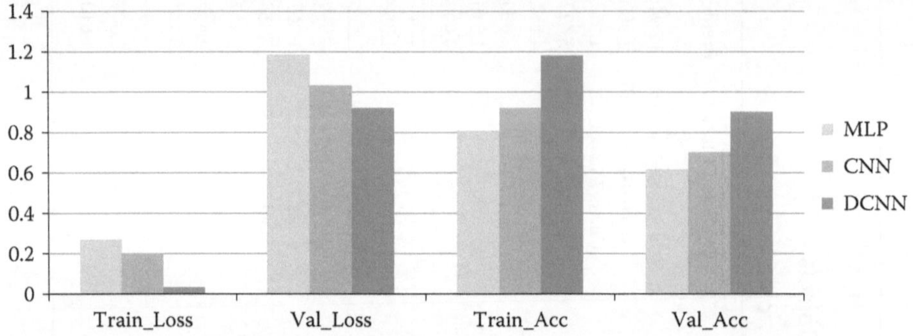

FIGURE 1.20 Graphical illustration for training and validation history for CIFAR-10.

REFERENCES

[1] Lilles, T.M., Kiefer, R.W. and Chipman, J.W., in "Remote Sensing and Image Interpretation", 5th edition, Wiley, 2004.

[2] Li Deng and Dong Yu, "Deep Learning: methods and applications" by Microsoft research [Online]. Available at: http://research.microsoft.com/pubs/209355/NOWBook-Revised-Feb2014-online.pdf.

[3] Ali, Z., Hussain, I., Faisal, M., Nazir, H.M., Hussain, T., Shad, M.Y., MohamdShoukry, A. and Hussain Gani, S., "Forecasting drought using multilayer perceptron artificial neural network model", *Advances in Meteorology*, 2017.

[4] Balamurugan, S.P. and Arumugam, G., "A novel method for predicting kidney diseases using optimal artificial neural network in ultrasound images", *International Journal of Intelligent Enterprise (IJIE)*, 2020, Vol. 7, Issue-1/2/3, pp. 37–55.

[5] Agarwal, M., Singh, A., Arjaria, S., Sinha, A. and Gupta, S., "ToLeD: Tomato leaf disease detection using convolution neural network", *Procedia Computer Science*, 2020, Vol. 167, pp. 293–301.

[6] Karthik, R., Hariharan, M., Anand, S., Mathikshara, P., Johnson, A. and Menaka, R., "Attention embedded residual CNN for disease detection in tomato leaves", *Applied Soft Computing*, 2020, Vol. 86, pp. 105933.

[7] Shin, H., Roth, H.R., Gao, M., Lu, L., Xu, Z., Nogues, I., et al., "Deep convolutional neural networks for computer-aided detection: CNN architectures, dataset characteristics and transfer learning", *IEEE Trans Med Imaging*, 2016, Vol. 35, Issue-5, pp. 1285–1298.

[8] Balamurugan, S.P. and Duraisamy, M., "Deep Convolution Neural Network with Gradient Boosting Tree for COVID-19 Diagnosis and Classification Model", *European Journal of Molecular & Clinical Medicine*, 2020, Vol. 7, Issue-11, pp. 2459–2468.
[9] https://deepai.org/dataset/mnist.
[10] https://www.cs.toronto.edu/~kriz/cifar.html.

2 An Efficient Technique for Image Compression and Quality Retrieval in Diagnosis of Brain Tumour Hyper Spectral Image

V.V. Teresa and J. Dhanasekar
Associate Professor, Department of ECE, Sri Eshwar College of Engineering, Coimbatore, India

V. Gurunathan and T. Sathiyapriya
Assistant Professor, Department of ECE, Dr. Mahalingam College of Engineering and Technology, Pollachi, India

CONTENTS

2.1 Introduction........27
2.2 Literature Survey........29
    2.2.1 Proposed System........31
    2.2.2 Data Latches with D-flip Flops........34
    2.2.3 Discussion and Results of the Simulation........34
2.3 Conclusion........43
References........43

2.1 INTRODUCTION

The movability of electronic elements has increased in recent years, and low-power arithmetic circuits have become increasingly significant in the VLSI industry. Adders are the most important circuits in VLSI designs, which have risen in demand for low-power arithmetic circuits. The Multiplier-Accumulator (MAC) unit is found in the DSP essential construction section. The Full Adder is a component of the Macintosh unit [1]. The Macintosh unit includes a Full Adder component, which can have a substantial impact on the overall system's performance. Because of the lower power consumption, the complete Adder circuit is crucial for decreasing

DOI: 10.1201/9781003217497-2

power consumption. The crucial procedure CSLA is computed in parallel. CSLA produces many carriers and a partial total. The sum and carry of extremes are chosen using multiplexers. Within the CSLA architecture, the addition operation is a vital arithmetic function that frequently rattles up the performance of digital systems. Adders are most commonly used in electrical applications. A novel type of adder, known as hybrid adders, was introduced in 2002. These adders are utilized to improve the speed of the adding procedure. Artificially CSLA/carry look-ahead style is provided by the adders. Low power multiplier planning is aided by improved artificial FAs. The speed of addition in digital adders is primarily supported by propagation delay, which is limited by the adder's propagation delay. The space and power optimized knowledge path log is one of the most important researches in VLSI design.

If we want to construct multipliers, we'll need to consider adders as an output. Adders are a part of the multipliers model. Microprocessors conduct a certain, endless number of directions every second. The size of the semiconductor device and its power consumption are the most important factors to consider when designing multipliers and adders. In general, an adder is used to add two numbers, and it is also an important component of the ALU. In a computer, the adder operation is used to determine the address and indices, as well as operation codes. Within the filtering process, a different DSP algorithm is also utilized adders. Adder's primary requirement is speed, and it is also the most important constraint. Minimum power, maximum speed, and knowledge logic style are all important aspects of VLSI. Knowledge systems have become an essential analytical space because of their efficient use of power and space with high-speed paths.

CSLA is designed to use an RCA, Binary to Excess-l converter circuit in this region of analysis, with an electronic device stage that picks the carry. The AOI then takes the place of the BEC, reducing the realm and latency. During this project, the altered SQRT CSLA with AOI is achieved by removing electrical devices, which minimizes the realm consumption over time (Figure 2.1).

In microprocessors, power consumption and space should be kept to a minimum. Computers, mobile phones, laptops, and other similar devices benefit from additional battery backup. As a result, a VLSI design must produce great these parameters in a very efficient manner. These are severe constraints, thus achieving them will be tough. Demand or the circuit's application in the trade will need the creation of constraints.

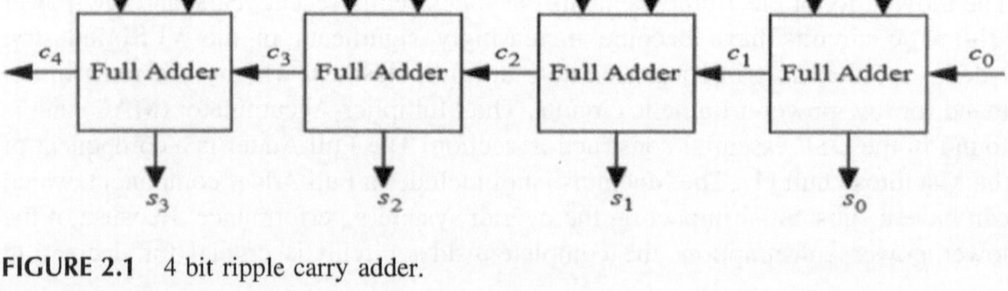

FIGURE 2.1 4 bit ripple carry adder.

This research is ordered and arranged in following sections: The second section provides the survey associated with CSLA. Section three mentioned regarding the adder blocks methodology of AOI and RCA. In section four the improved style of CSLA while not using multiplexers is mentioned. Section five deals with the stimulation result analysis of the planned circuit. Section six deals with the conclusion of the bestowed work.

2.2 LITERATURE SURVEY

Sasamal, T. N., & Ghanekar, U. et el., [2] Presented ideal quantum-speck cell automata (QCA) structure for full viper (FA) in light of an ideal three-input selective OR (XOR) door is exhibited. This structure of XOR uses another design of cells dissimilar to conventional door level methodologies. The coplanar QCA FA ranges and deferrals of clock cycles with cells. It accomplishes absolute vitality scattering as low vitality level. The functionality of the designed entryway is employed to create a swell convey conveyor (RCA) as a specialized application. Traditional cost metrics and QCA-explicit cost work are used by the developers to analyse execution. The proposed n-bit RCA outperforms the vast majority of currently available cutting-edge solutions. The low dimension coplanar RCA configuration results. Also, by considering the new cost measurements, it is discovered that the proposed snake performs genuinely well when contrasted with the past adders as well. These structures are acknowledged and mimicked utilizing QCADesigner.

Williams, A. C., & Zwolinski, M. et el., [3] analysed the worry over power scattering, combined with the proceeding with ascend in framework size and multifaceted nature, implies that there is a developing requirement for abnormal state configuration devices equipped for naturally improving frameworks to consider control dissemination, notwithstanding the more customary measurements of the zone, deferral, and test ability. Current methods for reducing power consumption will be specifically designated: for example, turning off or killing inactive components of the system, or a controlled reduction in a power supply. The conduct combination framework shown here includes an integrated steady power estimation capability, which makes use of movement profiles created organically through structure recreation on any standard VHDL test system; precise circuit-level cell models (again, created using SPICE reproduction); and a comprehensive framework control demonstration. This information, alongside comparative estimators for zone and deferral, manages the streamlining of the plan towards free client indicated goals for a conclusive zone, delay, clock speed, and vitality utilization. Likewise, a scope of intensity lessening highlights is incorporated, enveloping: Clock gating, input hooking, input gating, low-control cells, and pipelined and multicycle units are all examples of supply voltage scaling. As a result, they're often misused as part of the territory/delay/control dissemination switch-off method during development. The subsequent framework is equipped for decreasing the evaluated vitality utilization of a few benchmark plans by variables of somewhere in the range of 3.5 and 7.0 occasions. Besides, the plan investigation capacity empowers a scope of option auxiliary usage to be created from a solitary conduct depiction, with contrasting zone/delay/control exchange offs.

Ramkumar, B., & Kittur, H. M et el., [4] The proposed CSLA is one of the fastest adders currently in use for fluctuating data, allowing computers to perform quick calculations. Pass on the Select Adder configuration; evidently, the CSLA's size and power consumption can be reduced. This study employs a basic and master entrance level fix to drastically reduce the CSLA's domain and force. The standard SQRT CSLA building is made and differentiated as a result of this alteration square-root CSLA (SQRT CSLA) style is made and differentiated. The arranged to organize has a little area and power as differentiated and along these lines the typical SQRT CSLA with a slight delay augmentation. Using authentic drudge and uncommon art and configuration, this study evaluates the hand-carried out execution of pre-arranged plans relating to postponement, area, control, and their items in zero. An 18-m CMOS technology is being developed. The organized CSLA structure outperforms the normal SQRT CSLA, according to the results.

Ying, Z., Dhar, S. et el., [5] Photonic integrated circuits with small footprints and low power consumption have cleared the way for ultrafast and energy-efficient optical computing in a system similar to CMOS-based electrical integrated circuits in many ways. Directed logic is a novel optical computing paradigm that takes full advantage of both electronics and photonics. In this paper, we propose alternative designs for directed-logic-based electro-optic ripple-carry adders in integrated silicon photonics, in which optical equivalents replace electrical components in the critical path. Due to the use of ultralow-power microdisk modulators, all control signals are applied simultaneously, resulting in a significant reduction in propagation latency. As a proof of concept, a two-bit thermal-optic complete adder based on microdisk modulators is demonstrated, coupled with a prediction of high-speed performance. The proposed electro-optic full adder paves the way for future integrated silicon photonics optical computing that consumes less power and has higher bandwidth.

Wang, Z. R., Li, et el., [6] The presented memory registering design is advancing a progressive processing world view that has the potential to break the von Neumann bottleneck. The CMOS excellent 1T1R resistive irregular access memory (RRAM) connecting structure is demonstrated in this research. It is proposed that the capacity for comprehensive Boolean logic and math be supplied. Each of the 16 twofold rationales can be recognized in two rationale ventures with an additional readout venture for falling with a single 40-nm CMOS process 1T1R unit, demonstrating realistic reconfiguration and low computational complexity. To assure consistency and reliability, up to 10.7 cycles of NAND and XOR logic actions are done. In addition, as proof of the 1T1R registering engineering principle, a few important snake circuits are developed and tentatively illustrated in 1T1R devices. A swell convey snake and its updated plan, as well as a convey select viper, are among the adders investigated in this study, and they all show promise in terms of nonvolatility, calculation speed, and circuit territory. This document lays a solid foundation for future in-memory processing research by describing the most confusing but fruitful RRAM-based 8-bit expansion work to date.

Tan, Y., Xu, W et el., [7] Proposed memory figuring configuration is a rising progressive processing worldview that may break the Neumann bottleneck. In this study, the CMOS superb 1T1R resistive arbitrary access memory (RRAM) co-ordination structure is used to construct a reasoning door codesign processing technique. Experimentation has shown that total emblematic reason and number-crunching abilities are unquestionable. Everything about sixteen double rationales will be acknowledged in two rationale ventures with an additional readout venture for falling with one 40nm CMOS strategy 1T1R unit, indicating helpful re-configuration and low method multifarious nature. Up to ten seven cycles of NAND and XOR logic actions are conducted to ensure correctness and accountability. Furthermore, in light of the proof of the 1T1R processing structure's genesis, several rudimentary snake circuits are developed and proven in 1T1R gadgets by experimentation. The adders anticipated amid this paper exemplify a swell convey viper and its streamlined style and a convey select snake, All of these features show promise in terms of nonvolatility, computation speed, and rationale door space. This research presents the first experimentally verified entangled RRAM-based 8-bit expansion and creates a strong basis for developing a long-term in-memory figure strategy.

Balaji, N., & Kumar, G. K et el., [8–17] The patient's blastemal pathology was presented. In every study and clinical review, the measurement of magnetic resonance imaging (MRI) data is critical. MRI images are usually incredibly buzzing. As a result, diagnosing and concluding any illness is difficult for doctors. Various image de-noising techniques have been proposed in a recent study. Noise reduction alone will not be enough because brain illnesses are involved. Doctors who read the MRI images finally come to a conclusion about the illness once they have all of the information they want. This study aims to improve an affordable VLSI system that can aid clinical export to prognosis and conclusion on a certain neurological disorder. For feature extraction and neurological ailment identification utilizing MRI images, the suggested system employs a modified Daubechies algorithmic technique. On the FPGA, the VLSI processor is used because it provides reprogrammability, reconstruction robustness, and real-time resolution.

2.2.1 Proposed System

The design starts with the aim of reducing the area of the CSLA adder. Thus to reduce the area, we take a big action to eliminate the multiplexer in the CSLA which selects the sum and carry outputs of the adder. Actually, we cannot just modify the design simply; specifically the elimination of the mux is to be studied in detail. Because it can change the whole operation of the adder and in turn affect the performance of the adder. The CSLA without mux can be designed by giving the carry input directly to the AOI block. The AOI of the CSLA for the elimination of mux is shown in Figure 2.5. The AOI that includes another set of AND, OR and inverter gates to receive carry the input from the previous block. The AOI obtains the carry and computes it with the block's sum and carry. As in previous work, the

CSLA is separated into groups here. The full 16-bit CSLA in groups and its interconnections are shown in Figure 2.6. Except for the least-significant, Each sector of a carry-select adder conducts two adds in parallel, one with a carry-in of zero and the other with a carry-in of on. Two ripple carry adders and a multiplexer make comprise a four-bit carry select adder. The carry-select adder is simple but fast, with an O(n) gate-level depth. When using a carry select adder to add two n bit values, two adders (two ripple carry adders) are utilized, one with the carry supposed to be zero and the other with the carry assumed to be one. Where,

$$S = A + B + Cin$$

The equations below describe the sum and carry expressions.

Si = ai xor bi, where ai = Ci + 1 and bi = Ci + 1 are the variables.

Where,

Pi = Xi xor Yi – Carry Propagation
Gi = Xi and Yi – Carry Generation
Ci + 1 = Gi or (Pi and Ci) – Next Carry
Carry = A.B + B.Cin + A.Cin
Sum = A.B.Cin + CARRY(A+B+Cin)

The suggested system CSLA is based on the principle particularization shown in (1-bit Adder) in Figure 2.2: One HSG unit, one Carry Generation unit, one Carry total unit, and one total Generation unit are all included. For conveying the integers '0' and '1', the convey age unit is made up of two metric systems (CG0 and CG1). To aggregate word s0 of size n bits and half communicate word c0 of length n bits, the entire section uses two n-bit operands. Each CG0 and CG1 receive s0 and c0 from the HSG unit and construct two n-bit full-convey the words c10 and c11 about merged with convey '0' and '1', according to the HSG unit's foundation. The CG0

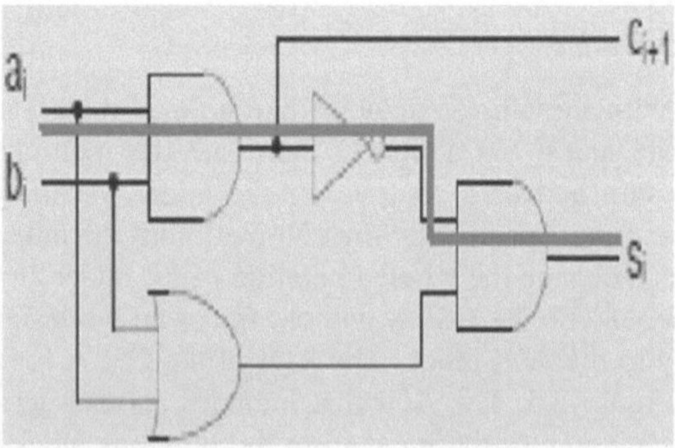

FIGURE 2.2 1 bit half adder.

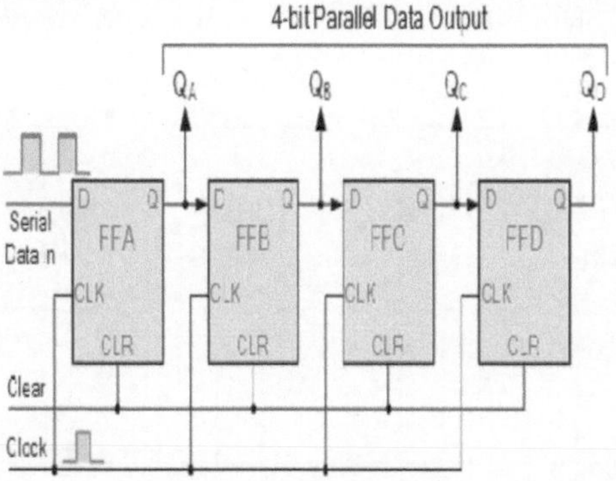

FIGURE 2.3 4- bit data latch serial-in to parallel out shift register.

and CG1 primary circuits have been updated to use fixed data transfer bits. The strategies of CG0 and CG1 have been fine-tuned. The Cs unit selects one last convey word from the two convey words accessible at its info line using the management flag Cin. It chooses c0 if cin = 0; otherwise, it chooses c11. The Cs unit is dead when using an n-bit two-to-one MUX. Regardless, the Cs units. This component is used to promote the notion of the Cs unit. The improved setup of the Qa, Qb, Qc, and Qd units is shown in Figure 2.3, which is made up of n AND–OR doors. The Q unit provides the last convey word, c. The c mutual savings bank is delivered to yield as cout, and (n 1) LSBs are XO. To collect (n1) MSBs of definite combination, red with (n 1) most significant half-whole (s0) within the complete generation (FSG). The least significant bit (LSB) of s0 is XORed with Cin to generate the LSB of s. Due to the multiple speed limits in any dynamic sector, various producers have addressed the expansion issue in the construction of conveys. This concept is present when Carry selects the Adder and uses D Latch to achieve management good and quick information ways principle frameworks. The CSLA and Regular 4-bit Carry Choose Adder, as well as the BEC 4-bit CSLA, were compared to the proposed 4-bit Carry Choose Adder. However, the goal of rapid expansion is achieved using BEC alongside an electrical device (mux), and one contribution of the multiplexer receives of the BEC yield is due to the multiplexer's contribution (B3, B2, B1, and B0) and input (B3, B2, B1, and B0). As a result, the Muxes are used to determine whether the BEC yield or the immediate contributions are to be employed as per the management flag. Cin, The 4-bit BEC's Boolean articulations are recorded here (Note: utilitarian pictures, ~ NOT, and AND,^ XOR) Figure 2.4.

a. **THE D-FLIP FLOP**

Except that D Flip Flop waits one clock cycle for the condition of the D contribution at the stage of a positive edge at the clock stick, the duty of D flip failure is

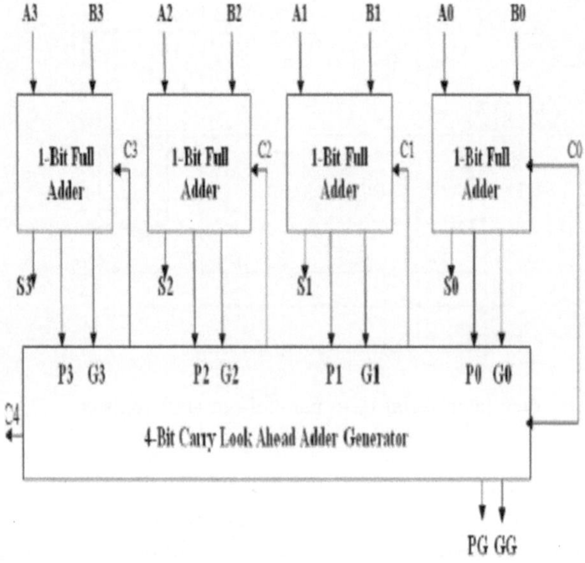

FIGURE 2.4 Carry look ahead adder 4- bit.

essentially equal to that of D lock (or a negative edge if the clock input is dynamic least). It is known as a postpone flip-flop because of this. To make a circuit or a zero-request hold, utilize the D Flip Flop. To make a circuit or a zero-request hold, utilize the D Flip Flop. The D-F-F 'straight forward lock' among the D-samples has The advantage is that the D input stick's flag captures the stage at which the flip-flop is timed, and subsequent modifications to the D input are disregarded until the next clock event.

2.2.2 Data Latches with D-flip Flops

A data latch is another interesting application of the D flip failure, comparable to recurrence division. The TTL 74LS74 or the CMOS 4042 are ideal for this purpose and are available in Quad group. An information lock is used as an instrument to convey or recall the information blessing on its information input, so serving as a touch kind of a single piece stockpiling gadget. A simple '4-bit' data hook is created by linking four 1-bit information locks together so that all of its clock inputs are associated together and 'timed' at the same indistinguishable moment. LATCH FOR 4-BIT DATA: Figures 2.7–2.10.

2.2.3 Discussion and Results of the Simulation

The proposed structure in this study was constructed in Verilog-HDL and blended in the Synopsys RTL plan compiler. All usual altered and proposed SQRT CSLAs

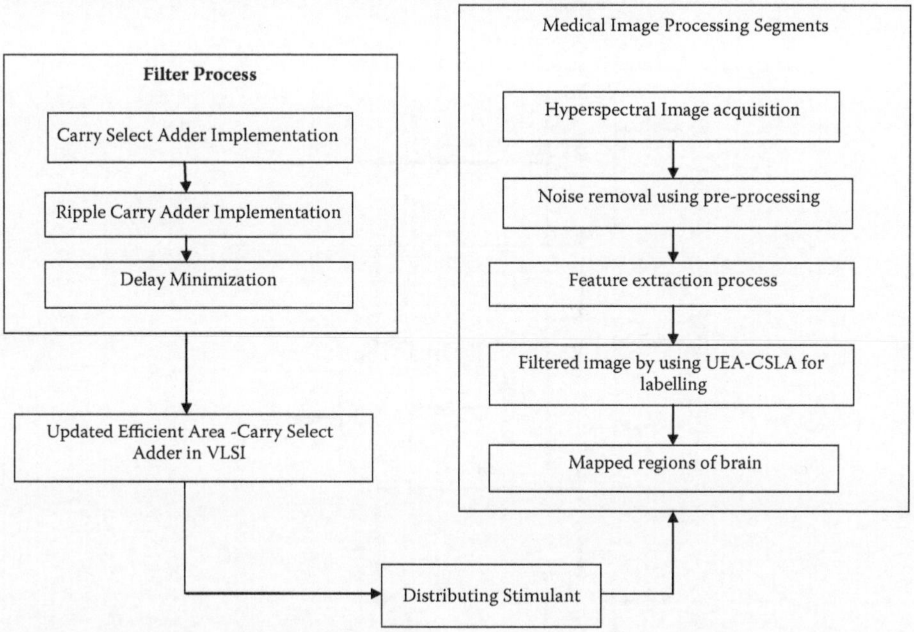

FIGURE 2.5 Research work flow model.

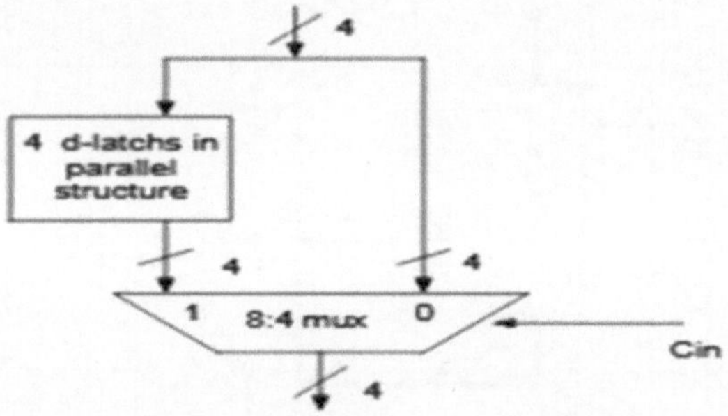

FIGURE 2.6 4- bit D-latch with a multiplier.

were included in the comparative plan. In terms of deferral, zone, and authority. Figures 2.1 to 2.4 indicate the reproductive consequences of all CSLA arrangements. The area represents the plan's all-out cell zone, with all-out power equaling the sum of spillage control, inner power, and exchanging power. As an element, the rate of reduction in the cell region, all-out power, all-out deferral, control postpone

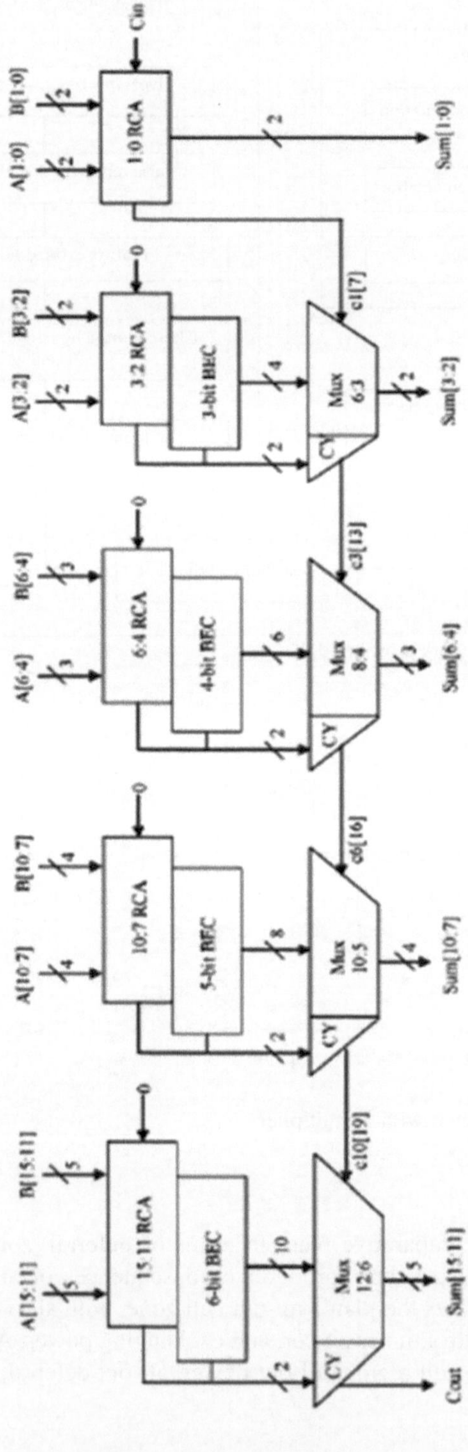

FIGURE 2.7 CSLA by using BEC.

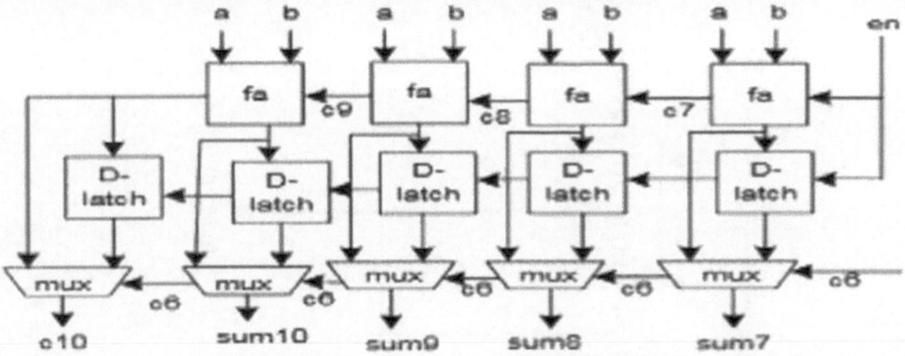

FIGURE 2.8 Internal structure of 5 D latches in parallel block.

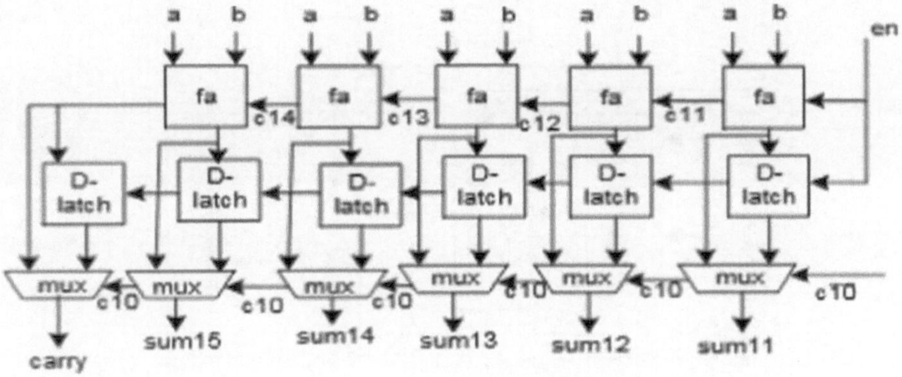

FIGURE 2.9 Internal structure of proposed CSLA by using D-latch.

item, and region postpone item and the region postpone item as an element of the bit size appeared underneath the table. Additionally plotted is the rate postponement and power diminished (Figures 2.11 and 2.12).

Nowadays, brain tumour is one of the most dangerous diseases, hence this investigation-based mapping of the districts of the cerebrum is done inside the bundle. The component extraction is authorized to abuse the help capacities and VLSI design is prepared and tried upheld the alternatives separated from the extraction technique following results are presented based on the VLSI Updated Efficient Area - Carry Select Adder propagation result dependent on Matrix Laboratory in the adaptation of R2018b following result wise diagnosis the brain

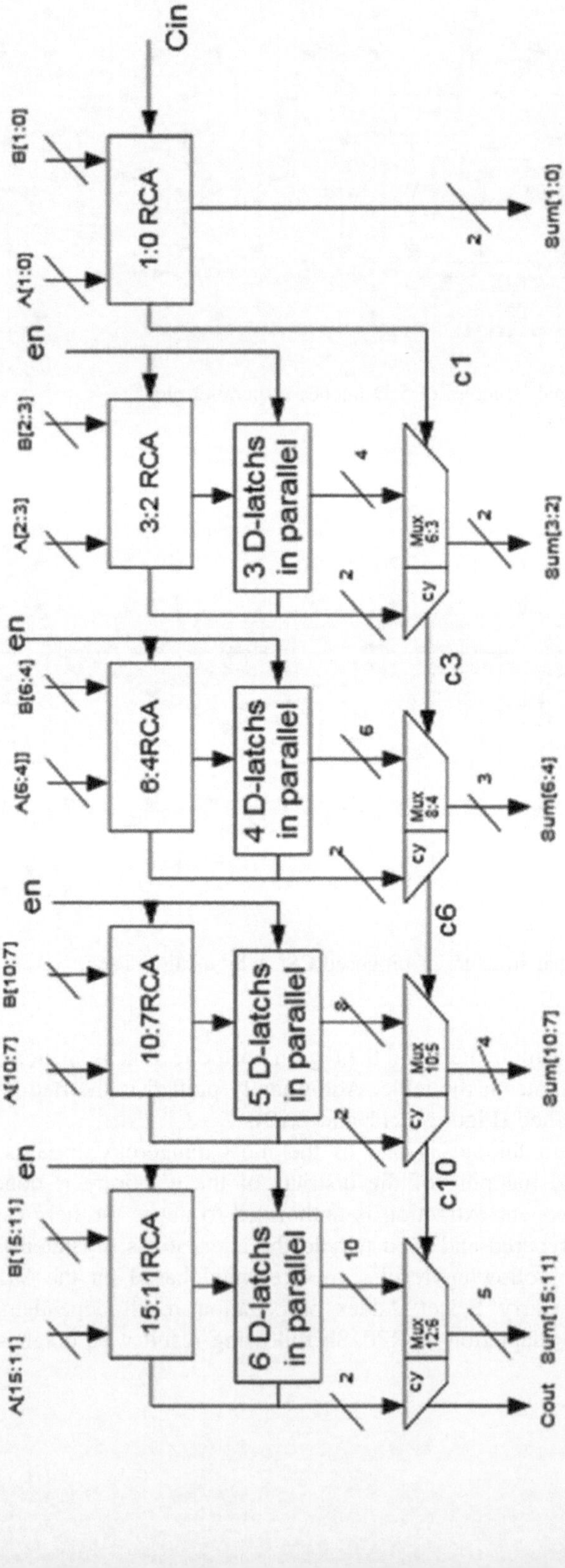

FIGURE 2.10 Presented D-latch.

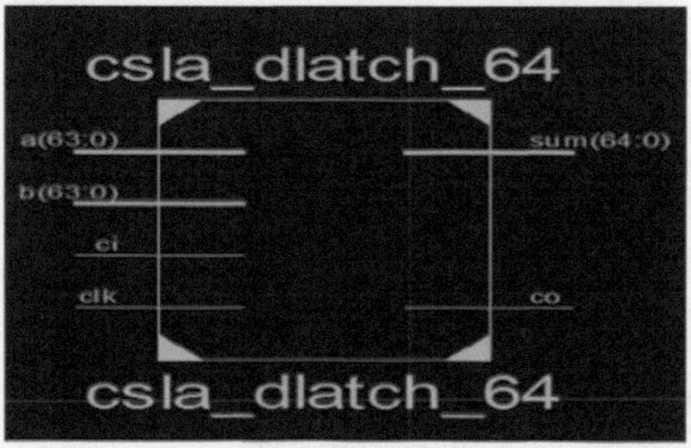

FIGURE 2.11 View of a 64-bit CSLA with D-latch in RTL.

tumour by using image dataset configuration. This image is collected by the patient clinical treatment dataset (Figures 2.13–2.17).

- **Mean Absolute Error**

The mean absolute error is that the distinction between the first and detected labelled values. MAE=original_pixel_valuedetected_pixel_value;

Mean absolute error gift following equation

$$\text{MAE} = \frac{\sum_{i=1}^{n} |y_i - x_i|}{n} = \frac{\sum_{i=1}^{n} |e_i|}{n}$$

Where,

X and y are variables of paired observation.

Mean Error is given following statement,

$$ME = \frac{\sum_{i=1}^{n} y_i - x_i}{n}$$

- PSNR

The image standard is calculated using the height signal to noise quantitative relationship. The difference between the first and detected labelled image is calculated. The amount of noise in the output is compared to the amount of noise in the input Tables 2.1 and 2.2.

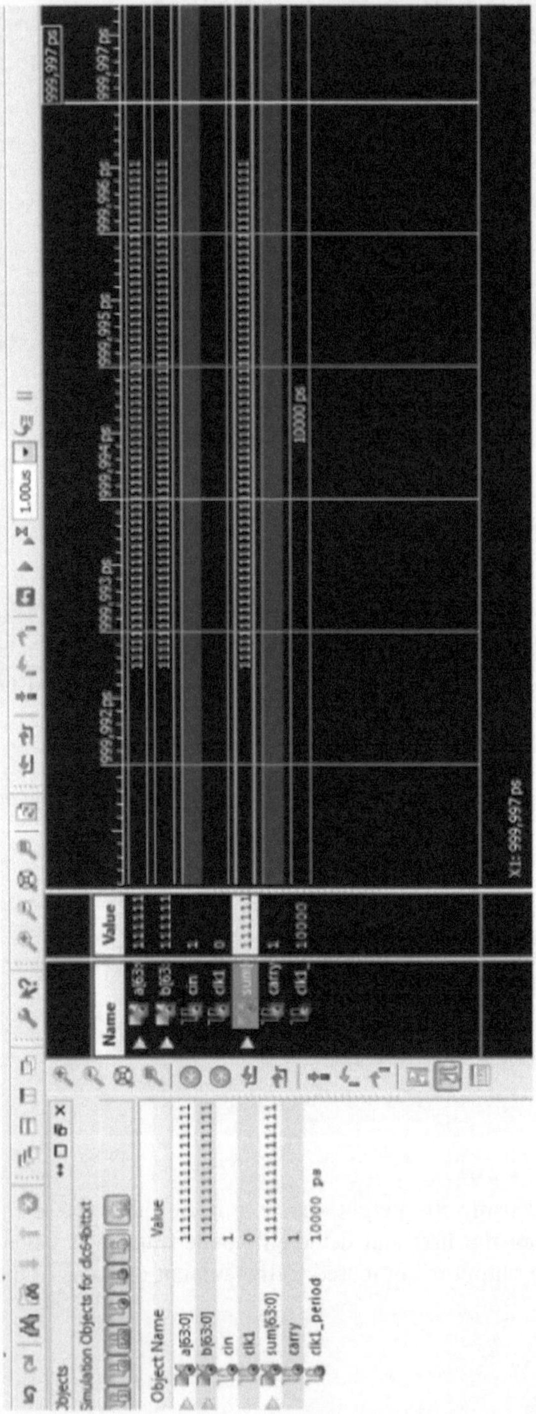

FIGURE 2.12 D-flip flop latch used to simulate the output of a carry select adder.

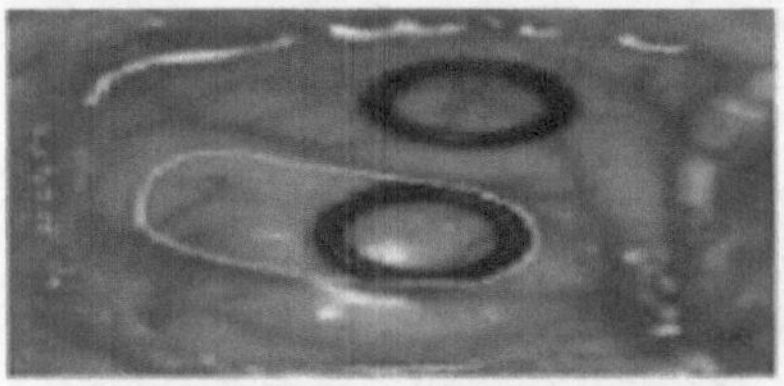

FIGURE 2.13 Input of hyper spectral image.

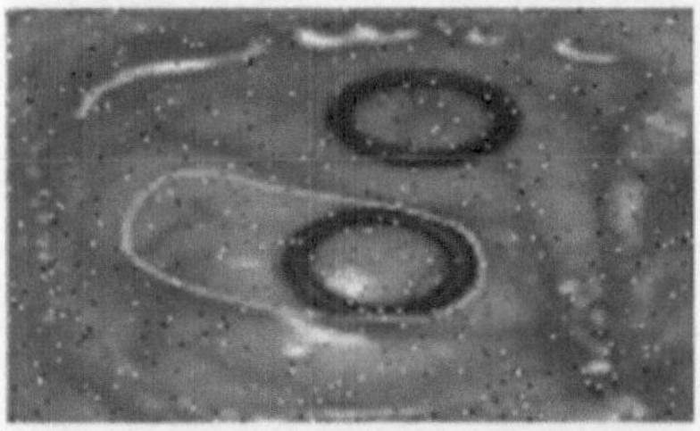

FIGURE 2.14 Noisy image.

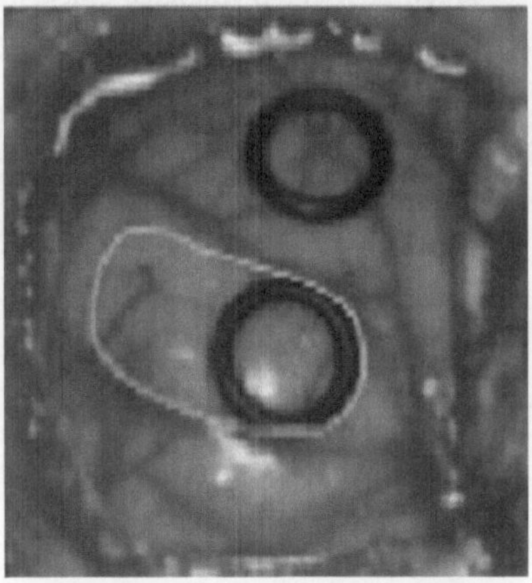

FIGURE 2.15 Gray scale image.

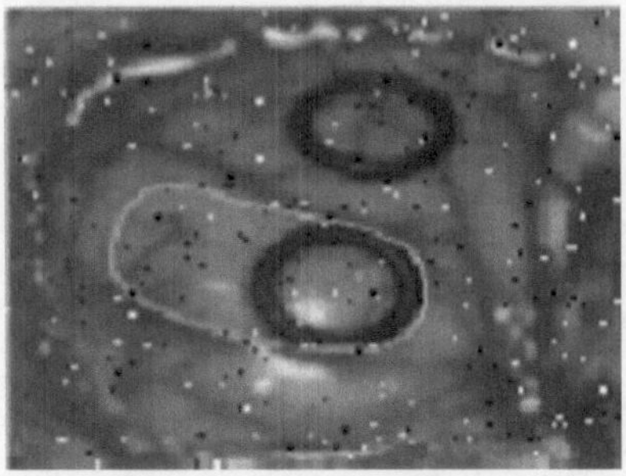

FIGURE 2.16 Noisy image.

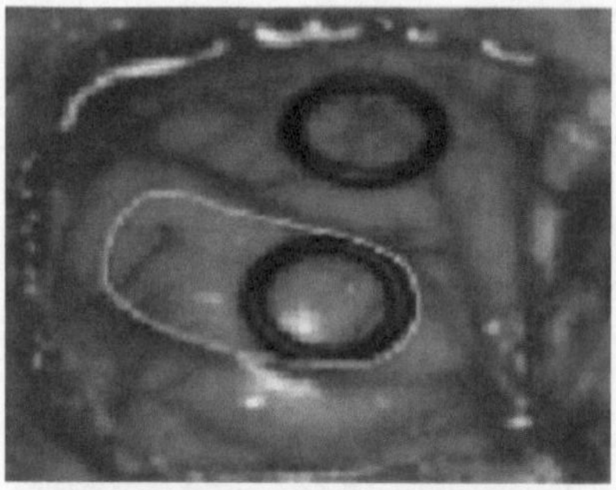

FIGURE 2.17 Filtered image.

TABLE 2.1
Performance Section Comparison

Performance Section	Existing Method (Modified Area Efficient Carry Select Adder)	Proposed Method (Updated Efficient Area - Carry Select Adder propagation)
Number of 4 input LUTs used	43	44
Available LUTs	9312	9313
Delay	37.772	14.73
Total Supply Power	76	72
Power Utilized	2.351	1.231

TABLE 2.2
Image Performance Comparison

Metric/method	Hyper spectral image		Filtered image	
	Existing Method	Proposed Method	Existing Method	Proposed Method
Mean absolute error value	75	65	70	40
Peak signal to noise ratio	72	80	75	50

2.3 CONCLUSION

In this work, the Updated Efficient Area-Carry Select Adder is proposed by disposing of the multiplexer, which chooses the yield depending on the convey input. Pressure frameworks are increasingly being implemented on a single chip. Here's a working CSLA that reduces delay and power usage by using a D-latch approach. On a Spartan XC3S500E FPGA device, the results of each of these adders are analysed. The power and area are calculated using RTL-based design. This paper has better outcomes when contrasted with CSLA and adjusted systems. The R2018b adaptation of MATLAB was used to construct a VLSI version of a modified UEA-CSLA architecture for brain disease detection and diagnosis. We will utilize new techniques and optimization algorithms in the future to minimize Area and Power parameters without using assets, based on the specified unique strategy.

REFERENCES

[1] Anand, B., & Teresa, V.V. (2017). Improved modified area efficient carry select adder (MAE-CSLA) without multiplexer. *Journal of Computational and Theoretical Nanoscience*, *14*(1), 269–276.

[2] Sasamal, T.N., Singh, A.K., & Ghanekar, U. (2018). Efficient design of coplanar ripple carry adder in QCA. *IET Circuits, Devices & Systems*, *12*(5), 594–605.

[3] Williams, A.C., Brown, A.D., & Zwolinski, M. (2000). Simultaneous optimisation of dynamic power, area and delay in behavioural synthesis. *IEE Proceedings-Computers and Digital Techniques*, *147*(6), 383–390.

[4] Ramkumar, B., & Kittur, H.M. (2012). Low-power and area-efficient carry select adder. *IEEE Transactions on Very Large Scale Integration (VLSI) Systems*, *20*(2), 371–375.

[5] Ying, Z., Dhar, S., Zhao, Z., Feng, C., Mital, R., Chung, C.J., … & Chen, R.T. (2018). Electro-optic ripple-carry adder in integrated silicon photonics for optical computing. *IEEE Journal of Selected Topics in Quantum Electronics*, *24*(6), 1–10.

[6] Wang, Z.R., Li, Y., Su, Y.T., Zhou, Y.X., Cheng, L., Chang, T.C., … & Miao, X.S. (2018). Efficient implementation of Boolean and full-adder functions with 1T1R RRAMs for beyond von Neumann in-memory computing. *IEEE Transactions on Electron Devices*, 65 (10), 4659–4666.

[7] Tan, Y., Xu, W., Huang, T., & Wang, L. (2018). A multilevel code shifted differential chaos shift keying scheme with code index modulation. *IEEE Transactions on Circuits and Systems II: Express Briefs*, *65*(11), 1743–1747.

[8] Balaji, N., Bodasingi, N., & Kumar, G.K. (2014, February). VLSI implementation of modified daubechies architecture for brain disease detection and identification. In *2014 International Conference on Electronics and Communication Systems (ICECS)* (pp. 1–6). IEEE.

[9] Wu, Y., Yang, X., Plaza, A., Qiao, F., Gao, L., Zhang, B., & Cui, Y. (2016). Approximate computing of remotely sensed data: SVM hyperspectral image classification as a case study. *IEEE Journal of Selected Topics in Applied Earth Observations and Remote Sensing*, *9*(12), 5806–5818.

[10] Kumar, G.K., & Balaji, N. (2017, February). Reconfigurable delay optimized carry select adder. In *2017 International Conference on Innovations in Electrical, Electronics, Instrumentation and Media Technology (ICEEIMT)* (pp. 123–127). IEEE.

[11] Prasad, G., Nayak, V.S.P., Sachin, S., Kumar, K.L., & Saikumar, S. (2016, May). Area and power efficient carry-select adder. In *2016 IEEE International Conference on Recent Trends in Electronics, Information & Communication Technology (RTEICT)* (pp. 1897–1901). IEEE.

[12] Kinsman, P.J., & Nicolici, N. (2013). Noc-based FPGA acceleration for monte carlo simulations with applications to spect imaging. *IEEE Transactions on Computers*, *62*(3), 524–535.

[13] Shi, C., & Luo, G. (2018). A compact VLSI system for bio-inspired visual motion estimation. *IEEE Transactions on Circuits and Systems for Video Technology*, *28*(4), 1021–1036.

[14] Müller, J., Wittig, R., Müller, J., & Tetzlaff, R. (2018). An improved cellular nonlinear network architecture for binary and grayscale image processing. *IEEE Transactions on Circuits and Systems II: Express Briefs*, *65*(8), 1084–1088.

[15] Hsieh, J.H., Shih, M.J., & Huang, X.H. (2018). Algorithm and VLSI architecture design of low-power SPIHT decoder for mHealth applications. *IEEE Transactions on Biomedical Circuits and Systems*, *12*(6), 1450–1457.

[16] Maamoun, M., Bradai, R., Meraghni, A., & Beguenane, R. (2010, September). Low cost VLSI discrete wavelet transform and FIR filters architectures for very high-speed signal and image processing. In *2010 IEEE 9th International Conference on Cyberntic Intelligent Systems* (pp. 1–6). IEEE.

[17] Cusinato, P., Bruccoleri, M., Caviglia, D.D., & Valle, M. (1998). Analysis of the behavior of a dynamic latch comparator. *IEEE Transactions on Circuits and Systems I: Fundamental Theory and Applications*, *45*(3), 294–298.

3 Classification of Breast Thermograms using a Multi-layer Perceptron with Back Propagation Learning

Aayesha Hakim and R. N. Awale
Veermata Jijabai Technological Institute, Mumbai, India

CONTENTS

3.1 Introduction....45
3.2 Related Works....47
3.3 Methods & Materials....48
 3.3.1 Pre-processing of Thermograms & Region of Interest (ROI) Segmentation....49
 3.3.2 Feature Extraction & Selection....49
 3.3.3 Designing Steps of a Multi-Layer Perceptron with Back Propagation Learning....51
  3.3.3.1 Phase I: Feedforward Computations....52
  3.3.3.2 Phase II: Back Propagation of the Error....54
  3.3.3.3 Phase III: Update Weights and Error in the Output and Hidden Units....54
3.4 Performance Evaluation Parameters....56
3.5 Classification Results & Discussion....59
 3.5.1 ANN Model with 5 Neurons in Hidden Layer....59
 3.5.2 ANN Model with 10 Neurons in Hidden Layer....62
 3.5.3 ANN Model with 15 Neurons in Hidden Layer....62
3.6 Conclusion & Future Work....66
References....71

3.1 INTRODUCTION

Breast cancer is the irregular, unruly, rapid growth of cells in the breast tissue [1]. It is cure-less and life-threatening. Early screening can improve the patient survival rate. Many imaging technologies [2] have been developed continuously to assist early diagnosis, like mammography, Magnetic Resonance Imaging (MRI) and

DOI: 10.1201/9781003217497-3

ultrasound. Mammography is the gold method to screen breasts for abnormalities but is disadvantageous for the patient due to radiation exposure, along with being invasive and painful. It misses cancer in women with dense glandular breasts. Ultrasound is often used in conjunction with mammography to screen pregnant women. It gives structural information about the breast lump. Like mammography, it fails to work well in dense breast cases giving low-resolution images. MRI gives high false-positives and uses a contrast agent that might be harmful to pregnant women. Due to the inherent negative characteristics of the currently existing imaging techniques, it is important to investigate upcoming technologies that can prove advantageous. One such screening technique is thermography that can detect vascular level changes occurring in breasts years before they get caught on any of the existing diagnosis methods. Thermography does not emit ionizing radiation, is a cost-effective, non-invasive, painless and private procedure. It is approved by Food & Drugs Administration (FDA) to be used in tandem with mammography for screening breasts [3]. A thermal image gives the colour-temperature profile of breasts where each colour maps a temperature. The analysis of this colour image helps to determine where the cancer is most active in the breast tissue [4]. Several past studies [4–6] have substantiated that the temperature of an abnormal/malignant region is higher than the normal region by 2-3°C due to an occurring phenomenon called angiogenesis [3]. Hence, a large number of research works have explored the thermal asymmetry between the contralateral breasts for breast cancer detection. The asymmetric breast patterns that get caught on a thermal camera open the possibility for infrared imaging to be used for safe screening of breasts as shown in Figure 3.1(a) & (b).

Computer-assisted analysis of thermograms with Artificial Intelligence (AI) can further help radiologists to improve diagnostic accuracy as human interpretation can be erroneous [4]. The novelty and contribution of this work are as follows:

i. Building a 2D vector of statistical image features representing breast region of interest (ROI) that includes three types of features (total 15): first order, second order and texture features,
ii. Using feature selection to optimize the number of features to be fed as input to artificial neural network (ANN) for prediction of malignancy,
iii. Designing a Multi-Layer Perceptron (MLP) using back propagation to recognize and differentiate between patterns of benign and malignant thermograms,
iv. Evaluating the model's decision-making ability using a public dataset [8,9] consisting of 214 patient thermograms,
v. Based on the quantitative results obtained, establishing the choice of most proficient neural network model (with respect to the number of neurons in the hidden layer as a hyperparameter) that classifies thermograms into one of its appropriate class.

This work is a step towards automating the screening of breasts and discriminating thermograms as malignant or benign using image statistical features and back propagation multi-layer perceptron. The remaining paper is organized as follows -

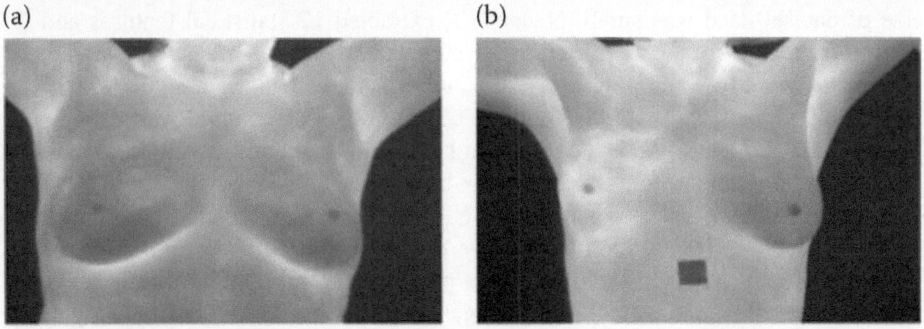

FIGURE 3.1 Sample thermograms (a) healthy, (b) sick [7].

past works related to neural networks are discussed in section 3.2; the methods and materials used to conduct the study are outlined in section 3.3. It also explains the design of MLP step-by-step. The performance evaluation metrics of neural network are briefly described in section 3.4. Results of experiments for classification are discussed in section 3.5. Section 3.6 concludes the paper by highlighting the importance of using thermograms coupled with a well-designed MLP for breast abnormality detection and summarizing the main findings of this work.

3.2 RELATED WORKS

Artificial Intelligence (AI) techniques reduce errors that occur due to manual interpretation and allow computers to perform tasks that require high accuracy, especially in cancer detection where decision making is extremely crucial. AI tools greatly help in improving the healthcare system and thus simplifying the detection of life-threatening diseases. There is a scarcity of radiologists in comparison to the number of cancer cases in India. Reports are read differently by different radiologists at a given time. Thus, good use of computers and AI tools can help sort thermograms into benign and malignant classes efficiently. This will help the clinicians save manual efforts and flag those most in need of the radiologist's attention (i.e., malignant cases) and medical aid. The objective of this study is to determine with a high degree of certainty if a hotspot in a thermal image is malignant or benign using AI.

Acharya et al. [10] extracted five higher order spectra features from thermograms and fed them to a feedforward artificial neural network (ANN). They achieved a sensitivity of 92%. Authors in [11] analysed 60 breast thermograms post extracting the breast region of interest using Canny operator. Employing a multilayer perceptron neural network coupled with biostatistical features, they classified the thermal images into three classes – normal, benign and malignant with an accuracy of 80%. Pramanik et al. [12] proposed Block Variance (BV) technique to extract asymmetry features from thermograms. Using gradient descent error correction rule with a feed-forward ANN, they evaluated 40 malignant and 60 benign thermograms from the Database of Mastology Research (DMR). The number of people who did not have cancer but were identified as having it were less than 0.1%. However, the size of dataset used was small. Nader [13] extracted 12 statistical features and 20 texture features from the thermograms of 206 patients using MATLAB. Using these features as input to a neural network, the author achieved an accuracy of 96.12% in classifying thermograms. In [14], a deep neural network was employed to segment tumour area and classify thermograms. In [15], neural network was used to classify vascular patterns in thermal images on the basis of Marseille system, i.e., TH1-TH5 category. In [16], a back propagation ANN was used to match ANN output with clinical outcome. The ANN successfully predicted the outcome of 18 out of 19 images correctly with the Resilient Back propagation training algorithm, however the dataset used was too small, with images of resolution 128x128. In [17], genetic algorithm was employed in addition to an ANN. Using 8 features collected from each of the 200 thermal images, the accuracy, sensitivity and specificity obtained were 70%, 50% and 75%, respectively. Studies like [18] used Complementary Learning Fuzzy Neural Network (CLFNN) to classify breast thermograms. In another research work [19], the authors used wavelet transformation to extract multidimensional features from 40 breast thermograms. These were downsized and fed to a multilayer perceptron (MLP) to classify images as healthy or pathological. In a similar study [20], Discrete Wavelet Transform (DWT) was applied on the segmented breast ROI to calculate the Initial Feature point Image (IFI). Then, 15 features were fed forward to a Multilayer Perceptron network (MLP). The achieved accuracy, sensitivity and specificity were 90.48%, 87.6% and 89.73%, respectively. Researchers in [21] worked upon estimating the location and dimension of a tumour in the numerically modelled cancerous breast in COMSOL software using Pennes bio-heat equation. They trained the ANN with tumour parameters and reported accuracies of 90% and 95% for predicting location and dimension of tumour, respectively. Authors in [22] used various machine learning algorithms like KNN, logistic regression, SVM and Naïve Bayes with and without Principal Component Analysis (PCA) on the DMR images and reported an overall accuracy of 92.74%. They obtained improvised results using tree-based classifiers in a further study [23]. An overall accuracy of 94.4% with 5-fold cross-validation was reported using random forest classifier. In [24], fractal texture features, namely Hurst coefficient, fractal dimension and lacunarity were extracted from the segmented breast region for abnormality identification. These features were fed to classification algorithms like Support Vector Machine (SVM), logistic regression, k-Nearest Neighbours (KNN) and Naïve Bayes to classify thermograms as healthy or sick. The best accuracy reported was 94.53% for Naïve Bayes classifier. All these studies indicate that there is evidence of using thermography along with neural networks and AI to automate the process of breast abnormality identification.

3.3 METHODS & MATERIALS

The objective of this study is to automate the process of determining if a suspicious region in thermogram is malignant or benign using multi-layer perceptron. We employed the Database of Mastology Research (DMR) [9] developed by Silva et al. [8]. It consists of unhealthy and healthy case images of women aged between 29–85 years. Experiments were conducted using MATLAB R2015b on HP system, Intel

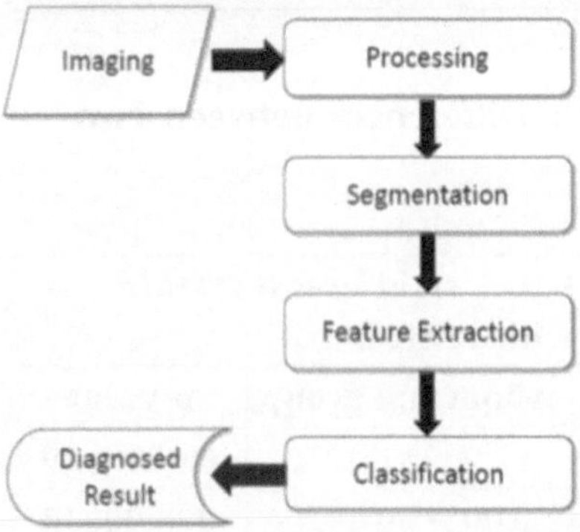

FIGURE 3.2 Flowchart of the proposed methodology.

(R) Core (TM) i5- 1035G1 CPU @ 1.00 GHz and 1190 MHz with 4.00 GB memory (RAM) on 64-bit Windows Operating System, x64- based processor. The flowchart of the proposed methodology is presented in Figure 3.2.

3.3.1 Pre-processing of Thermograms & Region of Interest (ROI) Segmentation

The Database of Mastology Research (DMR) comprises RGB breast thermal images. They are converted into grayscale images, G_{gray}, using the National Television System Committee (NTSC) conversion formula [25] as shown below:

$$G_{gray} = (0.299 * red_{component}) + (0.587 * green_{component}) + (0.114 * blue_{component})$$

The breast region of interest (ROI) is separated and the boundaries are delineated. Other warm areas like armpits, neck and area below the breasts are eliminated using a threshold and breast mask as discussed in detail in [26]. The process of ROI extraction is shown in Figure 3.3.

3.3.2 Feature Extraction & Selection

First-order statistical features, namely, mean, variance, standard deviation, skewness, kurtosis, entropy; second-order features, namely, contrast, correlation, energy,

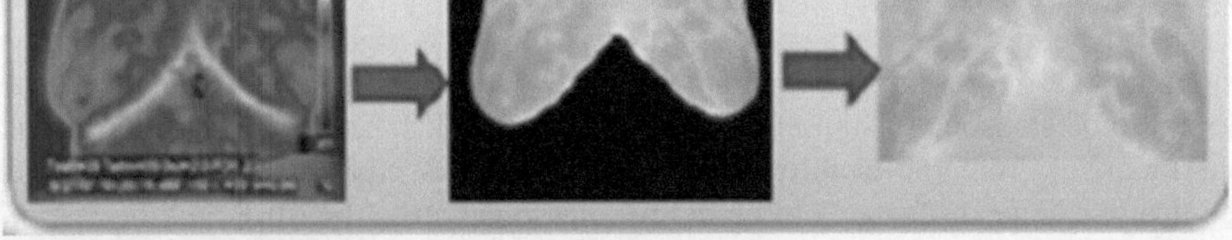

FIGURE 3.3 Segmentation of breast region (ROI).

TABLE 3.1
Test of Significance of Mean of Feature Value Differences Between Two Breasts [26]

		Average of left & right breast feature differences		
	Features	**Normal group**	**Abnormal group**	**p-value**
First Order Features	Mean	4.535±2.4067	11.969±1.4936	**0.0000819**
	Variance	0.0003±0.0025	0.0083±0.0096	**0.0000035**
	Standard Deviation	0.008±0.0076	0.0231±0.0143	**0.0000038**
	Skewness	0.176±0.1154	0.7115±0.256	**0.000334**
	Kurtosis	0.8045±0.234	0.1686±0.3651	**0.0002018**
	Entropy_1	0.186±0.1285	0.2251±0.198	0.0334
Second Order Features	Energy	0.014±0.0014	0.0241±0.0218	**0.00427**
	Contrast	0.018±0.013	0.0031±0.016	**0.00122**
	Correlation	0.004±0.0038	0.0085±0.0073	**0.0002539**
	Cluster Shade	7.021±2.115	8.116±1.215	0.089
	Cluster Prominence	18.51±2.091	15.116±4.129	0.075
	Entropy_2	0.05±0.0357	0.1093±0.0714	**0.0002398**
	Homogeneity	0.005±0.0029	0.0084±0.0049	**0.0001561**
	Dissimilarity	0.196±0.1121	0.312±0.009	0.051
	Maximum Probability	0.00004±0.00002	0.00005±0.00001	0.075

homogeneity, entropy, cluster shade, cluster prominence, dissimilarity, maximum probability is extracted from the segmented thermal breast region. Their mathematical formulae and descriptions are discussed at length in [26–29]. We test the significance of these features using the Mann-Whitney-Wilcoxon test [26]. The corresponding p-values are listed in Table 3.1.

When the means between values of the two classes is high, the test is statistically significant, as represented in bold in Table 3.1. Out of 15 features, 10 features are found to be statistically significant, i.e., with $p < 0.01$ in distinctly separating sick thermograms from the healthy ones. A feature set is created comprising of the clinically significant features to be fed for classification to the MLP and the rest of them are skipped. This helps to minimize the computation cost and time, increase the accuracy of neural network, represent the images using low dimension space and only the most relevant visual aspects are emphasized. We also normalize each of these 9 variables using the formula below such that all values range between 0 and 1. This helps in speeding up the training time.

$$X_{normalized} = \frac{X - X_{min}}{X_{max} - X_{min}}$$

where, $X_{normalized}$ is the normalized value of input, X is the observed value, X_{max} and X_{min} are the minimum and maximum observed values.

3.3.3 Designing Steps of a Multi-Layer Perceptron with Back Propagation Learning

The breast thermal images exhibit minute vascular patterns which are difficult to be identified by human vision. Artificial Neural Network (ANN) [7,30] is a supervised learning method that uses processing elements called neurons to recognize patterns that aid in medical diagnosis. These neurons are arranged in layers and are interconnected with synaptic weights [31]. The most effective 9 features of each thermal image are fed to the MLP for training and classification. The training data learns the association between features and the outcome, while the test data assess the classifier's generalization ability [32]. The quantity of neurons in the output layer is 2 corresponding to the 2 classes in the target vector, i.e., benign and malignant. Due to the presence of one hidden layer, this network is a shallow neural network. Figure 3.4 illustrates the system architecture to classify thermograms into predefined discrete binary classes, benign and malignant.

We apportion the data randomly as: 70% training data (150 samples), 15% validation data (32 samples) and 15% test data (32 samples). Figure 3.5 gives an illustration of the designed feed-forward, fully connected Multi-Layer Perceptron (MLP) using the back propagation learning algorithm. The training of this designed neural network comprises three phases which are repeated iteratively until the stopping condition is met. Once a solution is found, the network is said to have converged. The interconnection weights are selected during the training procedure

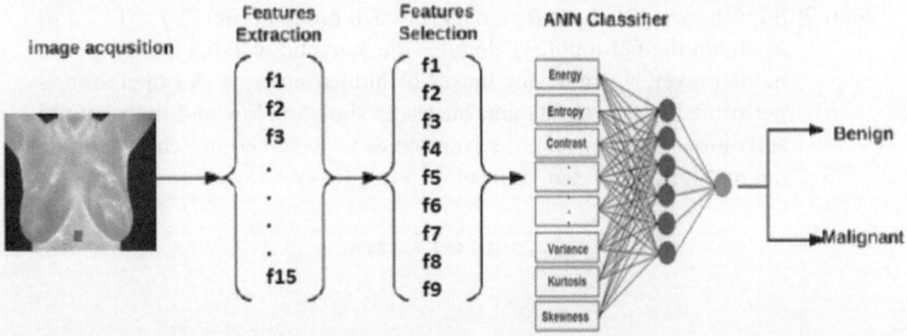

FIGURE 3.4 Neural network system architecture using 9 statistically significant features.

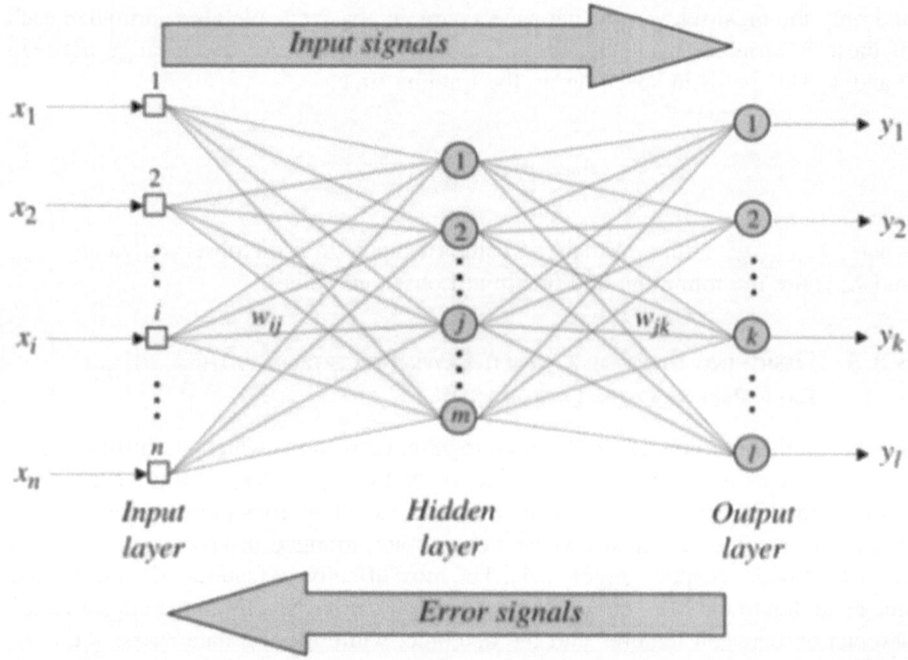

FIGURE 3.5 An illustration of the multi-layer perceptron with back propagation mechanism.

with the provided input-output pairs. Using them the MLP should be able to generate reasonable output for input that was not included in the training sets, i.e., unseen test data. After the network is trained, only feedforward happens. Figure 3.6 gives the pseudocode of the back propagation learning mechanism.

3.3.3.1 Phase I: Feedforward Computations

Step 1. Random set of weights and biases are generated for the neurons initially. The scaled input signal (x_i, $i = 1, \ldots, n$) is broadcasted to all the hidden layer units.

Step 2. Sum the weighted input signals for each hidden unit (Z_j, $j = 1, \ldots, p$) to obtain the net input. v_{ij} denotes the synaptic weights from input to hidden layer, v_{0j} indicates biases of hidden layer. A dot operation is performed with weights and biases as shown below and the required activation function (f), i.e., sigmoid is executed to calculate the output signal for each neuron.

$$z_{in\,j} = v_{0j} + \sum_{i=1}^{n} x_i v_{ij}$$

$$Z_j = f(z_{in\,j})$$

```
Assign all network inputs and output

Initialize all weights with small random numbers, typically between -1 and
1

repeat

  for every pattern in the training set

    Present the pattern to the network

//    Propagated the input forward through the network:
      for each layer in the network
        for every node in the layer
          1. Calculate the weight sum of the inputs to the node
          2. Add the threshold to the sum
          3. Calculate the activation for the node
        end
      end

//    Propagate the errors backward through the network
      for every node in the output layer
        calculate the error signal
      end

      for all hidden layers
        for every node in the layer
          1. Calculate the node's signal error
          2. Update each node's weight in the network
        end
      end

//    Calculate Global Error
      Calculate the Error Function

  end

while ((maximum number of iterations < than specified) AND
      (Error Function is > than specified))
```

FIGURE 3.6 Pseudocode for the multi-layer perceptron (MLP) with back propagation mechanism.

$$f(z_{in\,j}) = \text{sigmoid}(z_{in\,j})$$

Step 3. The weighted inputs for output units (Y_k, $k = 1, \ldots, m$) is summed and an activation function, i.e., SoftMax is applied to calculate the output signal for each neuron.

$$y_{in\,k} = w_{0k} + \sum_{k=1}^{p} z_j w_{jk}$$

$$Y_k = f(y_{in\,k})$$

where w_{jk} denotes the synaptic weight from hidden layer to the output layer, w_{0k} denotes the biases of hidden layer.

3.3.3.2 Phase II: Back Propagation of the Error

To minimize the discrepancy between the actual (clinical) & desired outcome for every training data point, training error must be minimally minimum. This error is sent back through the network and weights are changed at every step to have the steepest descent in error value using the gradient descent back propagation algorithm [33,34] as follows.

Step 4. Compute the error gradient term for each output unit (Y_k, $k = 1, \ldots, m$). The output unit receives a target and computes the error correction term as follows,

$$\delta_k = E(y, S(z))\, f'(y_{in\,k})$$

Step 5. Send δ_k to the hidden layer backwards and update the weights (increase or decrease) & biases between the hidden and output layer. The learning rate (α) is a multiplier, which determines the magnitude of change in the network weights and biases during each training cycle. The weights are trained to predict the right category for an incoming sample image. With a low learning rate, the algorithm takes smaller steps when updating the weights and biases, and thus may take longer to converge. However, a learning rate that is set too high may result in an unstable network. We chose a learning rate of 0.01 to reach the minima, i.e., negative gradient direction.

$$\Delta w_{jk} = \alpha \delta_k z_j; \quad \Delta w_{0k} = \alpha \delta_k$$

Step 6. Each hidden unit sums its delta inputs back propagated from the output units using,

$$\delta_{in\,j} = \sum_{k=1}^{m} \delta_k w_{jk}$$

Step 7. The weights and biases are updated between hidden and input layer using,

$$\delta_j = \delta_{in\,j} f'(z_{in\,j})$$

$$\Delta v_{ij} = \alpha \delta_j x_i; \quad \Delta v_{0j} = \alpha \delta_j$$

3.3.3.3 Phase III: Update Weights and Error in the Output and Hidden Units

If the output is incorrect, weights and errors have to be updated to reach the global loss minimum.

Step 8. Update the biases and weights ($j = 0, \ldots, p$) for each output unit using,

$$w_{jk}(\text{new}) = w_{jk}(\text{old}) + \Delta w_{jk}$$

$$w_{0k}(\text{new}) = w_{0k}(\text{old}) + \Delta w_{0k}$$

Step 9. Each hidden unit also updates its weights and biases using,

$$v_{ij}(\text{new}) = v_{ij}(\text{old}) + \Delta v_{ij}$$

$$v_{0j}(\text{new}) = v_{0j}(\text{old}) + \Delta v_{0j}$$

Step 10. Any of these stopping conditions [35] can cease the training of the MLP:

1. The limit of 50 epochs is reached.
2. The upper limit for the training errors is reached.
3. The gradient of performance falls below min_grad, i.e., 10^{-6}.
4. Validation performance has increased more than 6 times since the last time it decreased.
5. When the cross-entropy error of validation samples increases.

The activation function used at the output for the nth data sample is SoftMax transfer function that normalizes its input into 2 probabilities. This ensures that the sum of the probabilities of the output vector S(Z) is 1. The MLP will output the class with highest measure of certainty as the true class (benign or malignant). The SoftMax function and its derivative are expressed as follows,

$$S(Z_k) = \frac{e^{Zk}}{\sum_{i=1}^{H} e^{Zi}}$$

$$S'(Z_k) = S(Z_k) * [1 - S(Z_k) \text{ if } i = k$$

$$= - S(Z_k) * S(Z_i) \text{ if } i \neq k$$

Cross entropy (log loss) is used with SoftMax layer and is calculated using the following expression,

$$E(y, S(Z)) = -\sum_{i=1}^{H} y_i \times \ln(S(Z_i))$$

where, y_i is the probability of the class as per the ground truth. For an I-H-O net, the number of unknown weights & biases to be estimated is calculated using the

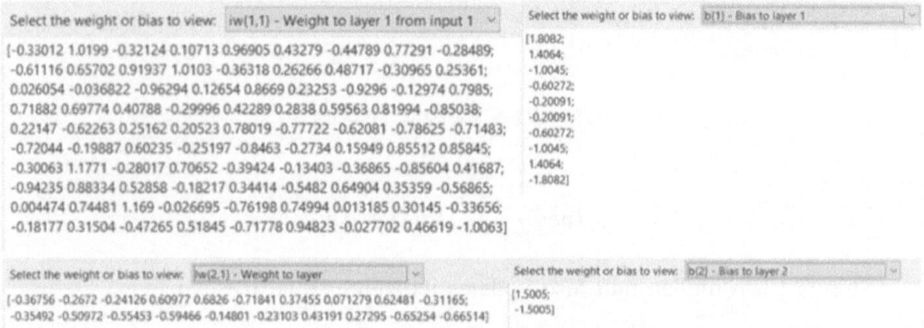

FIGURE 3.7 Estimated weights and biases for the MLP with 10 hidden neurons.

equation below. Figure 3.7 shows the estimated weights and biases for a model with 10 hidden neurons.

$$N_w = (I + 1) * H + (H + 1) * O = (9 + 1) * 10 + (10 + 1) * 2 = 122$$

3.4 PERFORMANCE EVALUATION PARAMETERS

Comparison of the performance of a classifier with other classifiers to categorize thermograms is done using various evaluation metrics. Accuracy, sensitivity,

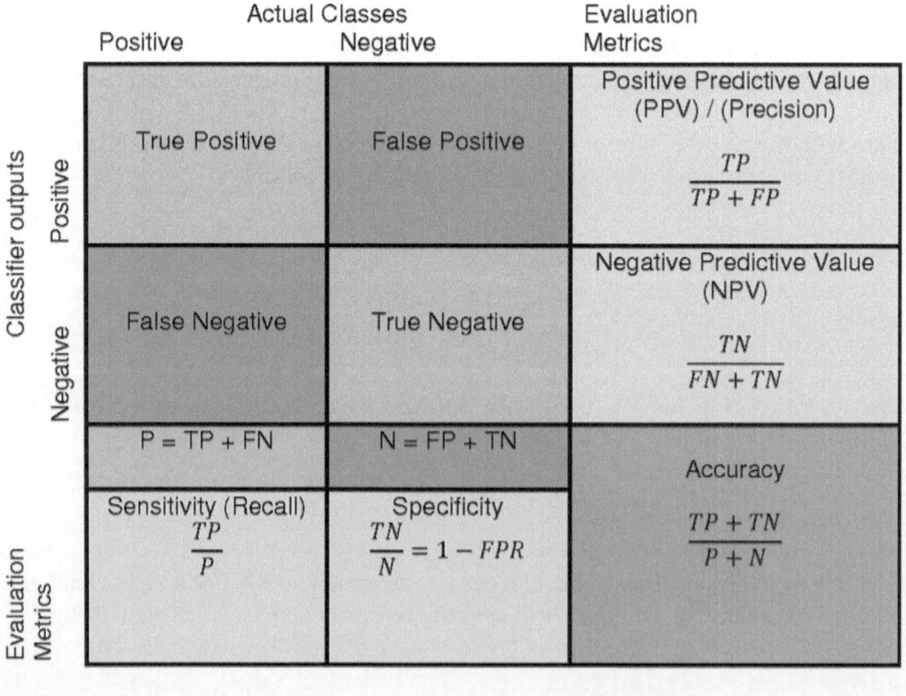

FIGURE 3.8 Confusion matrix and evaluation metrics of a classifier.

specificity, PPV and NPV are calculated using the data in the confusion matrix, which uses the values of - True-Positive (TP) True-Negative (TN), False Positive (FP) and False Negative (FN). True-Positive: malignancy is correctly classified; True-Negative: benign cases correctly identified as benign; False-Positive: benign cases incorrectly classified as malignant; False-Negative: malignancy incorrectly identified as benign. The confusion matrix is a 2 × 2 matrix that helps to evaluate the performance of supervised classification algorithms. The diagonal

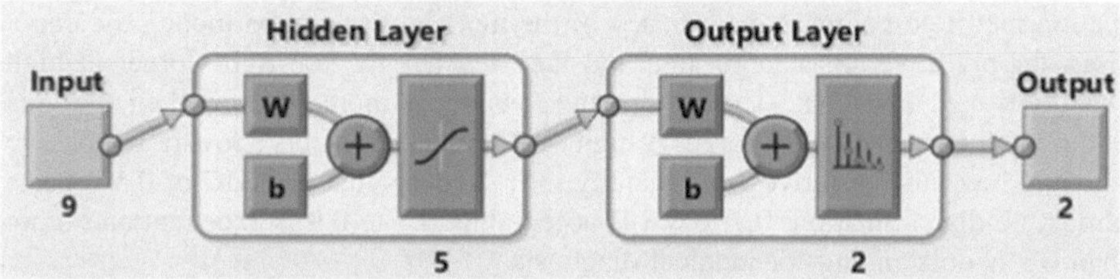

FIGURE 3.9 Design of ANN with 5 neurons in hidden layer.

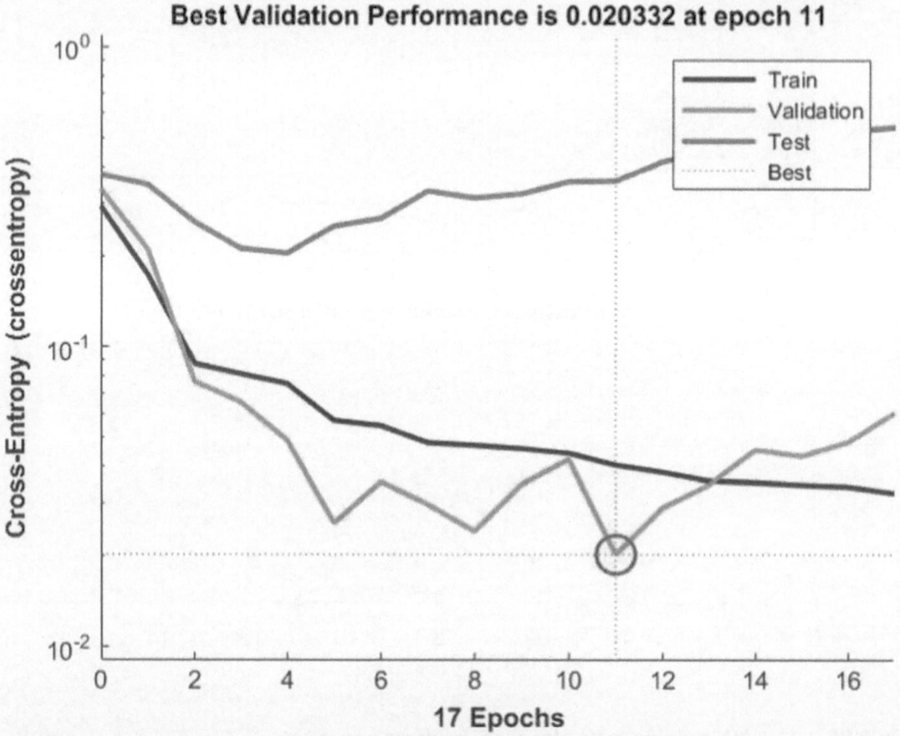

FIGURE 3.10 NN training performance plot for 5 hidden neurons.

grid values in the matrix show the number of cases that are correctly classified and the off-diagonal values show the falsely classified cases. Accuracy gives the percentage of correct classification. However, it is not enough alone to reveal how well the model predicted 'benign' and 'malignant' cases independently. Sensitivity is the ability of a classifier to detect malignancy while specificity is the ability to detect benign cases. PPV reflects the malignant possibility of positive result while NPV reflects the benign possibility of a negative result as shown in Figure 3.8.

The area under the Receiver Operating Characteristics (ROC) curve is an evaluation metric to compare the efficacy of the models. For a good model, the curve rises sharply covering a large area and then reaches the top-right corner at high sensitivity and low FPR. The results are considered more precise when the area under ROC curve (AUC) is large. A high AUC value represents a low false positive rate and low false negative rate. A study [36] suggests that an AUC of 0.5 reflects almost no discrimination, 0.7 to 0.8 is acceptable, 0.8 to 0.9 is excellent and more than 0.9 is outstanding for medical diagnosis.

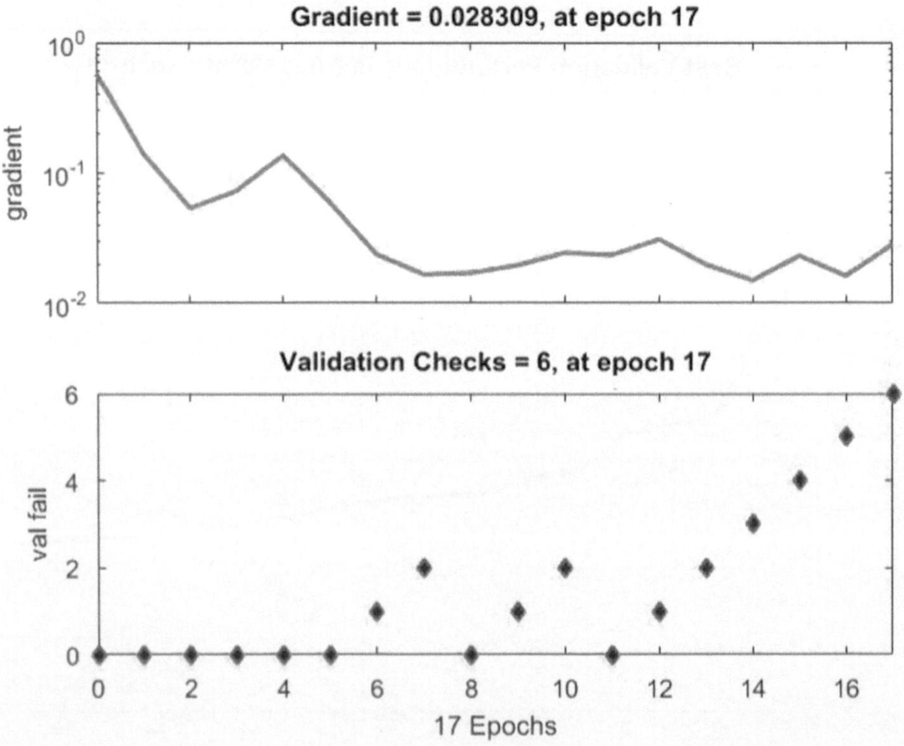

FIGURE 3.11 NN training state plot for 5 hidden neurons.

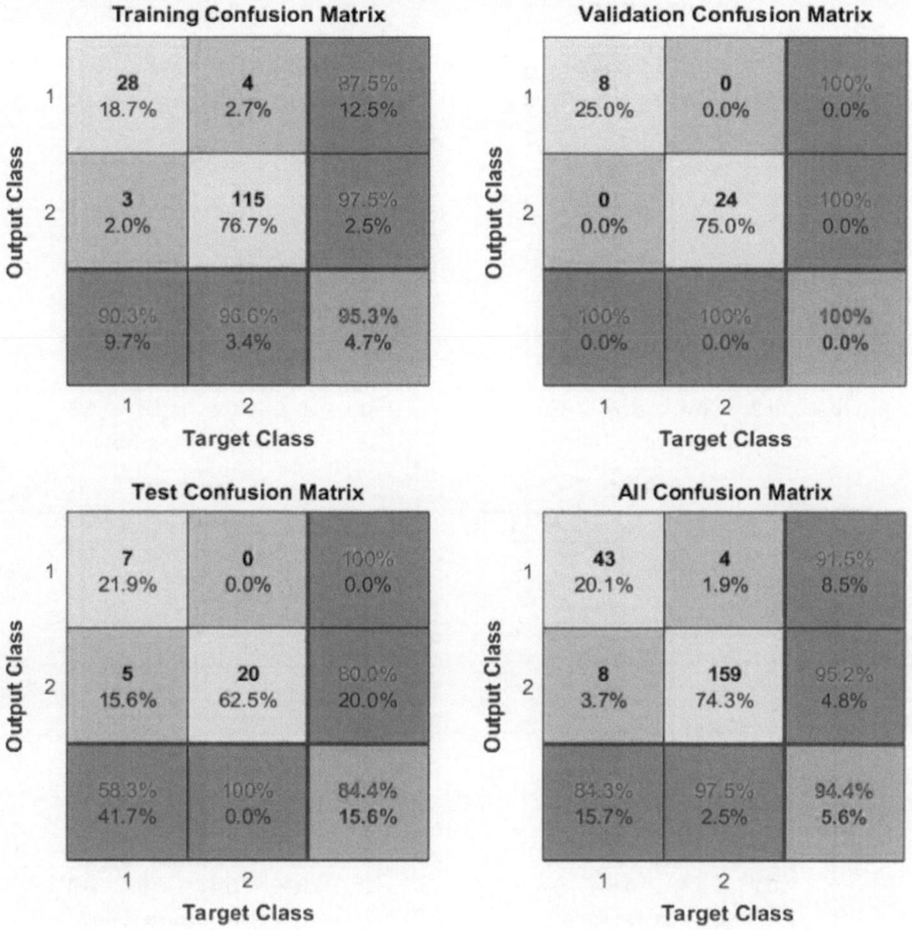

FIGURE 3.12 Confusion matrices for training, test and validation data for NN with 5 hidden neurons.

3.5 CLASSIFICATION RESULTS & DISCUSSION

3.5.1 ANN Model with 5 Neurons in Hidden Layer

We built a multi-layer perceptron with a back propagation mechanism using Neural Network Toolbox [35,37] in MATLAB to estimate the malignancy from breast thermal images. The layers include an input layer of 9 significant image features (shown in Table 3.1), a hidden layer with a number of neurons (hyperparameter) varied from 5 to 15 and an output layer classifying a certain thermogram as benign or malignant. The ANN models with 5, 10 and 15 hidden neurons are shown in Figures 3.9, 3.14 and 3.20, respectively. Many nodes in the hidden layer may lead to an increase in the computation time, whereas few nodes in the hidden layer can

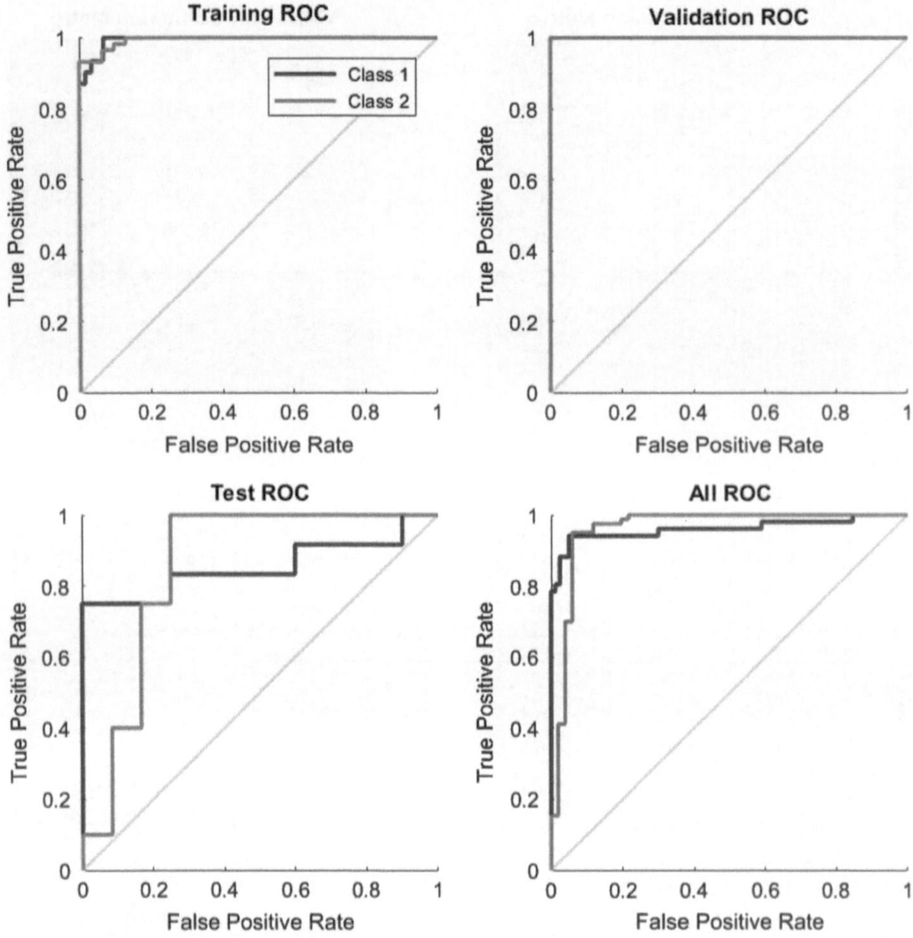

FIGURE 3.13 Training, test and validation data ROC Curves for NN with 5 hidden neurons.

hamper the learning capacity of the model. Usually, the hidden layer size is close to the size of input vector. An epoch is a single pass through all training inputs and target vectors. As the number of epochs increase, the desired output gets closer to actual outcome and cross-entropy rapidly decreases. Performance plot shows the state of training and pinpoints when the cross-entropy error of validation samples increases in green, i.e., stopping of training. Training, validation and test set performance plots for various models are shown in Figures 3.10, 3.16 and 3.21, respectively. The minimum gradient is a stopping criterion used to discontinue the training cycles if the gradient of the error function falls below a specified value. When the gradient decreases to a very small value, change in network weights and biases is not significant enough to produce any appreciable effect on the overall network performance. Training state plot shows the lowest gradient value at the corresponding epoch. For various models, they are shown in Figures 3.11, 3.17

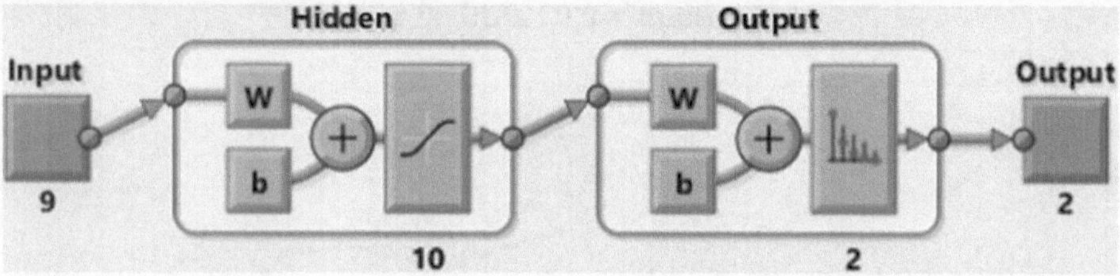

FIGURE 3.14 Design of ANN with 10 neurons in hidden layer.

Results

	Samples	CE	%E
Training:	150	6.35281e-1	6.66666e-0
Validation:	32	1.66789e-0	3.12500e-0
Testing:	32	1.69694e-0	6.25000e-0

FIGURE 3.15 Training, test and validation sample-wise cross-entropy and % error values.

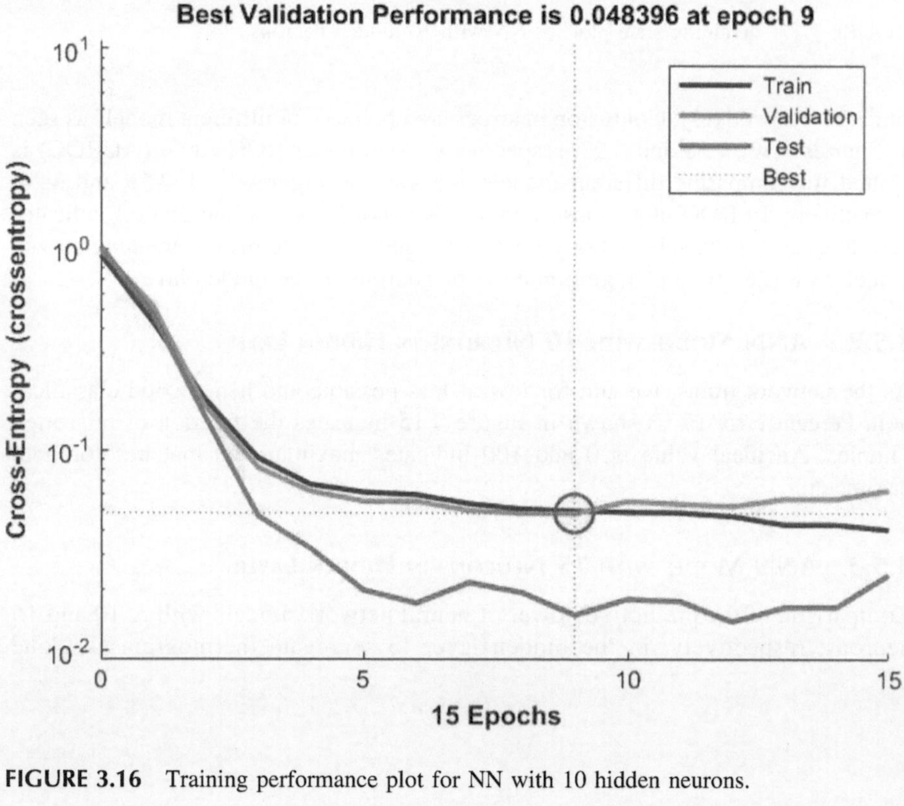

FIGURE 3.16 Training performance plot for NN with 10 hidden neurons.

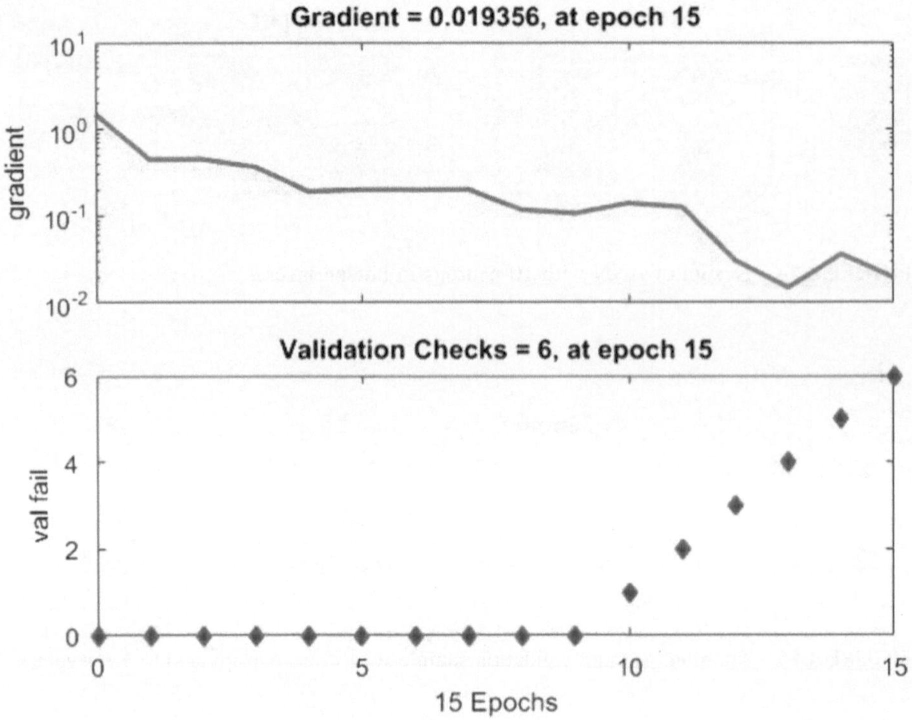

FIGURE 3.17 Training state plot for NN with 10 hidden neurons.

and 3.22, respectively. Confusion matrices are obtained for different models as seen in Figures 3.12, 3.18 and 3.23, respectively. Area under ROC curve (AUROC) is plotted for comparing different models as shown in Figures 3.13, 3.19 and 3.24, respectively. In ROC plots, class 1 indicates abnormal cases and class 2 indicates normal cases. In the sub-sections 3.5.1, 3.5.2 and 3.5.3, the results are summarized model-wise (i.e., w.r.t changing number of neurons in the hidden layer).

3.5.2 ANN Model with 10 Neurons in Hidden Layer

As the network trains, we aim for lowest loss possible and hence good classification. Percent error (%E) shown in Figure 3.15 indicates the fraction of missorted samples. An ideal value is 0 and 100 indicates maximum mismatches for both parameters.

3.5.3 ANN Model with 15 Neurons in Hidden Layer

Comparison of the predictive power of neural network models with 5, 10 and 15 neurons, respectively, in the hidden layer to segregate thermograms is done

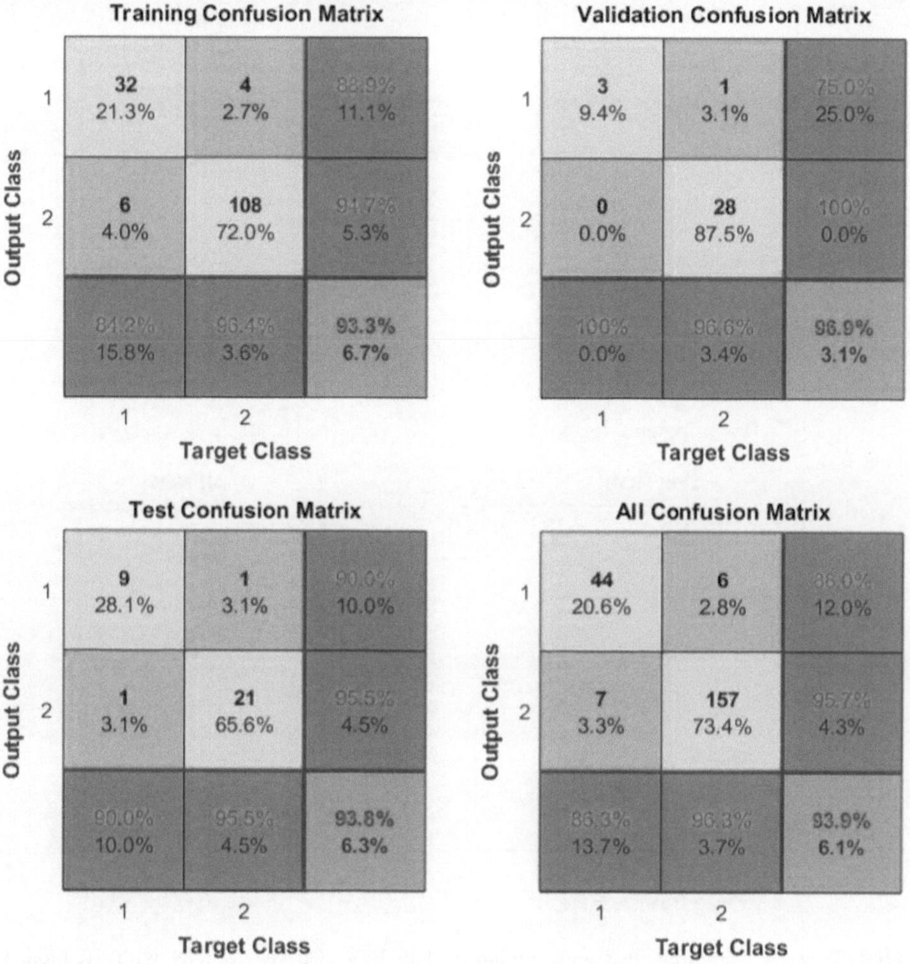

FIGURE 3.18 Confusion matrices for training, test and validation data for NN with 10 hidden neurons.

using accuracy, sensitivity, specificity, PPV and NPV, cross-entropy, gradient and training time. This data is summarized in Table 3.2. For comparison purposes, the number of neurons in hidden layer is varied from 5 to 15 to confirm the best performance of MLP. The accuracy and training time are noted in Table 3.3. The accuracy for test data is maximum for 10 hidden neurons and the MLP performance degrades as the number of hidden neurons are further increased.

In our study, the model with 10 hidden neurons gives the highest accuracy of 93.8% and reaches the target error 0.048396 at 9th epoch. High rates of sensitivity (90%) and specificity (95.5%) were obtained. Networks were sufficiently trained to

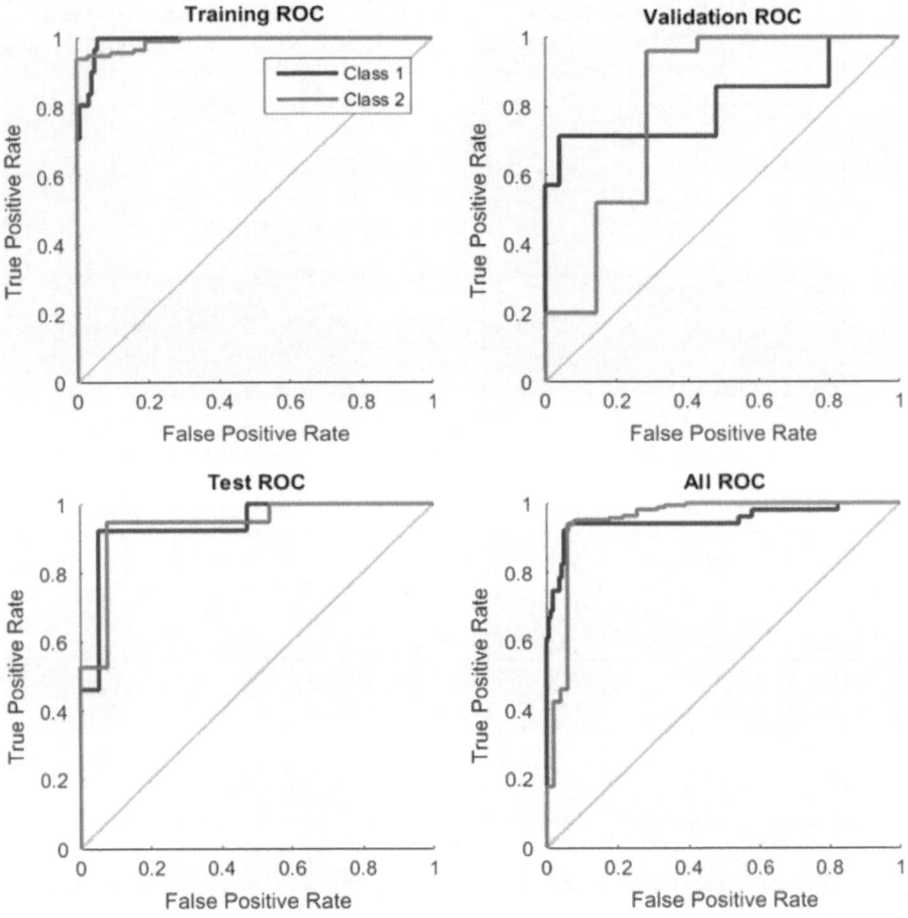

FIGURE 3.19 Training, test and validation data ROC Curves for NN with 10 hidden neurons.

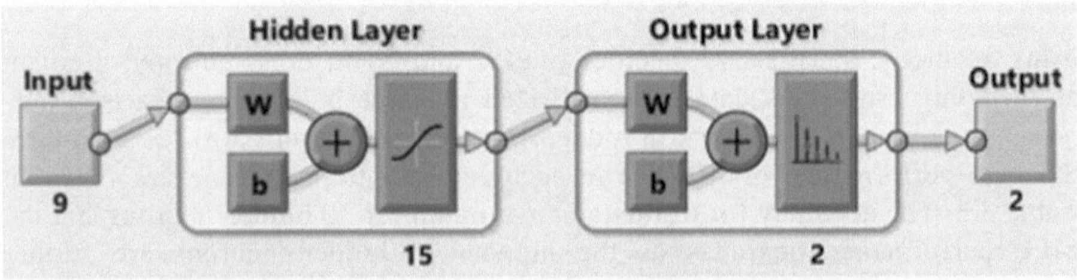

FIGURE 3.20 Design of ANN with 15 neurons in hidden layer.

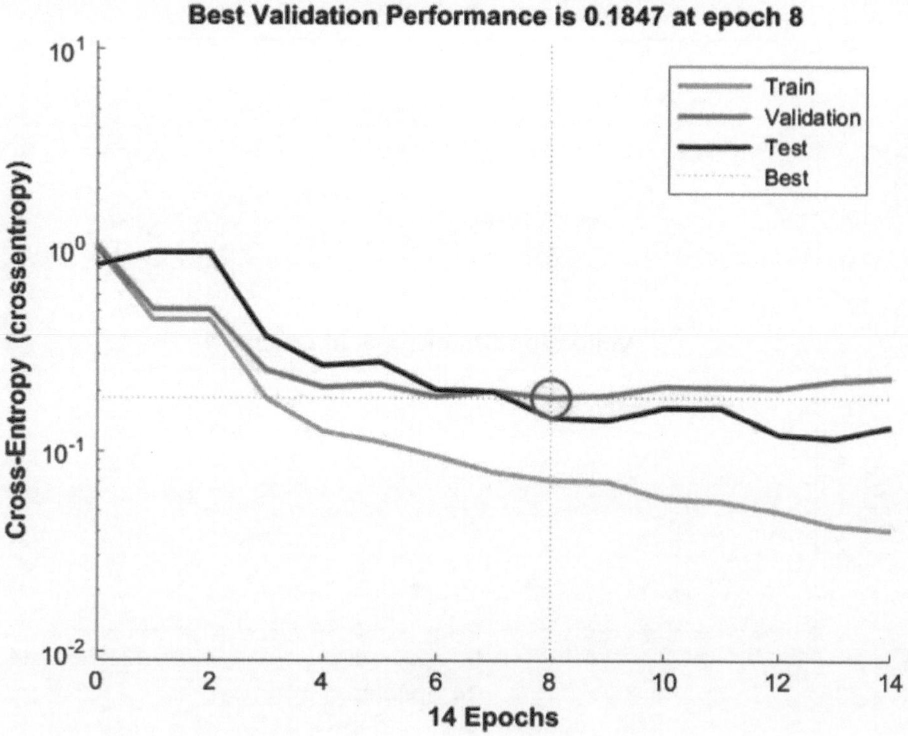

FIGURE 3.21 Training performance plot for NN with 15 hidden neurons.

recognize features used to differentiate the abnormal images from the normal images as the values for PPV are high. When the error of the validation set increases and train set decreases, it implies that the network is overfitted, hence training stops. If we train the network again or increase the number of neurons to 15, the training set performance improves, but the test set performance drastically drops, indicating an overfitted model. A model lacks generalizability when overfitting occurs, i.e., the model 'memorizes' the patterns unique to the training data set but fails to generalize the unseen data and results in low accuracy. Also, the lowest cross-entropy of 0.020332 was produced by the network with 5 hidden neurons but the accuracy was only 84.4%. After varying the number of hidden neurons from 5 to 15, accuracy still remains best for 10 hidden neurons as seen from Figure 3.25. Hence, the number of hidden nodes is chosen as 10 (optimum) in order to obtain the smallest network achievable and address the overfitting problem.

Comparative analysis of our results with the results obtained in past ANN works is tabulated in Table 3.4. The accuracy, sensitivity and specificity of this study are markedly higher as compared to past works with a greater number of images used.

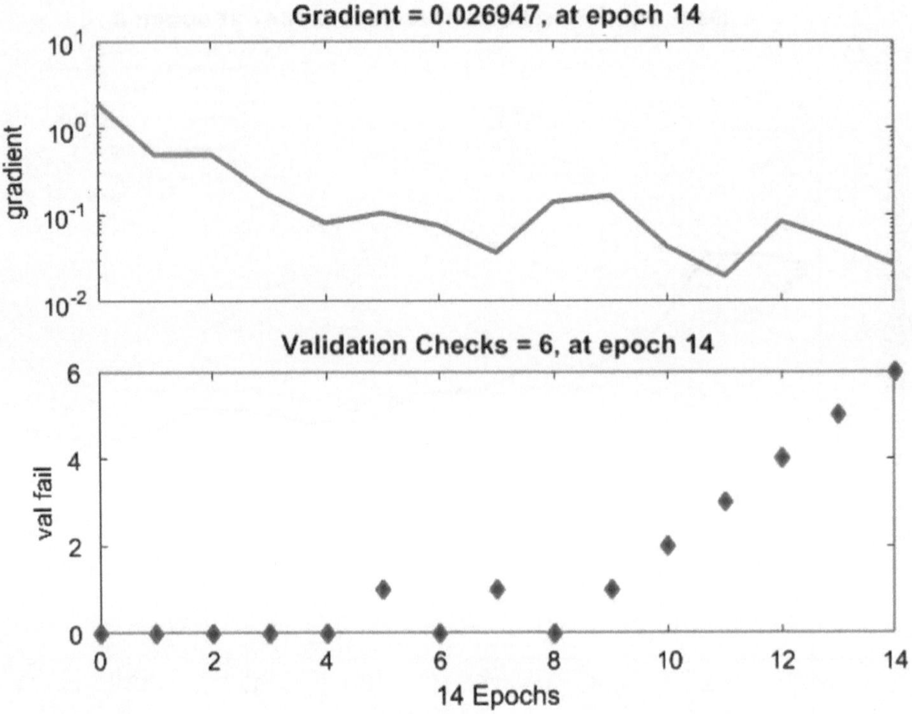

FIGURE 3.22 Training state plot for NN with 15 hidden neurons.

3.6 CONCLUSION & FUTURE WORK

Breast cancer is the cause of maximum female mortality globally. Despite the existence of imaging technologies, due to their inherent inconveniences and disadvantages, research in infrared imaging for breast screening is a necessity. Thermal imaging is an upcoming, non-invasive modality that is capable of screening breasts without exposing the patient to radiation. The manual analysis of thermograms is however sluggish and its perception depends on the level of expertise of the thermographers. This work attempts to segregate breast thermal images based on biostatistical image features using a multi-layer perceptron with back propagation learning. We compared the performance of the designed MLP by varying the number of neurons in the hidden layer as a hyperparameter. The model with 9-10-2 architecture (9 inputs, 10 neurons in the hidden layer and 2 outputs) outperforms the other models with an accuracy of 93.8% on testing data and 96.9% on validation data. The accuracy, sensitivity and specificity of this work are markedly higher as compared to other past works involving ANN. The outcome is promising with value of overall Area Under the Curve (AUC) greater than 0.9 for

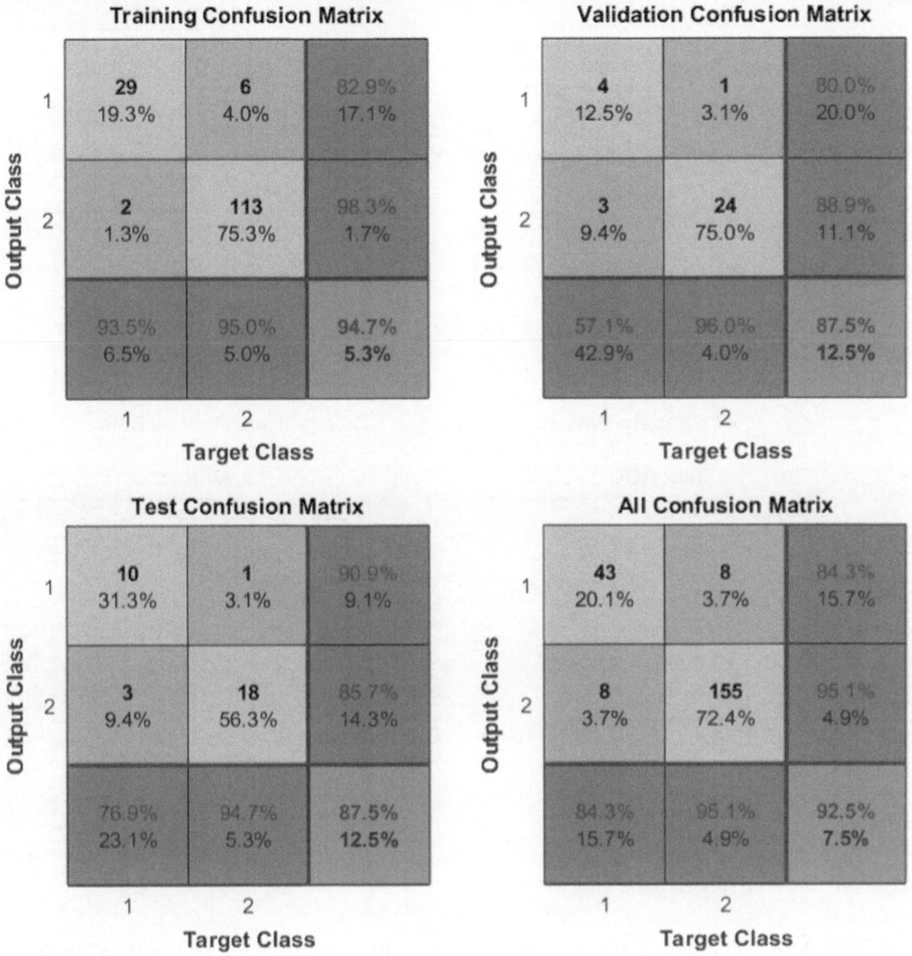

FIGURE 3.23 Confusion matrices for training, test and validation data for NN with 15 hidden neurons.

both classes. Results of the experiments conducted in this study show the potential of using statistical measures extracted from the breast thermograms coupled with well-designed neural networks to detect abnormalities. Thermography can probably be used in the near future in adjunct to ultrasound or mammography in clinical practice in tandem with AI tools. Future works including (a) consideration of fractal and Hurst features for analysing thermal asymmetry between the breasts, (b) use of deep learning AI approaches like Convolutional Neural Networks (CNN) to classify the thermal breast images, (c) localizing the actual size and quadrant-wise position

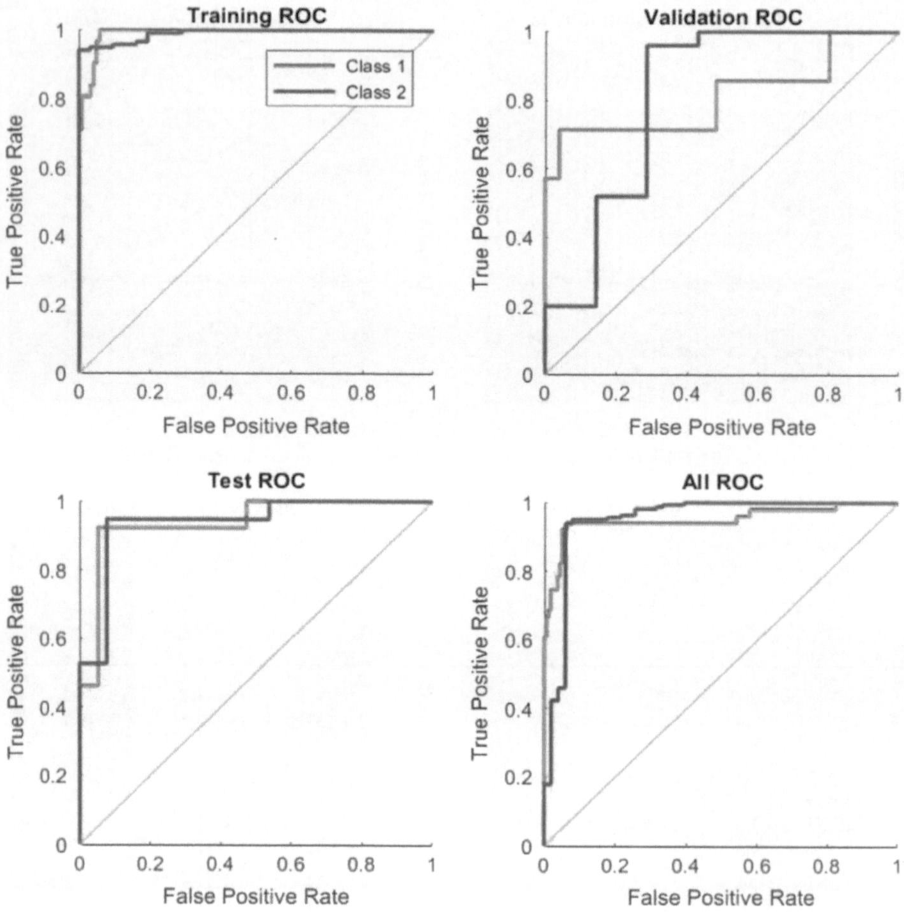

FIGURE 3.24 Training, test and validation data ROC Curves for NN with 15 hidden neurons.

of the tumour are already in progress. However, a larger database that is more inclusive of malignant cases will be helpful for training of robust deep learning classifiers. This work can be extended to employing real-time thermal images collected from various cancer hospitals and converted into an application so that the doctors can use thermography as a valuable supporting tool with AI for accurate breast cancer screening.

TABLE 3.2
Various Evaluation Metrics of the Designed BP-MLP for Varied Number of Neurons in the Hidden Layer

Evaluation metrics	Number of neurons in hidden layer = 10	Number of neurons in hidden layer = 5	Number of neurons in hidden layer = 15
Sensitivity (%)	90	58.3	76.9
Specificity (%)	95.5	100	94.7
PPV (%)	90	100	90.9
NPV (%)	95.5	80	85.7
Accuracy (%)	93.8	84.4	87.5
Cross-entropy	0.048396	0.020332	0.1847
Gradient	0.019356	0.028309	0.026947
Training time (s)	1.8208	0.7125	3.41603

TABLE 3.3
Accuracy and Training Time for Number of Neurons Varied from 5 to 15 in the Hidden Layer

No. of neurons in hidden layer	Accuracy (%)	Training time (s)
5	84.4	0.7125
6	85.6	0.9314
7	88.3	1.2063
8	90.4	1.4587
9	91.6	1.6214
10	93.8	1.8208
11	90.1	2.0012
12	89.6	2.4681
13	88.4	2.8124
14	88	3.1587
15	87.5	3.41603

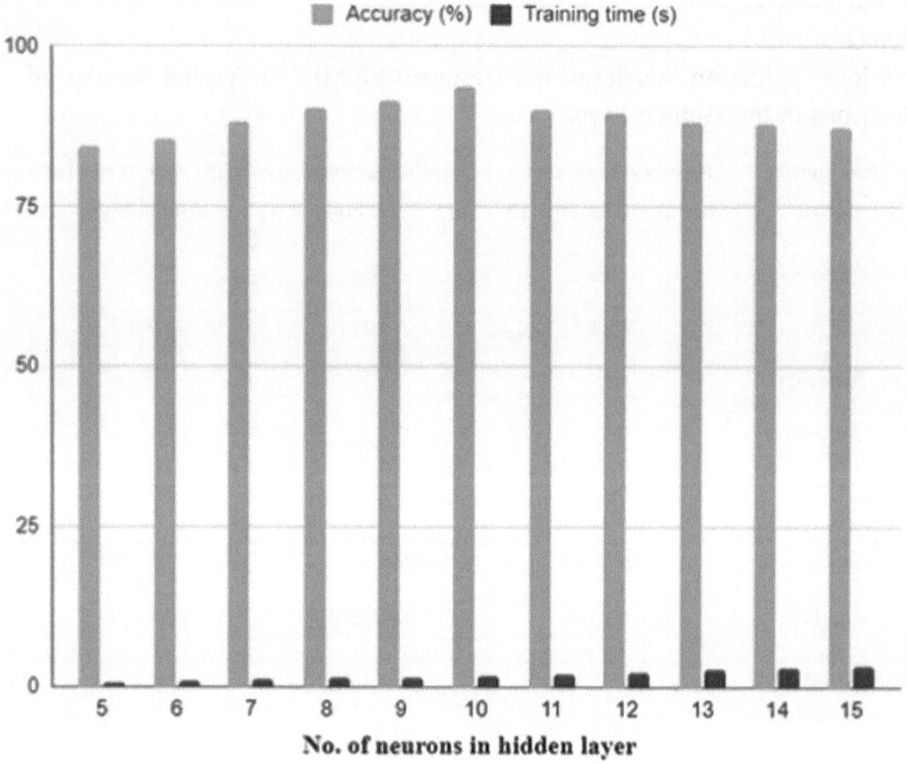

FIGURE 3.25 Accuracy and training time for a number of neurons varied from 5 to 15 in the hidden layer.

TABLE 3.4
Comparative Analysis of Results of this Study and Results of Past Work Involving ANN

Author(s)/ Method	Sensitivity (%)	Specificity (%)	Accuracy (%)	No of images used
Our results (BP-ANN)	**90**	**95.5**	**93.8**	**240 benign, 47 malignant**
G. Wishart et al. (2010) / Sentinel Breast Scan & Neural Network	48	-	-	65 benign, 41 malignant
Zadeh HG et al. (2012) / ANN & Genetic algorithm	50	75	70	200
N. A. Mohamed (2015) / Back propagation Neural Network	78.95	97.86	96.12	187 normal, 19 abnormal
Arora, Nimmi, et al (2008) / ANN	97	44	-	60 malignant, 34 benign
J. Koay, C. Herry, and M. Frize (2004) / Backpropagation 1-1-1 ANN	-	-	95	19

REFERENCES

[1] Breast Cancer India: Pink Indian Statistics. Available at: http://www.breastcancerindia.net/statistics/stat_global.html (accessed on 21 March, 2021).

[2] S. Prasad and D. Houserkova, "The Role of Various Modalities in Breast Imaging", *Biomedical Papers of the Medical Faculty of the University Palacky, Olomouc, Czechoslovakia*, 151(2):209–218, (2007). doi: 10.5507/bp.2007.036.

[3] U.S. Food and Drug Administration. Breast Cancer Screening|Thermography Is Not an Alternative to Mammography: FDA Safety Communication. Available at: https://www.fda.gov/NewsEvents/Newsroom/PressAnnouncements/ucm257633.htm. Date posted:6/2/2011. [Accessed March 3, 2019].

[4] A. Hakim and R. N. Awale, "Thermal Imaging–An Emerging Modality for Breast Cancer Detection: A Comprehensive Review", *Journal of Medical Systems*, 44, 136, (2020). doi: 10.1007/s10916-020-01581-y.

[5] R. N. Lawson and M. S. Chugtai, "Breast Cancer and Body Temperatures", *Canadian Medical Association Journal*, 88(2):68–70, (1963).

[6] A. Hakim and R. N. Awale, "Detection of Breast Pathology using Thermography as a Screening Tool", *15th Quantitative InfraRed Thermography Conference*, 2020. doi: 10.21611/qirt.2020.116.

[7] S. C. Fok, E. Y. K. Ng, and K. Tai, "Early Detection and Visualization of Breast Tumor with Thermogram and Neural Network", *Journal of Mechanics in Medicine and Biology*. 2:185–195, (2002).

[8] L. F. Silva, D. C. M. Saade, G. O. Sequeiros, A. C. Silva, A. C. Paiva, R. S. Bravo, and A. Conci, "A New Database for Breast Research with Infrared Image", *Journal of Medical Imaging and Health Informatics*, 4(1):92–100, (2014). doi: 10.1166/jmihi.2014.1226.

[9] [dataset] Visual Lab, A Methodology for Breast Disease Computer-Aided Diagnosis using dynamic thermography. Available online: http://visual.ic.uff.br/dmi Accessed on 15 April, 2020.

[10] U. R. Acharya, E. Yin-Kwee Ng, S. V. Sree, C. K. Chua, and S. Chattopadhyay, "Higher Order Spectra Analysis of Breast Thermograms for the Automated Identification of Breast Cancer", *Expert Systems*, 31(1):37–47, (2014).

[11] P. Kapoor, S. V. A. V. Prasad, and S. Patni, "Automatic Analysis of Breast Thermograms for Tumor Detection Based on Biostatistical Feature Extraction and ANN", *International Journal of Emerging Trends in Engineering and Development*, 2(7):245–255, (2012).

[12] S. Pramanik, D. Bhattacharjee, and M. Nasipuri, "Texture Analysis of Breast Thermogram for Differentiation of Malignant and Benign Breast", In Proceedings of the 2016 International Conference on Advances in Computing, Communications and Informatics (ICACCI), Jaipur, India, 21–24 September 2016; 8–14.

[13] N. A. Mohamed, "Breast Cancer Risk Detection using Digital Infrared Thermal Images", *International Journal of Bioinformatics and Biomedical Engineering*, 1(2):185–194, (2015).

[14] S. J. Mambou, P. Maresova, O. Krejcar, A. Selamat, and K. Kuca, "Breast Cancer Detection Using Infrared Thermal Imaging and a Deep Learning Model", *Sensors (Basel, Switzerland)*, 18(9):2799, (2018). doi: 10.3390/s18092799.

[15] A. Lashkari, F. Pak, and M. Firouzmand, "Full Intelligent Cancer Classification of Thermal Breast Images to Assist Physician in Clinical Diagnostic Applications", *Journal of Medical Signals and Sensors*. 6(1):12–24, (2016). doi: 10.4103/2228-7477.175866.

[16] J. Koay, C. Herry, and M. Frize, "Analysis of Breast Thermography with an Artificial Neural Network", *Annual International Conference of the IEEE*

Engineering in Medicine and Biology Society, 2:1159–1162, (2004). doi: 10.1109/IEMBS.2004.1403371.

[17] H. G. Zadeh, "Diagnosis of Breast Cancer using a Combination of Genetic Algorithm and Artificial Neural Network in Medical Infrared Thermal Imaging", *Iranian Journal of Medical Physics*, 9:265–274, (2012).

[18] T. Z. Tan, C. Quek, G. S. Ng, and E. Y. K. Ng, "A Novel Cognitive Interpretation of Breast Cancer Thermography with Complementary Learning Fuzzy Neural Memory Structure," *Expert Systems with Applications*, 33(3):652–666, (2007).

[19] S. Pramanik, D. Bhattacharjee, and M. Nasipuri, "Wavelet Based Thermogram Analysis for Breast Cancer Detection," in *Proceeding International Symposium on Advanced Computing and Communication (ISACC)*, Sep. 2015, pp. 205–212, doi: 10.1109/ISACC.2015.7377343.

[20] S. Mitra and C. Balaji, "A Neural Network-Based Estimation of Tumour Parameters from a Breast Thermogram," *International Journal of Heat and Mass Transfer*, 53(21-22):4714–4727, (Oct. 2010), doi: 10.1016/j.ijheatmasstransfer.2010.06.020.

[21] M. A. S. Al Husaini, M. H. Habaebi, S. A. Hameed, Md. R. Islam, and T. S. Gunawan, "A Systematic Review of Breast Cancer Detection using Thermography and Neural Networks", *IEEE Access*, 8:208922–208937, (2020).

[22] A. Hakim and R. N. Awale, "Harnessing the Power of Machine Learning for Breast Anomaly Prediction using Thermograms", *International Journal of Medical Engineering and Informatics (IJMEI)*, [in press], (2021).

[23] A. Hakim and R. N. Awale, "Predictive Analysis of Breast Cancer using Infrared Images with Machine Learning Algorithms", *Analysis of Medical Modalities for Improved Diagnosis in Modern Healthcare*, Taylor & Francis, CRC Press Book, (2020). [in press].

[24] A. Hakim and R. N. Awale, "Identification of Breast Abnormality from Thermograms Based on Fractal Geometry Features," 5th International Conference on Information and Communication Technology for Intelligent Systems (ICTIS-2021), 23-24 April, 2021 (virtual), India. [accepted].

[25] M. Gautherie, *Atlas of Breast Thermography with Specific Guidelines for Examination and Interpretation*. Milan, Italy: PAPUSA. (1989).

[26] A. Hakim and R. N. Awale, "Statistical Analysis of Thermal Image Features to Discriminate Breast Abnormalities", Fifth International Conference on Information and Communication Technology for Competitive Strategies (ICTCS-2020), 11th and 12th December, 2020 (virtual), India.

[27] Image Central moments computed using formulae given in: https://itl.nist.gov/div898/handbook/eda/section3/eda35b.htm (accessed on 24 April, 2020).

[28] R. M. Haralick, K. Shanmugam, and I. H. Dinstein, "Textural Features for Image Classification," *Systems, Man and Cybernetics, IEEE Transactions* on, SMC-3(6):610–621, (1973).

[29] E. Y. Ng, L. N. Ung, F. C. Ng, and L. S. Sim, "Statistical Analysis of Healthy and Malignant Breast Thermography", *Journal of Medical Engineering & Technology,* Nov-Dec, 25(6):253–263, (2001).

[30] T. Jakubowska, B. Wiecek, M. Wysocki, and et al., "Classification of Breast Thermal Images using Artificial Neural Networks", In The 26th Annual International Conference of the IEEE Engineering in Medicine and Biology Society. San Francisco, California: IEEE, 1155–1158, (2004).

[31] M. M. Mehdy, P. Y. Ng, E. F. Shair, N. I. Md Saleh, and C. Gomes, "Artificial Neural Networks in Image Processing for Early Detection of Breast Cancer", *Computational and Mathematical Methods in Medicine*, vol. 2017, Article ID 2610628, 15 pages, (2017). doi: 10.1155/2017/2610628.

[32] A. Arafi, Y. Safi, R. Fajr, and A. Bouroumi, "Classification of Mammographic Images using Artificial Neural Networks", *Applied Mathematical Sciences*, 7(89):4415–4423, (2013).
[33] Y. Hirose, K. Yamashita, and S. Hijiya, "Back-propagation Algorithm which Varies the Number of Hidden Units", *Neural Networks*, 4(1):61–66, (1991).
[34] G. Cauwenbergerghs, "A Fast Stochastic Error-descent Algorithm for Supervised Learning and Optimization", *Advances in Neural Information Processing Systems*, 5: 244–251, (1993).
[35] Statsoft, Model Extremely Complex Functions, Neural Networks, http://www.statsoft.com/textbook/neural-networks/apps (accessed on 25 February 2021).
[36] J. N. Mandrekar, "Receiver Operating Characteristic Curve in Diagnostic Test Assessment", *Journal of Thoracic Oncology*, 5(9):1315–1316, (2010).
[37] Neural Network Toolbox User's guide, R2015b, The Math Works, Natick, MA, 5-32–5-50, (2015).

4 Neural Networks for Medical Image Computing

V.A. Pravina
Assistant Professor, Department of Electronics and Communication Engineering, DMI College of Engineering, India

P.K. Poonguzhali
Assistant Professor, Department of Electronics and Communication Engineering, Hindusthan College of Engineering and Technology, India

A Kishore Kumar
Assistant Professor (SG), Department of Robotics & Automation, Sri Ramakrishna Engineering College, Coimbatore, Tamil Nadu, India

CONTENTS

4.1 Introduction....76
4.2 Structure of Neural Network....76
4.3 Learning Process in Neural Networks....77
4.3.1 Supervised Learning....78
4.3.1.1 An Overview of Supervised Learning....78
4.3.1.2 Supervised Learning in Medical Image Processing....79
4.3.2 Unsupervised Learning....79
4.3.2.1 Unsupervised Learning....79
4.3.2.2 Overview of Competitive Learning....80
4.3.2.3 Medical Analysis using Unsupervised Learning....81
4.3.3 Reinforcement Learning....81
4.3.3.1 Reinforcement Learning....81
4.3.3.2 Overview of Q-Learning....82
4.3.3.3 Adopting Reinforcement Learning in Health Sector....83
4.4 Types of Neural Networks....84
4.4.1 Perceptron....84
4.4.1.1 Perceptron....84
4.4.1.2 Perceptron in Medical Image Analysis....85
4.4.2 Radial Basis Function Network....86
4.4.2.1 Architecture of Radial Basis Function Network....86

DOI: 10.1201/9781003217497-4

4.4.2.2 Implementing Radial Basis Function in Medical Analysis ... 86
4.4.3 Convolutional Neural Network ... 87
4.4.3.1 Architecture of Convolutional Neural Network ... 87
4.4.3.2 Convolutional Neural Networks in Medical Diagnosis ... 88
4.4.4 Recurrent Neural Network ... 89
4.4.4.1 Introduction to Recurrent Neural Network ... 89
4.4.4.2 Types of Recurrent Neural Network ... 89
4.4.4.3 Medical Analysis using Recurrent Neural Network ... 90
4.4.5 Hopfield Neural Network ... 91
4.4.5.1 Overview of Hopfield Neural Network ... 91
4.4.5.2 Hopfield Neural Network in Medical Diagnosis ... 92
4.5 Conclusion ... 94
References ... 94

4.1 INTRODUCTION

Nowadays, neural networks are finding a steady place in the health care sector for the detection of diseases. In neural networks, there are a number of units being processed in parallel that are related to the characteristics of the human brain. Analyzing and processing digital images require complex algorithms that could extract information from images. These networks are trained using data supplied by the user and they provide the desired output. Healthcare industries are incorporating these algorithms to improve accessibility of care, meanwhile making it available at low cost. Neural networks are used to detect various diseases and help doctors make decisions regarding treatment options. These neural networks analyze medical images and help in classification of diseases like tumor and cancer, and can be applied across various medical imaging modalities. The health care industry provides immense opportunities to machine learning to make beneficial impact on human lives. These algorithms aid health care by early and faster diagnosis of diseases, assisting in surgical procedures, and making resource management more efficient.

4.2 STRUCTURE OF NEURAL NETWORK

The neural network contains algorithms that function in the same way as that of the human brain and helps in finding how the data are related to each other. They are inspired by the human brain, mimicking the way the human brain operates. The neural networks have numerous neurons similar to the biological neurons that transfer the signal to one another. These neural networks study the environment and adapt to it. Hence it could possibly analyze the different inputs and produce the outputs without modifying the entire structure.

The neural network functions similarly to the network model of the human brain. The comparison of Biological Neural Network and Artificial Neural Network is shown in Table 4.1. In the biological cell, the neuron performs the function of processing information. It has wires like structures through which the neurons transmit and receive information. There are huge numbers of neurons with

TABLE 4.1
Comparison of Biological Neural Network and Artificial Neural Network

Biological Neural Network	Artificial Neural Network
Axon	Output
Dendrites	Input
Synapse	Weight
Soma	Node

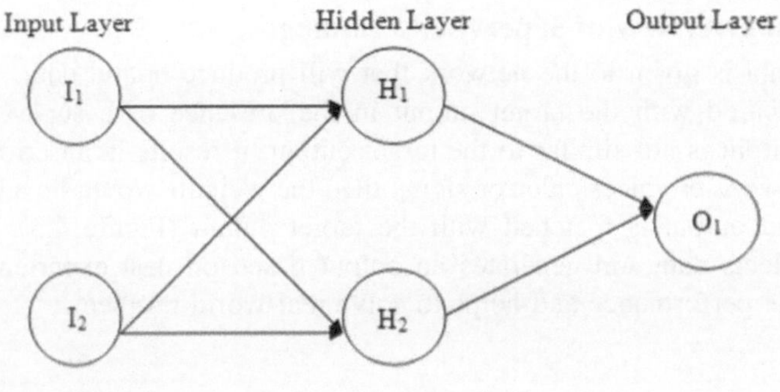

FIGURE 4.1 Simple neural network.

numerous interconnections. The biological neurons are comprised of soma, dendrites, synapses, and axon. The dendrites are those wire-like structures that receive information from various neurons that are present in a network. The soma receives the information from dendrites and passes it to the axon. The nerve fiber through which electrical signals travel from one neuron to another is called as axon. Synapses are small gaps that transmit signal between the neurons. It connects the axons to the dendrites. The neuron processes the information based on the architecture of the network.

Numerous nodes are connected with each other in different layers of the neural network (Figure 4.1). The activation function receives information from these nodes and yields the output. Based on the data collected from the input layer, the classification is performed. Hidden layers help in minimizing the errors by adding weights.

Neural networks are widely used in areas such as e-commerce, weather forecasting, customer research, biomedical analysis and natural language understanding.

4.3 LEARNING PROCESS IN NEURAL NETWORKS

The Neural Network trains itself by adopting learning algorithms and generates the output. The learning in Neural Network can be one of the following methods (Figure 4.2).

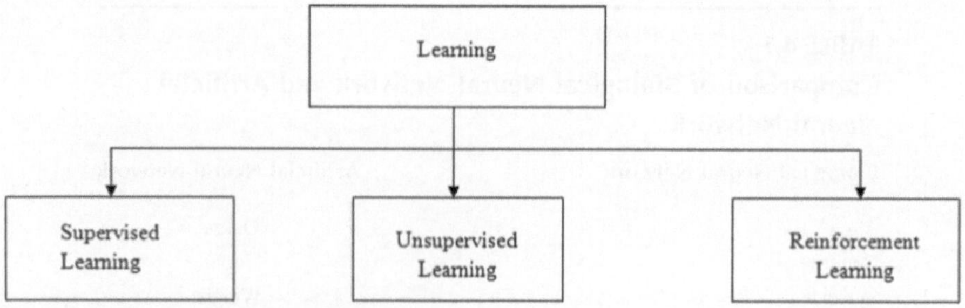

FIGURE 4.2 Learning in neural networks.

4.3.1 Supervised Learning

4.3.1.1 An Overview of Supervised Learning

The input data is given to the network that will produce output data. This output data is compared with the target output in the presence of a supervisor. If the generated output is not similar to the target output, it results in an error.

If the network produces an error signal then the weights would be adjusted until the generated output is matched with the target output (Figure 4.3). Supervised learning collects data and generates an output based on past experience. Thus it optimizes the performance and helps to solve real-world problems.

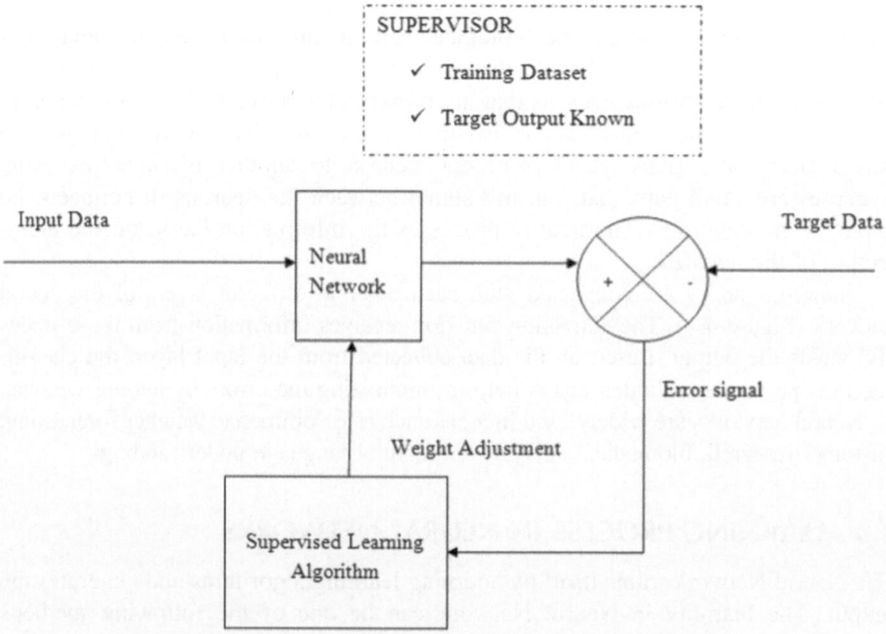

FIGURE 4.3 Supervised learning.

4.3.1.2 Supervised Learning in Medical Image Processing

Atherosclerosis is a type of cardiovascular disease that narrows the arteries and creates plaque as a result of cholesterol in the blood. Due to the accumulation of this plaque, the flow of blood reduces and the blood vessels get blocked, which may result in heart attack. Therefore, it is vital to detect the cardiovascular disease by developing a medical diagnostic support system (MDSS). It is developed using Artificial Neural Network, and Decision Tree algorithms [1]. They were applied on 835 samples which were collected from the UCI repository. The classification was done using the features that were obtained from the database. By computing different metrics the performance of the method was evaluated. Results showed that the model was able to achieve higher accuracy.

The images which were not labeled were utilized effectively by formulating an algorithm that uses self-supervised learning. The image features are helpful in image analysis. The context restoration is executed in ultrasound images, CT images, and magnetic resonance images [2]. During the analysis stage, feature maps were extracted from the input images. It consisted of convolutional units. There were downsampling layers in this stage. The reconstruction stage consisted of convolutional units. There were upsampling units present in this stage. It restored context information in the output images. Thus in all three cases, the algorithm yielded an improved performance.

4.3.2 Unsupervised Learning

4.3.2.1 Unsupervised Learning

In Unsupervised Learning, the input data that are similar are combined to form a cluster. Many clusters are formed based on the similarity of the data. When a new input is applied to the neural network, it gives an output indicating the cluster to which input data belongs (Figure 4.4).

This type of Neural Network takes no feedback from the environment and so the network must identify the patterns, features from the input data by itself.

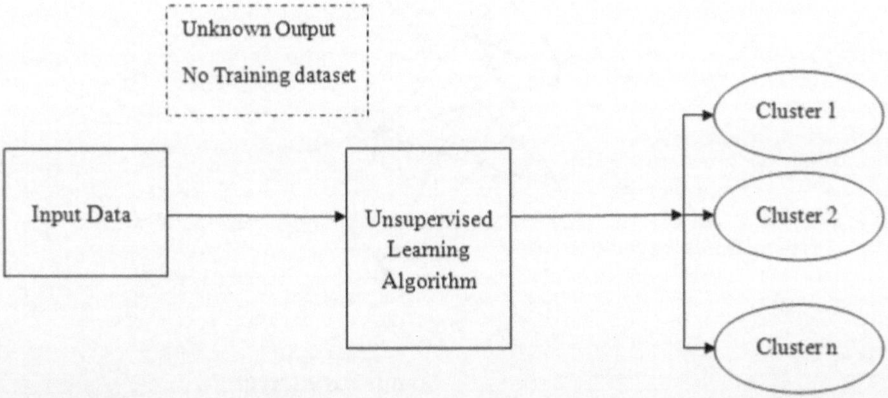

FIGURE 4.4 Unsupervised learning.

Unsupervised learning is able to locate the patterns that remain unknown in the data. It could extract features and help in clustering the data.

4.3.2.2 Overview of Competitive Learning

In competitive learning, the nodes in the network try to associate with a set of input. Here learning is unsupervised. In neural networks, neurons having activation functions acquire inputs and produce outputs but in competitive learning, the neurons compete to get fired. The activation function is given by measuring the distance between the data points. The highest activation is awarded to the neuron that is nearest to the data point. Therefore the neuron attracts some of its neighborhood and it becomes the winner neuron.

The elements involved in competitive learning are as follows:

- Neurons: The neurons with similar structures are initially attached to random weights. When input data is fed these neurons react differently.
- Limit: Each neuron in the network has its own limit.
- Mechanism: It allows the neurons to compete for the right to respond to the input data. Here one output neuron is active at a time. A "winner-take-all" neuron is the neuron that succeeds in this competition.

Competitive learning helps the neural network to group the data that are similar. During the learning process, samples are grouped based on data correlation. After being grouped, they are represented as a single artificial neuron (Figure 4.5).

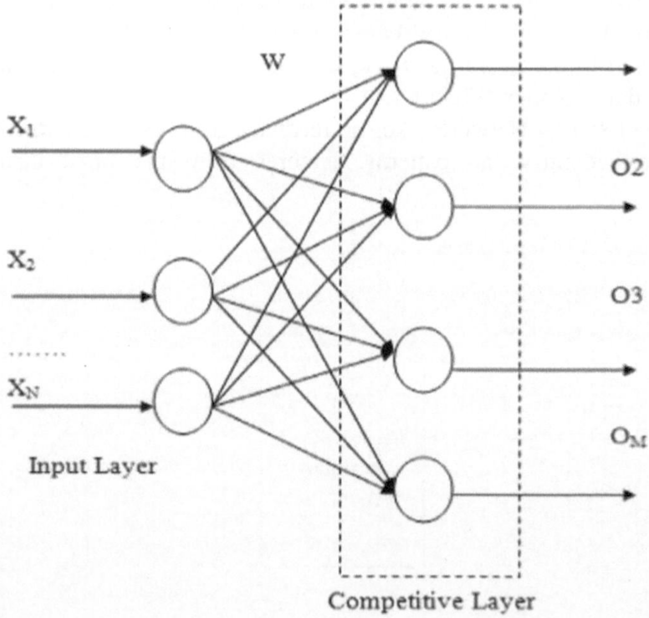

FIGURE 4.5 Competitive learning network.

4.3.2.3 Medical Analysis using Unsupervised Learning

The Unsupervised Learning algorithm can be effectively used to segment images when there is no training dataset available. An unsupervised image segmentation algorithm was developed based on local center of mass. The pixels of the one-dimensional signal were grouped and are used in an iterative process for two-dimensional and three-dimensional images. The method was applied on X-ray images, abdominal magnetic resonance (MR) images, and cardiovascular MR images [3].

The Unsupervised Learning algorithm was used to identify persons with dementia. Hierarchical clustering based on principal components was employed [4]. The Principal Component Analysis was used as it helps in dimensionality reduction while preserving the important information. Implementing Unsupervised Learning in the data obtained from population-based surveys helped in identifying individuals affected by dementia, so that they could get further clinical assessment.

The Unsupervised Learning algorithm is used to identify diseases by obtaining the data from social media [5]. The pre-processing stage involved extracting the social media messages with the user. The expressions of the individual about the symptoms were collected. Based on their expressions, the information related to the disease was acquired from symptom weighting vectors belonging to each individual. The data from Twitter was used to validate this method and the algorithm proved to be efficient in recognizing the diseases.

4.3.3 Reinforcement Learning

4.3.3.1 Reinforcement Learning

Reinforcement learning makes valuable decisions by adopting efficient training strategy. The agent learns to achieve an uncertain target through interaction and feedback (Figure 4.6). The learning uses a trial and error method to solve the given problem. Based on the solution and its target the artificial intelligence gets either

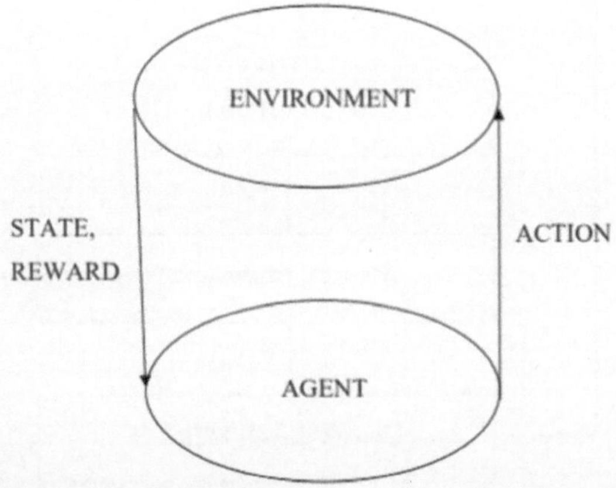

FIGURE 4.6 Reinforcement learning.

rewards or penalties. By employing more trails that are random, the learning algorithm tries to improve the rewards.

In reinforcement learning there is no supervisor. The reinforcement algorithm is developed based on three approaches. They are value-based approach, model-based approach, and policy-based approach. Learning algorithm maximizes the long-term reward in value-based approach. In policy-based approach, the agent decides the next state such that maximum reward is achieved. In model-based approach, the agent tries to behave in an environment which is created virtually. The reinforcement learning can either be positive or negative. In positive reinforcement learning, the performance is improved and is related directly to the decisions made by the agent. In negative reinforcement learning, improvement in the behavior occurs because of the condition that must have been avoided

4.3.3.2 Overview of Q-Learning

Q-Learning is a type of reinforcement learning algorithm that finds the best action to take for the current state. It looks for a better policy that maximizes the reward. A Q-table is created and then action is taken in the stated based on the Q-table (Figure 4.7).

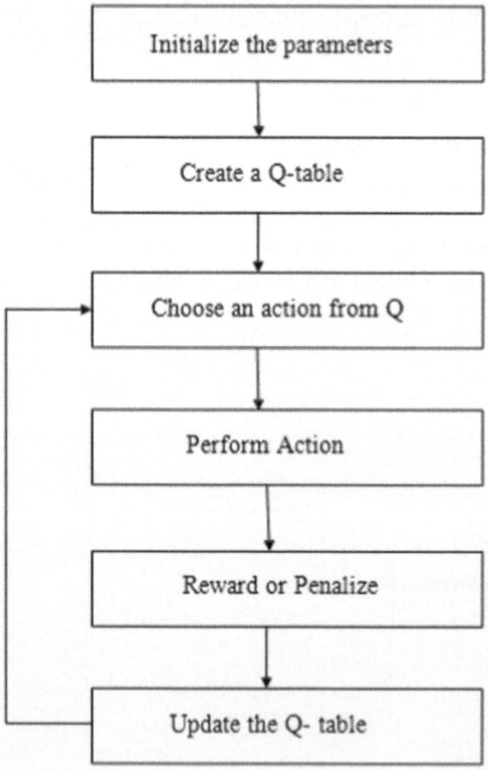

FIGURE 4.7 Q-learning.

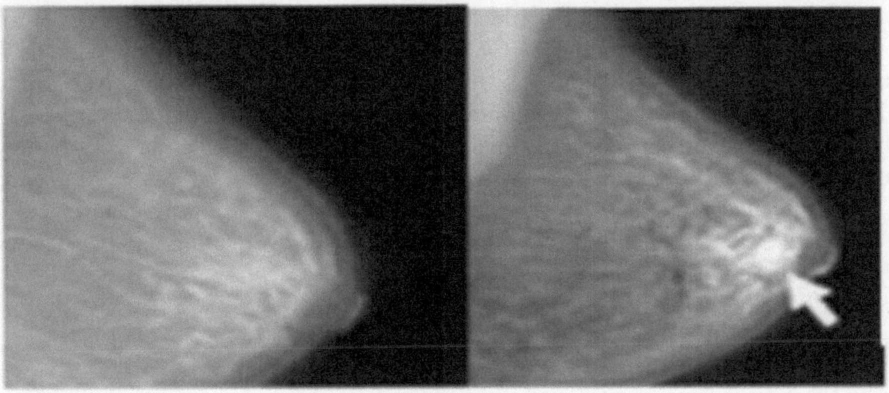

FIGURE 4.8 Normal and cancer affected breast mammogram.

After the action is taken and reward or penalty is obtained, the Q-table is updated. The Q-Learning helps the agent choose the best action in such a way that it maximizes the reward.

4.3.3.3 Adopting Reinforcement Learning in Health Sector

The Breast cancer cells form a tumor and it is crucial to determine if the lump is cancerous or not. If breast cancer is diagnosed at an early stage, there are higher chances of survival. Statistics reveal that out of overall deaths, 99.11 % of people die due to breast cancer.

Cancer can be classified as benign or malignant based on the mammogram obtained (Figure 4.8). With a better image classifier algorithm, the tumors are classified. The reinforcement algorithm and data augmentation in the classifier algorithms, handles large amount of data. Models are trained and better results are obtained [6]. Reinforcement learning methods are used in attaining efficient treatment for cancer chemotherapy. Q-learning is used for determining the dosage of drugs in chemotherapy [7].

Diabetes mellitus is a disease that increases the sugar levels in the blood as the body could not generate sufficient insulin. The International diabetes federation states that the number of adults having diabetes will rise to 700 million by 2045. Diabetes can affect various organs in the human body. Adults having diabetes are more prone to heart attacks and strokes. Reinforcement Learning is applied to regulate the glucose levels in Artificial Pancreas systems. Q-learning algorithm was used to measure the rate at which the insulin is delivered [8]. Anatomical landmark detection is very crucial in diagnosing Alzheimer's disease. For this purpose of detecting medical landmarks, reinforcement learning is applied [9].

Reinforcement learning finds its application in segmentation of medical images. The local threshold value is obtained and the prostate in ultrasound images is segmented. The agent uses the ultrasound images, performs actions, and behaves accordingly in the environment. Survey shows that the accuracy is improved when reinforcement learning methodology is adopted in medical image segmentation.

Epilepsy is a neurological disorder in which seizures occur in the nerve cell of brain. Electroencephalography (EEG) is more helpful in detecting epilepsy as it measures temporal and spatial information in the brain. Reinforcement learning allows direct optimizations of deep-brain stimulation based on the flow of ions in the brain that causes spikes. It reduces the number of stimulation and thereby minimizes the cell damage.

Reinforcement learning delivers better decision and finds a prominent place in heath care sector. It simplifies the tasks of physicians by providing good values for the decision model, thereby increasing the accuracy.

4.4 TYPES OF NEURAL NETWORKS

With the increasing use of machine learning, various neural networks keep emerging. Some of the neural networks that are most widely used are listed below.

- Perceptron
- Multilayer Perceptron
- Deep Convolutional Neural Network
- Support Vector Machine
- Kohonen Network
- Hopfield Network
- Markov Chain
- Radial Basis Functional Neural Network

4.4.1 Perceptron

4.4.1.1 Perceptron

Perceptron is an artificial neuron that classifies the input data. It is a supervised learning algorithm and it helps in feature detection. There are two types of perceptron. They are single layer perceptron and multi layer perceptron

The single-layer perceptron works based on the threshold function and is able to analyze binary targets (Figure 4.9). It has a feed forward network. The multi-layer

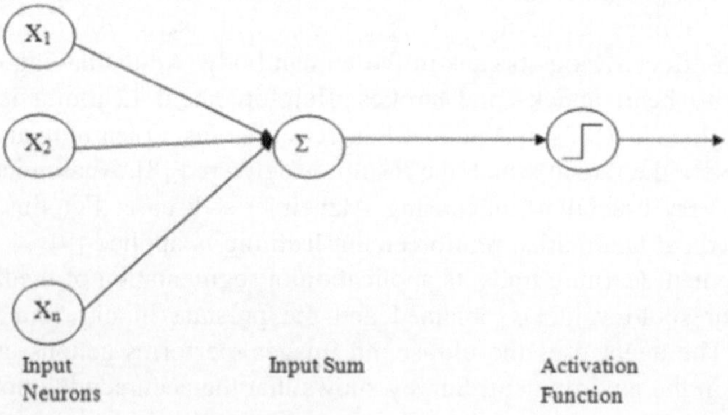

FIGURE 4.9 Structure of single-layer perceptron.

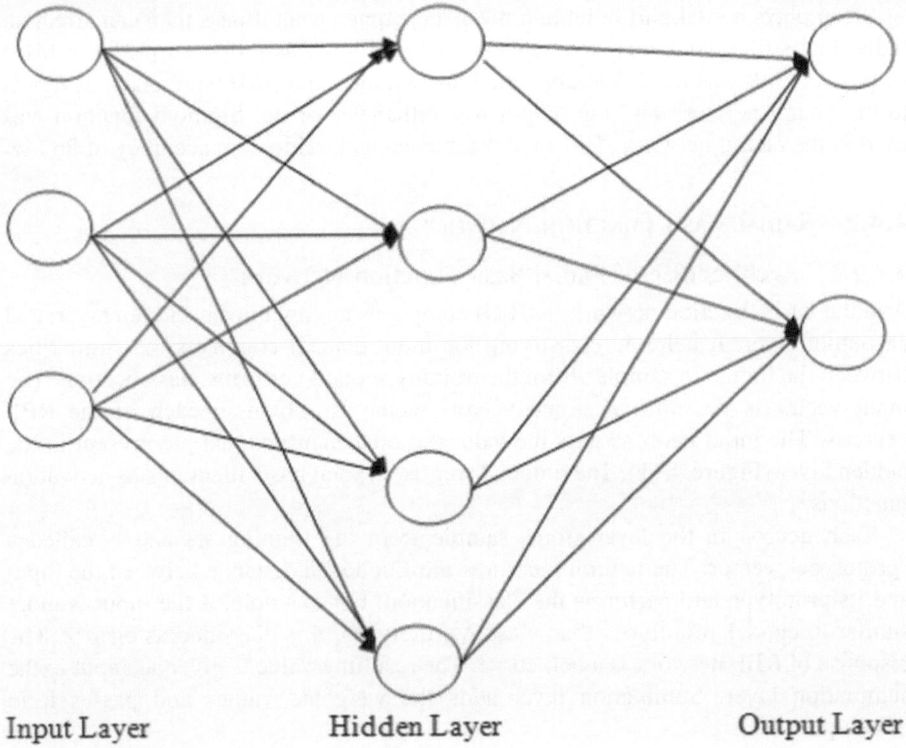

FIGURE 4.10 Multi-layer perceptron.

perceptron has multiple hidden layers and works on both forward and backward stages (Figure 4.10).

4.4.1.2 Perceptron in Medical Image Analysis

Classifying medical images is one of the most important problems in medical diagnosis. This requires a good classification algorithm that helps in detecting diseases. A Coding Network with Multilayer Perceptron is used to combine both high-level features and traditional features [10]. The high-level features are obtained using a deep convolutional neural network. And a MultiLayer Perceptron neural network model is trained such that it can map the features into the feature space. ReLus is used as an activation function. The multi layer perceptron comprises of softmax layer and fully connected layer. The model was applied on skin lesion dataset for classifying skin tumors into Melanoma and Nevus. It resulted in acquiring good discriminative features for medical images and resulted in 90.1% of accuracy.

The multi-layer perceptron model was applied on Wisconsin Breast Cancer dataset, SaHeart dataset, and Pima Indians Diabetes dataset [11]. The multi-layer perceptron model was used for both training and testing for predicting the diseases.

The multi-layer perceptron is used for detection of stress levels. The datasets were gathered from wrist-worn sensors that were attached to the human body. The model analyzed the data and classified the emotions into different states [12].

Sleep plays a vital part in human life. Sleep apnea is an illness than can affect an individual's life. To detect sleep apnea, an algorithm was proposed [13]. An MLP neural network was used. Variables such as sex, age, and BMI were taken as inputs to the neural network and the output was either yes or no. Sigmoid function was used in the neural network. This model achieved a classification accuracy of 86.8%.

4.4.2 Radial Basis Function Network

4.4.2.1 Architecture of Radial Basis Function Network

A radial basis function network (RBFN) comprises an input layer, hidden layer, and an output layer. It helps in classifying the input data. It compares the similarities between the inputs to samples from the training set and performs classification. The input vector is the n-dimensional vector, which is shown to each of the RBF neurons. The input neurons pass the values to other neurons that are present in the hidden layer (Figure 4.11). The hidden layer uses radial basis functions as activation functions.

Each neuron in the layer stores sample from the training set and is called a "prototype" vector. The neuron measures the Euclidean distance between the input and its prototype and performs the classification. For example, if the input is more similar to class 1 prototypes than class 2 prototypes, it is classified as class 2. The response of RBF network is a bell curve. The resulting value is given as input to the summation layer. Summation layer adds the weighted values and passes it to the output layer.

4.4.2.2 Implementing Radial Basis Function in Medical Analysis

RBFN is used for image denoising applications. The degraded image is given as input to the Radial Basis Function Neural Network Filter [14]. Back propagation algorithm is used as a training algorithm in the RBFN network. MRI images and X-ray images were used as input. The results showed that RBFNNF was able to

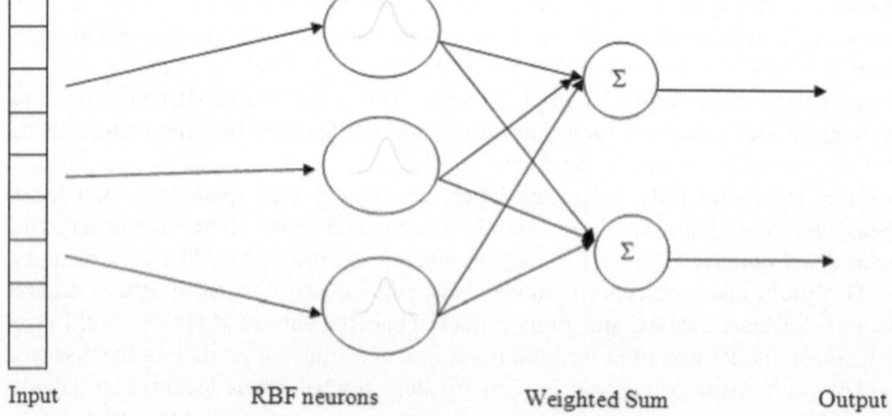

FIGURE 4.11 RBFN architecture.

remove noise and preserve more details. It had better image quality and was able preserve discontinuities, contrast, and edges.

The Radial Basis Function Neural Network can handle large dataset efficiently. It is applied for the classification of organs where identifying the specific organs has been a major issue in diagnosing medical images. Radial Basis Function Neural Network was able to classify organs effectively. It could segment abdominal magnetic resonance (MR) images. Four magnetic resonance sequences were given as input and three classifiers were used to classify liver, kidney, and other tissues [15]. The number of correctly classified samples was computed and the algorithm showed a better performance. Also the Radial Basis Function Neural Network was able to process large datasets with less computation time.

The Radial Basis Function Neural Network algorithm was applied to Computed Tomography images. Fourteen features were given as input and the Radial Basis Function Neural Network classified it into 5 tissue classes, such as skull, brain, calcifications, intra cerebral brain hemorrhage, and background [16]. Results showed that with the implementation of Radial Basis Function Neural Network, the segmentation error was minimized to a larger extent.

Selecting relevant features plays an important role in improving the accuracy of any algorithm. The Radial Basis Function is used for the detection of Graves disease [17]. Support vector machine hybridized with Radial Basis Function was incorporated in the classification. The thyroid disease dataset was used and its features were transformed to RBF Kernel space. The features having high F-scores were selected and better performance was achieved yielding a classification accuracy of 92.6.

4.4.3 Convolutional Neural Network

4.4.3.1 Architecture of Convolutional Neural Network

Convolutional neural network (CNN) is a feed forward neural network. It has less number of weights compared to a fully connected network. Convolutional neural networks have multiple layers of artificial neurons that compute the weighted sum of inputs and provide an activation value. It can process one-dimensional data, two-dimensional image data, and three-dimensional data.

The CNN allots weights to objects that are present in the input image.

The CNN consists of convolutional layer, pooling layer, and fully connected layer. They contain nodes that process the input data and yield an output. When the input image is given to the network, the convolutional layer locates the spatial features in the image (Figure 4.12). The convolution layer then performs convolution by multiplying the weights with the input. The kernel creates a feature map in its output.

These kernels are grids of values that slide over an image and produce an output. These kernels are able to detect intensity changes in the images. The convolutional layer acts as a feature extractor. Then an activation function is applied after which it is passed to the pooling layer. It helps in reducing the dimensionality of the input

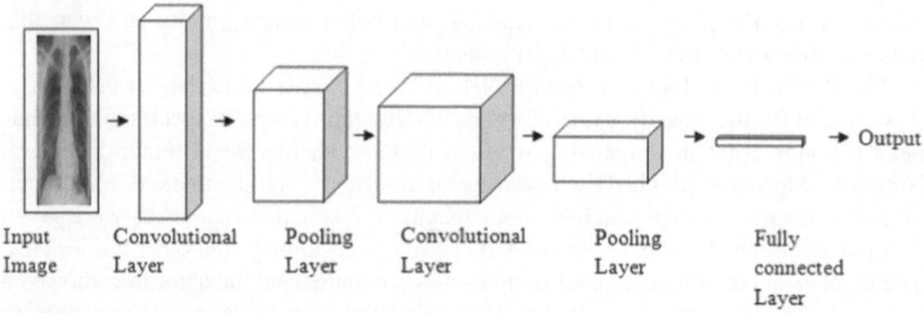

FIGURE 4.12 Architecture of convolutional neural network.

data. The output of the pooling layer is passed as an input to the fully connected layer. It classifies features and assigns class scores. The CNN finds optimal weights by the process of back propagation and changes weights that produce errors in classification.

4.4.3.2 Convolutional Neural Networks in Medical Diagnosis

The CNN is used in the field of drug discovery. Targets are proteins that make the tumors grow. In drug discovery, the molecules that interact with the target will be identified. An algorithm known as AtomNet was able to identify patients affected by Ebola virus. This algorithm could predict the interaction between the molecules and it is used in drug research programs.

The CNN is used for detecting diabetic retinopathy. It is a disease that damages blood vessels in the retina. These blood vessels create more new blood vessels that tend to bleed with the affected tissue. If not treated, this may lead to vision loss. Therefore, proper diagnosis is essential for detecting diabetic retinopathy. The detection is done by the CNN, which was applied to a dataset containing 3,662 pre-classified fundus images, with images of all stages of the disease. The CNN successfully classified fundus images into 5 classes and yielded better accuracy [18].

The convolutional neural network was used to detect pneumonia. The chest X-ray images were used as an input. It classified the input into two classes with 91% accuracy [19].

The CNN was used as a classification algorithm and it was applied to breast mass and brain tumor tissues. Multiple CNN having convolution kernel of different sizes and more feature maps were constructed [20]. Thus a multilayer CNN consisting of 10 layers was created and trained. Then the outputs of the 10-layer CNN are merged and the classification accuracy is measured. This CNN when applied to breast mass, the classification accuracy of 96.5% was achieved and it was able to classify brain tumor tissues with an average accuracy of 91.12%.

The CNN was used for detecting pulmonary nodule disease and the algorithm yielded better detection rate. CNN is used in detecting Alzheimer's disease. The network segmented the brain MRI images into hippocampus, cortical thickness, and brain volume providing an accuracy of 96.85% [21].

4.4.4 Recurrent Neural Network

4.4.4.1 Introduction to Recurrent Neural Network

Recurrent Neural Network (RNN) predicts the output based on the input data. It stores the output of a specific layer and uses it as an input to determine the output of the layer.

As shown in the above architecture, the input layer is denoted as "x", the output layer is denoted as "y", and the hidden layer is denoted as "h". RNNs deal with variables that change over time. The network parameters help improve the performance of a network and are denoted as A, B, and C in the above architecture (Figure 4.13). Thus the output of the network is improved using a feedback model.

4.4.4.2 Types of Recurrent Neural Network

The RNNs can be classified into four types:

- One to one
- One to many
- Many to one
- Many to many

The one to one RNN contains a single input and a single output (Figure 4.14). It is basic form of RNN.

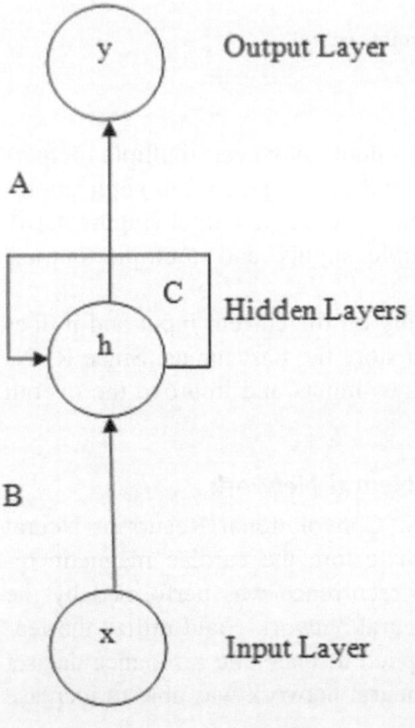

FIGURE 4.13 Representation of recurrent neural network.

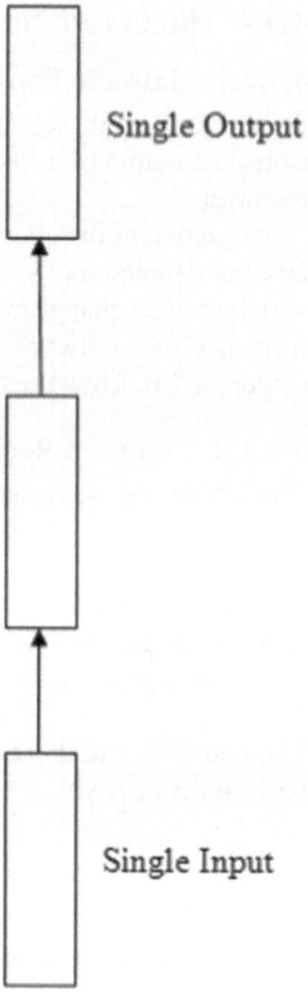

FIGURE 4.14 Architecture of one to one recurrent neural network.

The one to many RNN contains a single input, however multiple outputs (Figure 4.15). It can be used for image caption and music generation applications.

The many to one RNN contains multiple inputs and single output (Figure 4.16).

The many to many RNN contains multiple inputs and multiple outputs (Figure 4.17).

The feed forward neural network depends only on the current input and it does not store the previous inputs. But the RNN can store the past inputs. Since RNNs have internal memory, it could study the previous inputs and improve the overall performance of the network.

4.4.4.3 Medical Analysis using Recurrent Neural Network

Image reconstruction algorithms employ RNN. Convolutional Recurrent Neural Network (CRNN) architecture was modeled to restore the cardiac magnetic resonance images from undersampled data. The recurrence was performed by the vanilla RNN architecture [22]. The recurrent neural network could utilize the features with huge filter size. This method was applied to magnetic resonance dataset and the metrics were evaluated. The recurrent neural network was able to increase

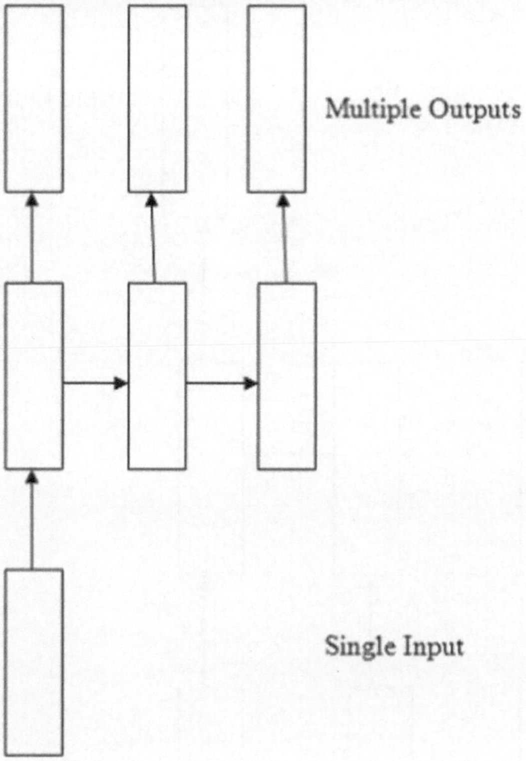

FIGURE 4.15 Architecture of one to many recurrent neural network.

the size of receptive field. It could pass information in temporal direction efficiently. This recurrent neural network was able to reconstruct images with higher reconstruction accuracy.

The recurrent neural network was modeled to create a label which could identify the fracture and non-fracture cases. Natural language processing system uses recurrent neural networks to recognize presence or absence of a fracture in the musculoskeletal radiography reports [23]. The RNN encoder-decoder with more hidden layers was used. The word error rate was computed and the performance of the RNN as a fracture classifier was evaluated. The model yielded a word error rate less than 3.57% and effectively identified fractures in musculoskeletal radiography reports.

4.4.5 Hopfield Neural Network

4.4.5.1 Overview of Hopfield Neural Network

The Hopfield neural network has neurons connected to each other. It is used in pattern recognition applications and in applications that require optimization. It has a single layer which comprises one or more fully connected recurrent neurons (Figure 4.18). The Hopfield network is capable of reconstructing the data even after the input data is corrupted.

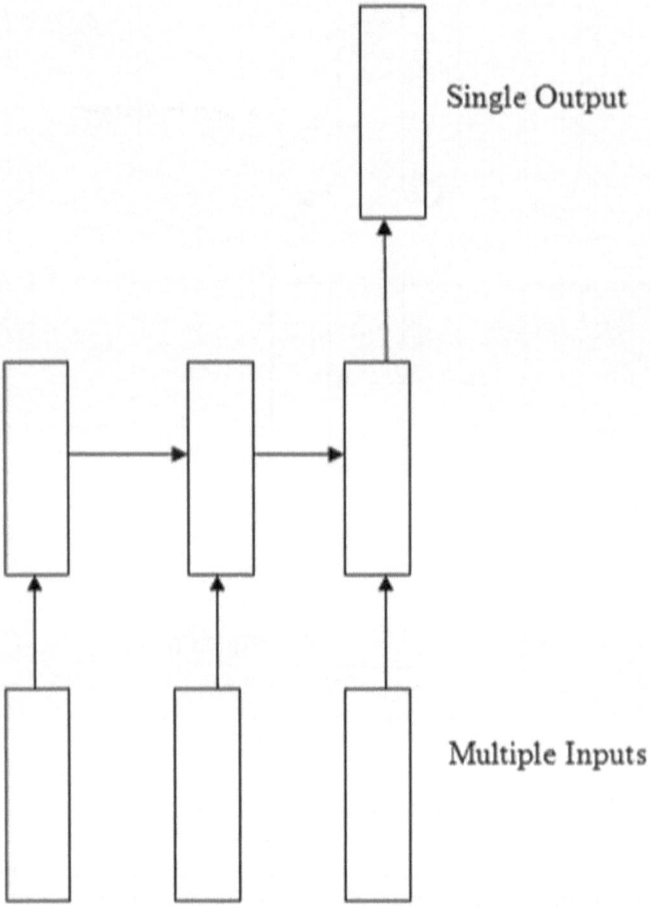

FIGURE 4.16 Architecture of many to one recurrent neural network.

The neurons in a Hopfield neural network are connected by links. The activation function initially equals the input vector. The weights are updated at the training phase. During the testing phase the activation is applied to the input and the output is computed. Then this output is broadcasted to all other nodes in the network.

4.4.5.2 Hopfield Neural Network in Medical Diagnosis

A fuzzy Hopfield neural network was proposed to segment medical images. It used both local and global gray-level information to segment images [24]. Global gray-level information was used for initial partition and local information was used to develop the Hopfield neural network. Each neuron relates to a pixel. The synaptic weights are fixed. The synaptic weight between two neurons is determined by calculating the Euclidean distance, which is based on the similarity of their image intensities. The outputs of the neurons are found and the relation of a pixel to a cluster is determined. The model was applied to CT images of a head scan. In

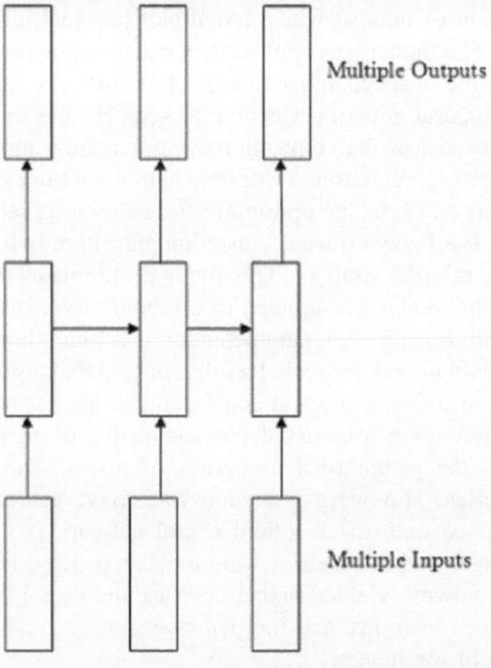

FIGURE 4.17 Architecture of many to many recurrent neural network.

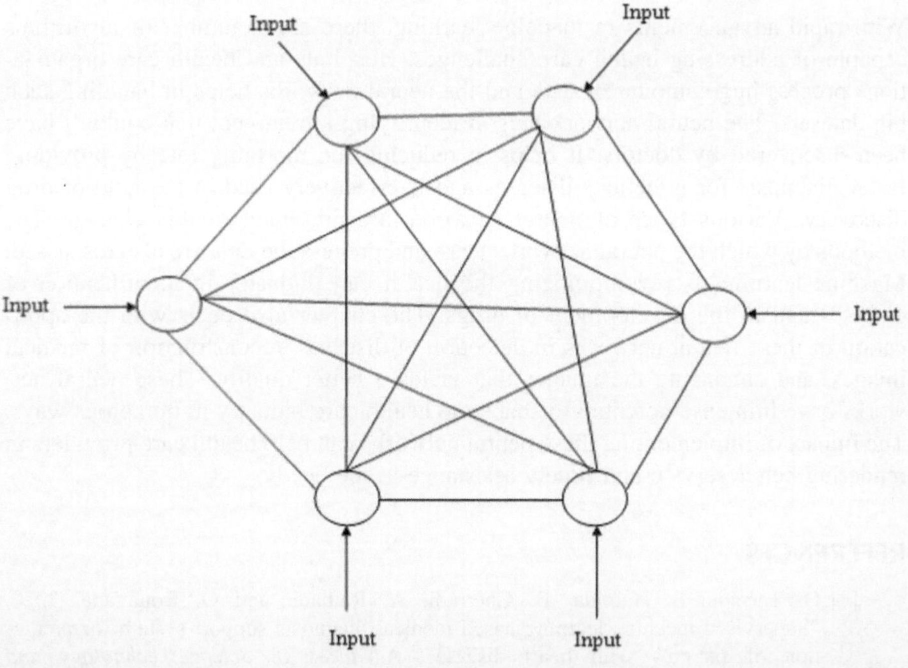

FIGURE 4.18 Representation of Hopfield neural network.

CT images, the region of interest was a blood clot that had higher intensity compared to soft tissue. The model was applied to echocardiographic images, where the region of interest is the heart chamber that has low intensity. Results showed that this fuzzy Hopfield neural network was able to segment the images with a higher accuracy better than most of the conventional segmentation methods.

For medical image segmentation, a Hopfield neural network employing Fuzzy C Means algorithm is used [25]. The optimum segmentation is selected based on the Euclidean distance. The fuzzy c-means clustering algorithm is formulated based on "within-class scatter matrix" strategy. This method eliminates the need to find the weighting factors. The model was applied to CT brain, liver images, MR of brain, and chest images with fuzzification parameter set to 1.2 and threshold value (E) set to 0.001 in the Hopfield neural network. Results showed that algorithm converges to the desired solution at a faster rate and could achieve greater performance.

Hopfield neural network is used to enhance the quality of images. The network is developed based on the geometrical properties of pixels. The patterns of pixels represent the memories. The energy function was converged and the intensity of each pixel was mapped onto the Hopfield neural network [26]. The method was applied to MRI images and the metrics were evaluated. Results demonstrated that the Hopfield neural network yielded higher contrast and visual information fidelity. This method improved visibility and the perceived image quality meanwhile preserving the features of the image.

4.5 CONCLUSION

With rapid advancements in machine learning, there are a number of algorithms capable of addressing health care challenges. Hospitals and health care organizations process huge amount of data and the neural networks helps in handling such big datasets. The neural network aids in identifying a treatment that couldn't have been discovered by doctors. It helps in reducing the mortality rate by providing faster diagnosis for infectious diseases and is effectively used in the field of drug discovery. Various types of neural networks are presented in this chapter. The methods by which the neural networks learn and process the data are also discussed. Machine learning is revolutionizing the health care industry in identification of diseases and in the development of drugs. The chapter also deals with the application of these neural networks in detection of diseases, reconstruction of medical images, and enhancing the images that yields a better quality. These neural networks have immense potential to shape the health care industry in numerous ways. The impact of implementing these neural networks can help health care providers in rendering better service and timely assistance to the needy.

REFERENCES

[1] O. Terrada, S. Hamida, B. Cherradi, A. Raihani, and O. Bouattane, 2020. "Supervised machine learning based medical diagnosis support system for prediction of patients with heart disease", *Advances in Science,Technology and Engineering Systems Journal*, vol. 5, no. 5, 269–277.

[2] L. Chena, P. Bentley, K. Mori, K. Misawa, M. Fujiwara, and D. Ruecket, 2019. "Self-supervised learning for medical image analysis using image context restoration", *Elsevier Journals*, vol. 58, Article ID 101539.
[3] I. Agani, M.G. Harisinghani, R. Weissleder, and B. Fischl, 2018. "Unsupervised medical image segmentation based on the local center of mass", *Scientific Reports*, vol. 8, Article ID13012.
[4] L.C..de Langavant, E.Bayen, and K. Yaffe, 2018. "Unsupervised machine learning to identify high likelihood of dementia in population-based surveys: Development and validation study", *Journal of Medical Internet Research*, vol. 20, no. 7, e10493.
[5] S. Lim, C. S. Tucker, and S. Kumara, 2017. "An unsupervised machine learning model for discovering latent infectious diseases using social media data", *Elsevier Journal of Biomedical Informatics*, vol. 66.
[6] A.-Al Nahid and Y. Kong, 2017. "Involvement of machine learning for breast cancer image classification: A survey", *Computational and Mathematical Methods in Medicine*, vol. 2017, Article ID 3781951.
[7] Y. Zhao, M. R. Kosorok, and D. Zeng, 2009. "Reinforcement learning design for cancer clinical trials", *Statistics in Medicine*, vol. 28, no. 26, 3294–3315.
[8] S. Yasini, M. B. Naghibi Sistani, and A. Karimpour, 2009. "Agent-based simulation for blood glucose", *International Journal of Applied Science, Engineering and Technology*, vol. 5, 89–95.
[9] A. Alansary, O. Oktay, Y. Li, L. L. Folgoc, B. Hou, G. Vaillant, K. Kamnitsas, A. Vlontzos, B. Glocker, B. Kainz, and et al., 2019. "Evaluating reinforcement learning agents for anatomical landmark detection", *Medical Image Analysis*, vol. 53, 156–164.
[10] Z. Lai and H.F. Deng, 2018. "Medical image classification based on deep features extracted by deep model and statistic feature fusion with multilayer perceptron", *Computational Intelligence and Neuroscience*, vol. 2018, Article ID 2061516.
[11] T. Bikku, 2020. "Multi-layered deep learning perceptron approach for health risk prediction", *Journal of Big Data*, Article ID 50.
[12] R. Li and Z. Liu, 2020. "Stress detection using deep neural networks", *BMC Medical Informatics and Decision Making*, vol. 20(Suppl 11), Article ID 285.
[13] Z. Kohzadi, R. Safdari, and K. S. Haghighi, 2020 "Determination of sleep apnea severity using multi-layer perceptron neural network", *Journal of the Korean Society of Sleep Medicine*, ISSN 2093- 9175/eISSN 2233-8853.
[14] M. Debakla, K. Djemal, and M. Benyettou, 2015. "A novel approach for medical images noise reduction based RBF neural network filter", *Journal of Computers*, vol. 10, no. 2, 68–80.
[15] M. Xu, P. Qian, J. Zheng, H. Ge, and R. F. Muzic, 2020. "A novel radial basis neural network-leveraged fast training method for identifying organs in MR images", *Computational and Mathematical Methods in Medicine*, vol. 2020, Article ID 4519483.
[16] D. Kovacevic and S. Kovacevic, "Radial basis function-based image segmentation using a receptive field",
[17] Babu P, Rajkumar N, Palaniappan S, and Pushparaj T, 2020. "Development of RBF image processing techniques for graves disease", *International Journal of Scientific & Technology Research*, vol. 9, no. 3.
[18] G. Rosati, "Medical Diagnosis with a Convolutional Neural Network",
[19] H. Deshmukh, "Medical X-ray image classification using convolutional neural network", *Medical Image Computing*.
[20] F.-P. An, 2019. "Medical image classification algorithm based on weight initialization-sliding window fusion convolutional neural network", *Hindawi Journals*, vol. 2019, Article ID 9151670.

[21] S. Sarraf and G. Tofighi, DeepAD: Alzheimer's disease classification via deep convolutional neural networks using MRI and fMRI. BioRxiv 2016. doi: 10.1101/070441.

[22] C. Qin, J. Schlemper, J. Caballero, A. N. Price, J. V. Hajmal, and D. Rueckert, 2019. "Convolutional recurrent neural networks for dynamic MR image reconstruction", *IEEE Transactions on Medical Imaging*, vol. 38, no. 1, 280–290.

[23] C. Lee, Y. Kim, Y. S. Kim, and J. Jang, 2019. "Automatic disease annotation from radiology reports using artificial intelligence implemented by a recurrent neural network", *American Journal of Roentgenology*, vol. 212, no. 4.

[24] C. C. Liang and C. Y. Tai, 2002. "Fuzzy hopfield neural network with fixed weight for medical image segmentation", *Optical Engineering*, vol. 41, no. 2, 351–358.

[25] J.-S. Lin, K.-S..Cheng, and C.-W. Mao, 1996. "A fuzzy hopfield neural netwolrk for medical image segmentation", *IEEE Transactions on Nuclear Science*, vol. 43, no. 4.

[26] F. Alenezi and K. C. Santosh, 2021. "Geometric regularized hopfield neural network for medical image enhancement", *International Journal of Biomedical Imaging*, vol. 2021, Article ID 6664569.

5 Recent Trends in Bio-Medical Waste, Challenges and Opportunities

S. Kannadhasan
Assistant Professor, Department of Electronics and Communication Engineering, Cheran College of Engineering, Tamil Nadu, India

R. Nagarajan
Professor, Department of Electrical and Electronics Engineering, Gnanamani College of Technology, Tamil Nadu, India

CONTENTS

5.1 Introduction 97
5.2 Waste Disposal 99
5.3 Health Care Industries 100
5.4 Conclusion 107
References 107

5.1 INTRODUCTION

The majority of the garbage created by health care facilities is non-hazardous trash (about 85%). It consists of food scraps, paper cartons, packing materials, fruit peels, and wash water, among other things. At different times over the years, the term "potentially contagious garbage" has been used in scientific literature, guideline manuals, and guidelines for infectious waste. Medical waste that is infectious, dangerous, red bagged, or contaminated, as well as regulated and non-controlled medical waste, are all instances. Although the designations used in legislation are usually more precise, they all relate to the same kind of trash [1–5]. Waste collects and is kept in the areas and stages between the point of garbage generation and the point of waste treatment and disposal. While accumulation refers to the temporary storage of small quantities of trash at the point of production, waste storage refers to lengthy storage periods and large waste volumes. A majority of the time, storage facilities are close to where the garbage is collected. Biomedical waste is described

DOI: 10.1201/9781003217497-5

as "any solid or liquid waste, including its container and any intermediate product, generated during the diagnosis, treatment, or immunisation of people or animals." Biological waste is generated in a variety of settings, including hospitals; nursing homes; clinics; laboratories; physicians, dentists, and veterinarian offices; home health care; and funeral homes. It must be treated with caution in order to safeguard the general public, especially healthcare and sanitation workers who are frequently exposed to biological waste as a job hazard. As a consequence, little study has been done on infection transmission via medical waste. According to the American Dental Association and the Centers for Disease Control, medical waste disposal must adhere to strict guidelines. Any health care management approach must include appropriate waste processing, treatment, and disposal. Protecting health care personnel, patients, and the surrounding community is easier with the right strategy [6–10].

Carts and containers that are not utilised for any other purpose may be utilised to transport bio-medical wastes. Every day, the trolleys must be cleaned. The name and address of the transporter should be clearly marked on the offsite carrying vehicle. It is recommended that the biohazard sign be coloured. It is necessary to ensure that a suitable mechanism for securing the weight during transportation is in place. With rounded sides, such a mode of transportation should be easy to clean. Before returning to the seller, all discarded plastic should be shredded. Unprocessed bio-medical waste should not be kept for longer than 48 hours [11–15]. Treatment refers to any process that alters waste in any manner before it reaches its final destination. The first step is to disinfect or sanitise the waste at the source, ensuring that harmful organisms are no longer present. The remains may then be appropriately handled, transported, and preserved after this treatment. Shred syringe nozzles and needles using syringe cutters and needle destroyers. Figure 5.1 shows how broken glass, scalpel blades, and Lancets should be stored in separate containers with bleach, then transferred to plastic/cardboard boxes and sealed to prevent leaking before being transported to incubators. Sterilisation, disinfection, and cleaning of glassware are all required. Potential cultures must be autoclaved, and the medium must be placed in suitable bags and discarded. After sterilisation, the plates may be reused. Before discarding gloves, they should be cut, torn, or

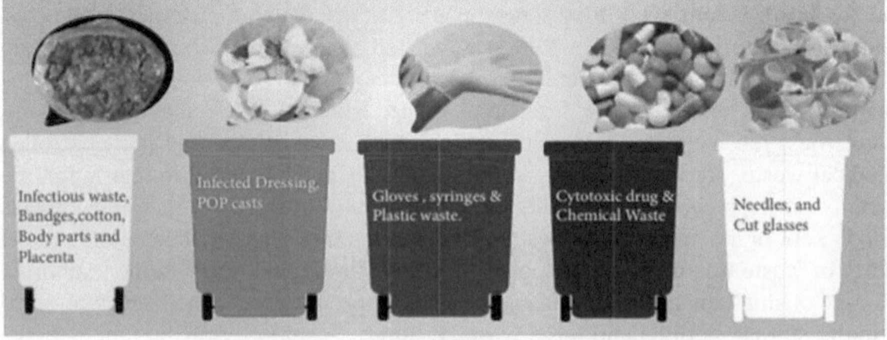

FIGURE 5.1 Biomedical waste in colour-coded bags.

disfigured. Chemical sterilisation should be followed by burning of swabs. They might be thrown away if they just had a little amount of blood that does not drop [16–18].

5.2 WASTE DISPOSAL

While typical solid and liquid trash does not need to be treated before being disposed of, practically all infectious trash should be handled beforehand. The expense of disposing of infectious garbage might be 10 times that of routine garbage disposal. Any approach that lowers the cost of infectious waste disposal lowers the quantity of infectious waste produced. syringes, blood, urine bags, catheters, and other things made of plastic are used in health care. A decrease in sperm count, genital abnormalities, and a rise in breast cancer incidences have all been related to plastic. When plastics are burnt, carcinogens such as dioxin and furan are produced. Because of its non-biodegradable nature, plastic has become a serious environmental and health hazard. Long-term, landfilling, or recycling are all ecologically sound ways to dispose of plastic garbage. Before returning to the seller, all discarded plastic should be shredded. The development of environmentally friendly, biodegradable polymers is urgently required. It is also critical to reduce the amount of plastic garbage produced. For medical practitioners, biomedical waste management is just as vital as a treatment strategy. All health care employees and auxiliary people from different health care institutions should be educated about the present state of scientific biomedical waste management systems, as well as their value and advantages to patients, staff, and the community as a whole.

Ongoing education and training, as well as continuing medical education and updates, should be done on a regular basis. For successful initiatives in health care waste management, a solid legal/ regulatory framework must be used in conjunction with scientific judgement. The safe management of health care waste systems should be reviewed on a regular basis, according to the experts. The occupational health and safety of health care employees should be prioritised since they are the ones who are most at risk if waste is poorly managed. Individual health care centres/units must develop and execute a plan that best suits them in order to comply with the notification of biological waste (handling and management) laws of 1998 in a strict and transparent manner. Every community member has a right to know about the harmful effects of medical waste. As a consequence, the general people must be educated in a thorough manner via mass media. To guarantee quality in the disposal of health care waste by health care centres/units, a clear comprehensive plan in medical services is needed. This should include environmentally sustainable and cost-effective waste management.

Garbage is produced in enormous quantities as a result of human activity. Garbage of this kind may be dangerous, requiring appropriate disposal. Industrial, sewage, and agricultural waste pollute water, land, and air, putting people's health and the environment in danger. Solid waste may be classified into a variety of categories depending on where it originates from. Garbage from the home, industry, biological waste, medical trash, and infectious waste are all included. Waste generated during the diagnosis, testing, treatment, research, or manufacturing of biological products for humans or animals is referred to as biomedical waste. It's also known as medical waste or infectious waste. Biomedical waste includes syringes, live vaccines, body parts, waste, sharp needles, cultures, and lancets. Improper waste management at health care facilities has a direct impact on the health of the community, as well as the health of health care workers and the environment. Hazardous, infectious, and non-infectious solids and liquids make up the bulk of the waste generated at these institutions.

Furthermore, garbage that is not separated and processed properly will pollute the environment, thereby impacting the community's health. Any infection control programme in a health care office must include appropriate handling, treatment, and disposal of biological wastes. Correct process will aid in the protection of health care staff, patients, and the surrounding community. Waste management, if correctly conceived and implemented, maybe a reasonably effective and efficient compliance-related activity. Biomedical waste must be properly collected and separated. At the same time, the amount of trash produced is critical. A lower volume of biological waste equals less labour for waste disposal personnel, lower costs, and a more effective waste disposal system.

Liquid wastewater is spread across land even after treatment. As a consequence, pollution of the land is inevitable. The open dumping of bio-medical waste is the most important cause of soil pollution. Executives in hospitals must be aware of the gravity of the issue and be able to differentiate between hospital and general garbage. They must ensure that Bio-Medical Waste is correctly recognised, separated at the time of manufacture, collected in colour-coded containers, transported securely, processed appropriately, and disposed of in an environmentally friendly way. Health education and training should be provided to everyone involved in the management and disposal of bio-medical waste. Last but not least, effective rule enforcement by competent authorities via surprise visits and inspections is critical. As well as holding everyone involved in the management of bio-medical waste responsible. If hospital management wants to keep our environment and community healthy, it must raise awareness of this important issue, not only for the benefit of health care professionals, but also for the general public's benefit.

5.3 HEALTH CARE INDUSTRIES

The health care sector includes a broad range of organisations, from large general and specialty hospitals to small municipal clinics and D-type institutions. All of these facilities are critical components of our society, with the aim of decreasing and eliminating health problems and dangers. In the course of treating health problems, the health care sector produces a significant amount of bio-medical waste, which may be hazardous to anybody who comes into contact with it. Hazardous waste management is a problem for every health care organisation. Health care waste management (HCWM) is a waste management (WM) process that aids in maintaining hospital cleanliness and the safety of health care workers and the general public. Workers in the health care sector have a unique opportunity to influence the environmental effects of their work. Their acts may seem little, yet they all contribute to the ultimate achievement by establishing a foundation of sound behaviour and thinking. The Ministry of Environment and Forests published the Bio-Medical Waste (Management and Handling) Rules, 1998, to guarantee that bio-medical waste is properly managed. These rules are designed to improve India's health care facilities' overall waste management. It has been emphasised that adopting regulations alone would not be enough in guaranteeing proper bio-medical waste disposal. It's essential that the general public be aware of these regulations, as well as the policies and enforcement that follow them. The goal of this study is to find out how well-informed, knowledgeable, and behaved health care workers are regarding BMW management in fourteen Agra medical institutions.

Any solid, or liquid waste, including its container and any intermediate product, generated during the diagnosis, treatment, or immunisation of humans or animals, in related research, or in the production or testing of biological and animal waste from slaughterhouses or other similar establishments, "according to the definition of bio-medical waste." Medical waste is described as "any waste generated in the diagnosis, treatment, or immunisation of people or animals, in associated research, or in the production or testing of biological products." Antibiotics, cytotoxics, caustic chemicals, and radioactive substances are all utilised in today's hospitals and health care institutions, including research institutes, and all of them end up in hospital garbage. In hospitals, the introduction of disposables has resulted in a host of issues, including incorrect recycling, unauthorised and illegal re-use, and an increase in waste volume. Medicine, Surgery, Orthopedics, Eye, Radiotherapy, Physiotherapy, and Electro Medical Diagnosis all have their own Outpatient Departments (OPDs) (which includes ECG, EEG, TMT, Endoscopic treatments, and other procedures). (Pathology/Microbiology/Biochemistry) are also close to the OPD blocks for the convenience of OPD patients. A separate blood bank and antirabic immunisation section are also available.

The CSSD, laundry, kitchen, morgue, and hospital store are all located on the premises. Infectious agents from research and industrial labs, waste from biology, toxins, dishes and equipment used for culture transfer are all examples of laboratory cultures, stocks or specimens of microorganisms, live or attenuated vaccines, human and animal cell culture used in research, infectious agents from research and industrial labs, human and animal cell culture used in research, infectious agents from research and industrial labs, waste from biology, Needles, syringes, scalpels, knives, glass, and other sharp items that may puncture or cut are prohibited. This category includes both used and unused sharps. Medicines that are no longer in use have become tainted and are being discarded. Items infected with blood and human fluids include cotton, bandages, solid linen, plaster casts, linen, beddings, and other blood-contaminated materials. Other disposable items, including tubing, catheters, and intravenous sets, generate waste. Laboratory activities such as washing, cleaning, housekeeping, and disinfection generate waste. Chemicals that are utilised in biological production, disinfection, insecticides, and other uses.

Unwanted materials produced during diagnostic, treatment, and surgical, immunisation, or research procedures, including the production of biologicals, are referred to as biomedical waste. Health care institutions generate a lot of biological waste, which may be a source of infection transmission, especially for hepatitis B and C, HIV, and tetanus. According to many Indian newspapers and magazines, rag

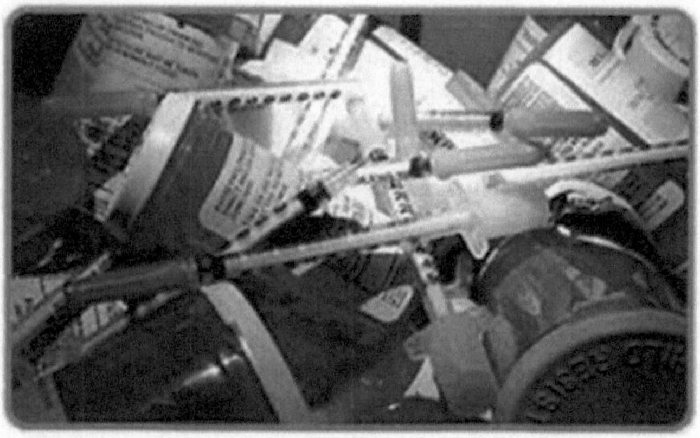

FIGURE 5.2 Biomedical waste in healthcare industries.

pickers collect disposable syringes, needles, catheters, bags, medicine vials, bottles, and intravenous drip sets, which are then sold to duplicators, recycled, and replaced without proper care. Highly polluted human tissues are simply thrown away in municipal garbage cans and subsequently disposed of in landfills, adding to air pollution. Some hospitals' incinerators pollute the environment because the wastes used in them are not adequately separated. Such garbage disposal practices put surrounding people at risk of disease.

In order to protect the environment and the health of the population, the Ministry of Environment and Forestry has issued a "Bio-medical Waste Notification" (management and handling). All hospitals, community health centres, primary health centres, slaughterhouses, and laboratories must offer safe disposal and environmentally sound management of waste produced by them, as stated in the standards for the disposal of bio-medical waste. Figure 5.2 illustrates the chief executive officer's responsibility for ensuring the health of employees involved in the processing, transportation, and disposal of biomedical waste, as well as the safety of the community and environment.

The management and disposal of medical waste from hospitals has been a subject of growing concern in recent years. This is due to the wastes' toxicity and the danger of disease transmission to humans and other living things. A study was carried out to establish how biological wastes from hospitals are created, as well as to characterise and quantify these wastes. Medical care is essential for our survival, health, and happiness. Waste gathered from medical practises, on the other hand, may be poisonous, hazardous, and even deadly owing to their high potential for disease transmission. Across the world, infectious disease outbreaks and indiscriminate trash disposal have been a source of concern for hospital waste management. Medical waste has been recognised by the US Environmental Agency as the third-largest known source of dioxin air emissions and a contributor to about 10% of mercury emissions to the environment from human activities. Biomedical waste production has increased in recent decades, and medical waste management remains a major issue.

Hospitals, health care educational institutions, research institutions, blood banks, clinics, laboratories, veterinary institutes, and animal shelters, among other locations, often collect biomedical waste. Incineration reduces the value of waste by burning it at a high temperature, eliminating hazardous elements, and turning it to ash. The incineration technique is appropriate for pathological and sharp trash. Biomedical waste is autoclaved to destroy bacteria and infectious material, rendering it non-infectious and acceptable for disposal. Syringes, scalpels, vials, glass, plastics, blades, and other similar objects are shredded in the shredding machine. It shreds or chops trash into little bits, making it unrecognisable and ideal for recycling and landfill disposal. The medical waste will be transported from a common storage site to a Bio-Medical Waste Treatment Facility's common storage location. In both private and governmental organisations, medical waste management has received inadequate attention, resulting in insufficient and inefficient biological waste separation, collection, transportation, and storage, according to this study. The Ministry of Health should pay more attention to waste disposal and suitable management policies in order to enhance and appropriate medical waste management processes.

Furthermore, regular worker training, continuous education, and management evaluation techniques for systems and people must be adopted. Every health care facility should have a waste management unit that takes garbage collection seriously. Cleaning crews, nurses, and sanitary workers should all get adequate training. Garbage sorting using a colour-coded scheme at the source should be treated seriously. The government should either ensure that hospital incinerators are in good operating condition or create a central incinerating facility to transport and treat these wastes before disposal. The storage and transportation of biological waste will be investigated further. Liability issues, landfill regulations, public outcry, and a huge increase in the cost of handling, transporting, and disposing of medical waste have all contributed to the current predicament. Garbage is produced by all living creatures on the earth in some form or another. In the past decade, public concern over medical waste disposal has skyrocketed. The high quantity of dangerous organisms and organic chemicals in hospital solid waste is the primary source of concern regarding medical waste. Poor waste management practices may endanger the general public's health.

Biomedical waste includes solids, liquids, sharps, and laboratory waste, which are all generated as a result of human and animal healthcare activities. It is dangerous because it has a high potential for damage, not only to people but also to the environment if it is not properly managed. As a consequence, sanitation of medical waste is an important step in minimising the risks of handling and transportation. This major advancement also provides assurance to hospital administrations in charge of hazardous waste for as long as it presents a threat. The four main kinds of biomedical waste are clinical garbage, laboratory rubbish, nonclinical trash, and kitchen trash. Despite the fact that infectious or hazardous hospital trash makes only a small proportion of total medical waste, it is a hot topic among the public owing to ethical issues and potential health risks. The bulk of hazardous and toxic waste is generated in hospitals and clinics. Domestic and industrial sources make up a small percentage of the total. At the very least, the first two categories should be a significant cause of concern for everyone engaged in healthcare operations. As a consequence, all medical institutions should have sufficient medical waste disposal equipment. If not, a variety of accidents may occur, and healthy people could get ill simply as a result of not being careful enough while handling medical waste.

Infections and pollutants may spread quickly and affect a large number of people this way. Hospital waste generation has become a major concern as a risk element for the health of patients, hospital workers, and the general public as a consequence of its many ramifications. Hospital trash refers to any biological and nonbiologic waste that is discarded and not intended for reuse. Medical waste is a subset of hospital waste that comprises materials generated as a result of patient diagnosis, treatment, or immunisation, as well as materials generated during biological research. BMW is manufactured at hospitals, research institutions, health care teaching institutes, clinics, labs, blood banks, animal shelters, and veterinary facilities. For every microorganism grown in culture, the bacteriological profile of biomedical waste was taken into account. The cost of constructing, operating, and maintaining a waste management system makes for a significant part of a hospital's overall budget if the BMW handling standards are followed to the letter. Self-contained on-site treatment processes may be desirable and feasible for large hospitals, but they are neither practical nor cost-effective for smaller hospitals. A constant supply of colour-coded bags, daily infectious waste collection, and safe transportation of garbage to an off-site treatment facility for final disposal utilising suitable technology should all be in place.

Garbage is produced in enormous quantities as a result of human activity. Garbage of this kind may be dangerous, requiring appropriate disposal. Industrial, sewage, and agricultural waste pollute water, land, and air, putting people's health and the environment in danger. Solid waste may be classified into a variety of categories depending on where it originates from. It consists of (a) domestic garbage, (b) industrial garbage, and (c) biomedical, hospital, or infectious waste. Hospital waste is categorised as hazardous waste because it includes harmful chemicals. This waste is generated during the diagnosis, treatment, or immunisation of humans or animals, as well as during research in these fields. Cleaning and washing water that is directed down the drain are divided into two categories: (a) wasted liquid reagents/chemicals, and (b) wasted liquid reagents/chemicals.

Previously, medical waste management was not considered a concern. In the 1980s and 1990s, concerns about human immunodeficiency virus (HIV) and hepatitis B virus (HBV) infection spurred investigations into the risks connected with medical waste. Hospital waste generation has become a major concern as a risk element for the health of patients, hospital workers, and the general public as a consequence of its many ramifications. Hospital trash refers to any biological and nonbiologic waste that is discarded and not intended for reuse. Medical waste is a subset of hospital waste that comprises materials generated as a result of patient diagnosis, treatment, or immunisation, as well as materials generated during biological research. Biomedical waste is generated at hospitals, research institutions, health care teaching institutes, clinics, labs, blood banks, animal homes, and veterinary institutes (BMW). Waste is defined as any substance (solid, liquid, or gas) that has no direct use and is discarded indefinitely. A waste is considered hazardous if it is flammable, reactive, explosive, corrosive, radioactive, infectious, irritating, sensitising, or bio-accumulative. Hospital trash refers to any rubbish that has been produced, abandoned, or is not intended for future use in the hospital. The risks are not limited to waste management; they also include the environmental risk connected with waste treatment and disposal. The effective handling of biological waste has now become a worldwide humanitarian problem. The risks of poor biomedical waste management have aroused worldwide concern, especially given their far-reaching effects on human health and the environment. Waste management techniques must be efficient, safe, and ecologically sustainable in order to protect people from voluntary and accidental waste exposure while collecting, processing, storing, transporting, processing, or disposing of trash. In addition, such decisions must be cost-effective in the Sri Lankan context, taking into account local logistical needs. Despite the fact that clinical waste management should be an integral part of the health care delivery system, it is mostly due to budgetary limitations. It's still tough for health care personnel to distinguish between medical waste and ordinary garbage. The main goals of biological waste management are to prevent disease transmission from one patient to another, disease transmission from patients to health professionals, and disease transmission from health professionals to patients and vice versa, as well as to protect personnel in health care units and support services. As a result, the adverse effects of cytotoxic, genotoxic, and chemical wastes in general that are generated in hospitals are reduced. Waste management, when properly planned, may be a fairly effective and efficient method that is linked to compliance. When it comes to the proper disposal of biological waste, it has become a humanitarian problem all over the world. Hazardous and insufficient biomedical waste management has been a subject of concern, particularly considering its far-reaching implications for human and animal health, as well as the environment.

The World Health Organization (WHO) recognises that improper clinical waste management and disposal remain a significant threat to a healthy working environment in many nations. Clinical waste, in general, has a huge volume, a long disposal procedure, and significantly higher costs than other waste categories. As a consequence, many hospitals are having financial difficulties dealing with clinical waste. Furthermore, at the municipal level, less specialised methods for handling clinical waste in a cost-effective manner have been developed. Finding cost-effective solutions for the disposal of clinical waste is a big issue for hospitals, according to the study, since it requires a considerable amount of technology and financial commitment.

Most hospitals lack cost-effective methods to dispose of clinical waste, despite the fact that only a few large hospitals employ innovative treatments or contract to the commercial sector. The goal of this page is to provide readers with an overview of medical waste management, including medical waste definitions, exposure issues, medical waste management procedures, and control mechanisms. One of the main issues with current biological waste management in many hospitals is the lack of compliance with Bio-Trash laws, since some facilities dispose of trash in a haphazard, wasteful, and thoughtless manner.

Hospital trash is intermingled with ordinary rubbish due to a lack of segregation methods, making the whole waste stream hazardous. Waste segregation that isn't done correctly leads to waste disposal that isn't done correctly. Inadequate bio-medical waste management will result in pollution, unpleasant odours, the development and proliferation of vectors such as insects, rodents, and worms, and the spread of illnesses such as typhoid, cholera, hepatitis, and AIDS via injuries from infected syringes and needles. Several infectious diseases transmitted via water, sweat, blood, body fluids, and diseased organs must be avoided. Flies, insects, rodents, cats, and dogs are attracted to bio-medical waste scattered about hospitals, contributing to the spread of infectious illnesses such as plague and rabies. Rag pickers who sort the garbage at the hospital are at risk of getting tetanus and HIV. Inadequate sanitation of disposable syringes, needles, IV sets, and other items such as glass bottles causes hepatitis, HIV, and other viral diseases. It is now the responsibility of hospital administrators to handle waste in the safest and most environmentally friendly manner feasible. Medical waste should be classified according to the source, kind, and risk factors associated with its management, storage, and disposal. Waste separation at the source is the most important step, and reduction, reuse, and recycling should all be handled in their proper settings. Some of the issues/limitations that must be addressed for proper biological waste management include a lack of concern and understanding, as well as economic concerns. As a consequence, the general public should be aware of the health hazards associated with biomedical wastes and be concerned about them. Finally, in order to protect the environment and our own health, we must educate ourselves. This research discusses the notion of medical waste, legislative acts governing medical waste treatment, exposure issues, medical waste management procedures, and control techniques.

In hospitals, there are two kinds of waste: risk waste and non-risk waste. Risk waste includes infectious waste, pathological waste, pharmaceutical waste, sharps waste, chemicals, genotoxic waste, and radioactive waste. Food leftovers and packaging generate non-hazardous waste, which includes garbage and ordinary trash. In developed countries, hospital waste disposal infrastructure is well-organised. A well-trained staff handles various waste disposal operational activities such as segregation, internal transportation, and final disposal. All human action generates waste. We are all aware that such waste may be dangerous and must be disposed of properly. The risks of poor biomedical waste management have aroused worldwide concern, especially given their far-reaching effects on human health and the environment. Health care workers, the general public, and surrounding flora and fauna are all in danger from hospital waste. Problems with waste disposal in hospitals and other health care facilities have been a major topic of concern. As a consequence of environmental pollution caused by pathological waste produced by increasing populations and the consequent rapid growth in the number of health care centres, the majority of nations across the world, especially developing countries, are facing a grave situation.

5.4 CONCLUSION

Industrial waste, sewage, and agricultural waste contaminate the water, land, and air. It's also possible that it'll be damaging to people and the environment. Similarly, hospitals and other health care facilities generate a lot of waste, which may transmit diseases such as HIV, hepatitis B and C, and tetanus to anybody who comes into contact with it. Biomedical waste management has recently become a significant issue for hospitals, nursing homes, and the environment. The effective handling of biological waste has now become a worldwide humanitarian problem. With the exception of a few large private hospitals in major cities, none of the smaller hospitals or nursing homes has a sufficient waste disposal infrastructure. These health institutions have been throwing trash into local municipal bins or, worse, out in the open, without regard for safety or the environment. For many years, such negligent disposal has encouraged the illicit reuse of medical waste by rag pickers. India generates approximately three million tonnes of medical waste each year, with an annual growth rate of 8% anticipated. The first step is the construction of large dumping sites and incinerators, which certain progressive states like Maharashtra, Karnataka, and Tamil Nadu are doing against the opposition. We must educate ourselves on this important subject not only for the benefit of health management, but also for the benefit of the community if we want to preserve our environment and community's health.

REFERENCES

[1] Sutha, A. I., "An analytical study on medical waste management in selected hospitals located in Chennai city", *Journal of Environmental Waste Management and Recycling*, Volume 1, Issue 1, Pages 5–8, 2018.

[2] Ravinder, S. T., "Management of bio-medical waste in Himachal Pradesh: A case study of Indira Gandhi Medical College and Hospital, Shimla, HP, India", *Indian Journal of Environmental Sciences*, Volume 13, Issue 4, Pages 1–13, 2017.

[3] Mishra, K., Sharma, A., Sarita, and Ayub, S., "A study: biomedical waste management in India", *IOSR Journal of Environmental Science, Toxicology and Food Technology*, Volume 10, Issue 5, Ver. II, Pages 64–67, May 2016.

[4] Barar, M. and Kulkhestha, A., "Biomedical waste management: Need of today, a review", *International Journal of Science and Research*, Pages 2417–2421, 2015.

[5] Tiwari, A. V. and Kadu, P. A., "Biomedical waste management practices in India-A review", *International Journal of Current Engineering and Technology*, Volume 3, Issue 5, Pages 2030–2033, December 2013.

[6] Melanen, M., Waste Management in Hospitals, Case project with Ecosir Oy and Eksote. Saimaa University of Applied Sciences, Faculty of Business Administration Lappeenranta, International. Bachelor's Thesis, Retrieved on March 06. 2019. from https://www.theseus.fi/handle/10024/116209, 2016.

[7] Pandey, A., Ahuja, S., Madan, M., and Asthana, A. K., "Bio-medical waste management in tertiary care hospital: An overview", *Journal of Clinic and Diagnostic Research*, Retrieved on March 12. 2019 from 10.7860/JCDR/2016/22595.8822, 2016.

[8] Rutberg, P.G., et al., "The technology and execution of plasmachemical disinfection of hazardous medical waste", *IEEE Transactions on Plasma Science*, Volume 30, Issue 4, Pages 1445–1448. 2002.

[9] Thornton, J., et al., "hospitals and plastics. Dioxin prevention and medical waste incinerators", *Public Health Reports*, Volume 111, Issue 4, Page 298. 1996.
[10] Katoch, S.S., "Biomedical waste classification and prevailing management strategies", in *Proceedings of the International Conference on Sustainable Solid Waste Management*, 2007.
[11] Park, K., "Hospital waste management", *Park's Textbook of Preventive and Social Medicine*. 20th edition. Jabalpur, India: M/s Banarasidas Bhanot Publishers, Pages 694–699. 2009.
[12] Seymour Block S. *Disinfection, sterilization and preservation.* 5th ed. Lippincott Williams and Wilkins publication. 2001.
[13] Tiwari, A. V. and Kadu, P. A., "Biomedical Waste Management Practices In India-A Review", *International Journal of Current Engineering and Technology*, Volume 3, Issue 5. 2013.
[14] Mosman, E. A., Peterson, L. J., Hung, J. C. and Gibbons, R. J., "Practical methods for reducing radioactive contamination incidents in the nuclear cardiology laboratory", *Journal of Nuclear Medicine Technology*, Volume 27, Issue 4, Pages 287–289. 1999.
[15] Kannadhasan, S., Mobile Phones Security Using Biometrics, Emerging trends in Computer Science and Information Technology, Organized by Bapurao Deshmukh College of Engineering (NCETCSIT 2013) Maharashtra on 2 January 2013, *Published for International Journal of Computer Applications*, ISBN(0975-8887) Special Issue on 2013.
[16] Rutala, W.A. and Sarubbi, F.A., "Management of infectious waste from Hospitals", *Infection Control*, Volume 4, Issue 4, Pages 198–204. 1983.
[17] Rutala, W.A. Odette, R.L. and Samsa, G.P., "Management of infectious waste by US hospitals", *JAMA*, Volume 262, Issue 12, Pages 1635–1640. 1989.
[18] Sharma, S. and Chauhan, S.V.S., "Assessment of bio-medical waste management in three apex government hospitals of Agra", *Journal of Environmental Biology*, Volume 29, Issue 2, Pages 159–162. 2008.

6 Teager-Kaiser Boost Clustered Segmentation of Retinal Fundus Images for Glaucoma Detection

P M Siva Raja and R P Sumithra
Amrita College of Engineering and Technology, Nagercoil, India

K Ramanan
Rohini College of Engineering and Technology,
Tamil Nadu, India

CONTENTS

6.1 Preamble 109
6.2 Methodology 110
6.2.1 Nonlinear Teager-Kaiser Filtering Technique 111
6.2.2 Teager-Kaiser Boost Clustered Segmentation 112
6.2.3 Clinical Feature Extraction 114
6.3 Results and Discussion 115
6.3.1 Quantitative Analysis 117
6.4 Conclusion 119
References 120

6.1 PREAMBLE

Glaucoma is an eye disease and it leads to blindness. The cruel vision-related diseases are ignored by early identification and accurate treatment of glaucoma. Many researchers are carried out for Glaucoma disease identification. However, segmentation plays a significant task that correctly detects glaucoma.

In [1], an end-to-end region-based convolutional neural network (Joint RCNN) technique was introduced for determining the glaucoma identification to improve the accuracy through the joint optic disc and cup segmentation. However, it failed to minimize the time consumption. In [2], to separate the optic disc and optic cup with higher accuracy, a Level Set Based Adaptively Regularized Kernel-Based Intuitionistic Fuzzy C means (LARKIFCM) technique was developed. But, the retinal structures were not provided in an accurate manner to enhance the glaucoma disease accuracy.

In [3], for the segmentation of the optic cup, the glowworm Swarm Optimization algorithm was introduced with the aid of retinal images. However, the clinical

DOI: 10.1201/9781003217497-6

features were not extracted namely the cup-to-disc ratio. In [4], a deep learning-based automatic segmentation was presented. However, it failed to carry out the filtering-based segmentation with lesser time for glaucoma identification.

In [5], to find glaucoma, an automatic segmentation method was designed with the retinal image. But, the disease detection time was not reduced. In [6], to correctly discover the optic disc and cup segmentation and the glaucoma disease, an Adaptive Region-based model was introduced. However, the filtering technique was not employed to enhance the accuracy.

In [7], a novel optic disk detection scheme was developed to determine glaucoma according to the k means clustering. But, the optic cup segmentation and the cup-to-disk ratio dimension were not addressed from the eye disease to correctly diagnosis glaucoma.

In [8], in order to determine the optic disc segmentation, a modified Dolph-Chebyshev matched filtering technique was developed. The designed technique failed to minimize the PSNR and MSE. In [9–12], a gradient boosting decision tree (GBDT) classifier was designed for attaining improved accuracy for glaucoma screening. However, the appropriate and reliable method was not utilized.

Our contribution:

- In order to solve the existing issues, a novel technique called NTKFIBC-IS is introduced and the contributions are listed below,
- To improve the glaucoma detection accuracy, a novel NTKFIBC-IS technique is introduced which includes different processes namely pre-processing, segmentation, and feature extraction.
- To improve the PSNR with lesser MSE, Nonlinear Teager-Kaiser filtering is applied in the preprocessing. Also, noise filtering is used for eradicating the noise in the input image.
- To extract the region of interest, NTKFIBC-IS technique uses an infomax boost clustering-based segmentation where it separates the image into dissimilar regions based on pixel characteristics. This helps to reduce disease detection time.
- From the segmented region, the different clinical features and the statistical analysis is performed to identify the Glaucoma affected eye or normal.
- Finally, a qualitative and quantitative analysis is carried out with the various related algorithms to discover the performance improvement of NTKFIBC-IS technique with the performance metrics

The organization of the paper is described as follows. In Section 6.2, the process of the NTKFIBC-IS technique is described for accurate glaucoma disease detection. In Section 6.3, the presented NTKFIBC-IS technique and other related works are evaluated in terms of qualitative and quantitative discussion with the help of charts and tables. At last, conclude the paper with a discussion is presented in Section 6.4.

6.2 METHODOLOGY

In medical diagnosis, medical imaging generates the image of the internal part of the individuals. It is employed for fast identifying the main diversity of eye diseases

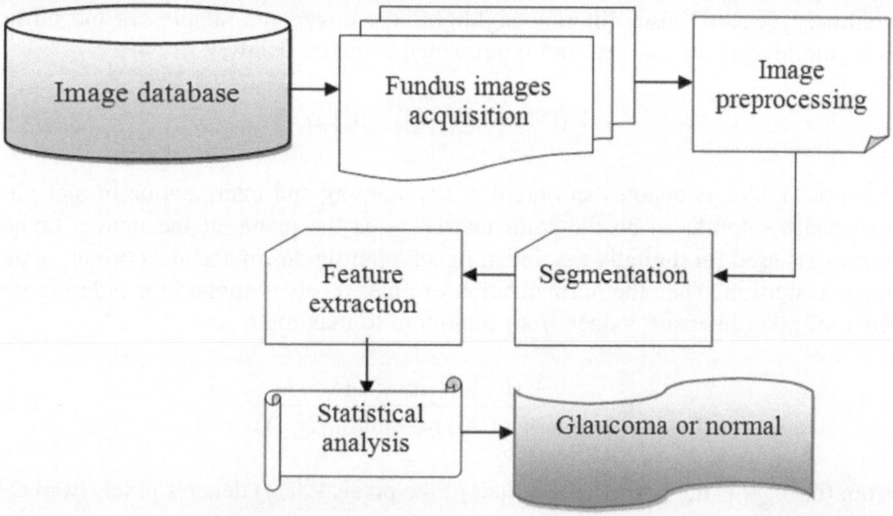

FIGURE 6.1 Proposed NTKFIBC-IS technique.

that happen on the retina with aid of the doctors. The fundus camera is utilized for catching the retinal images. Owing to the obliteration of the optic nerves, glaucoma is the most important disease that affects eye vision loss. Recovering the injured optic nerves are identified as a difficult task. Thus, it is very significant for discovering automated glaucoma disease. The dissimilar machine learning techniques are employed to discover the glaucoma diagnosis. However, the accurate detection of disease was not performed with lesser time. In order to overcome the issues, a novel NTKFIBC-IS is designed to discover glaucoma disease.

As shown in Figure 6.1, the architecture of the proposed NTKFIBC-IS technique is demonstrated for accurately discovering the disease by using image segmentation. Initially, gathers the number of fundus images as input in the dataset. After gathering the input images, the Nonlinear Teager-Kaiser filtering technique is employed for performing the image preprocessing to correctly detect the disease. This helps to enhance the image quality and eradicate noise artifacts. Lastly, the testing disease feature is used to match the extracted features. This detects the input fundus images as normal of glaucoma disease in an accurate manner. The proposed NTKFIBC-IS technique processes are explained as given below.

6.2.1 Nonlinear Teager-Kaiser Filtering Technique

NTKFIBC-IS technique is used in the initial process of image preprocessing to achieve contrast enhancement for accurate glaucoma disease detection. The contrast enhancement is obtained using the Nonlinear Teager-Kaiser filtering technique.

Let us consider the input fundus images '$\delta_i = \delta_1, \delta_2, \ldots \delta_N$' are collected from the Image Database. Each image consists of different pixels $\delta_i = b_1, b_2, \ldots b_n$ represented in the filtering windows in the form of rows (i) and columns (j). Then the

Nonlinear Teager-Kaiser filtering highlights the edges and suppresses the noise. Then the images are warped and interpolated as given below,

$$V(i, j) = (\sum_{i=1}^{n} \sum_{j=1}^{m} w_a b_{ij}) \tag{6.1}$$

From (6.1), $V(i, j)$ denotes an output of the warping and interpolation to make an image into smooth, w_a be the warp matrix, b_{ij} is the pixels of the image. Image warping is used for digitally manipulating an input fundus image and correcting the image distortion. Then the normalization of input pixels is applied for ordering the range of pixel intensity values from minimum to maximum.

$$N_{ij} = \frac{V(i, j) - \min(V(i, j))}{\max(V(i, j)) - \min(V(i, j))} \tag{6.2}$$

From (6.2), N_{ij} is the normalized output of the pixels $V(i, j)$ denotes pixels from the warped and interpolation, *minandmax* denotes a minimum and maximum value of pixels in the warping and interpolation. After the normalization, images are then applied to median denoising for smoothing the input image by removing the artifacts and obtaining the final super resolutions fundus image. The formula for denoising the input image is expressed as given below,

$$F(x) = med\{N(b_{ij})\} \tag{6.3}$$

In the above equation (6.3), $'F(x)'$ denotes an output of the median denoising and *Med* denotes a median, $N(b_{ij})$ denotes a normalized value of the pixels using warped and interpolation. The obtained normalized values are arranged in the ascending order and take a center value as the median. The center value of image pixels in the filtering window is replaced by the median value resulting in removal of the noisy pixels in the filtering window.

6.2.2 Teager-Kaiser Boost Clustered Segmentation

Image segmentation is employed to split the image into different parts based on similar pixel characteristics. In general, image segmentation is applied in different applications such as image compression, disease identification object recognition, and so on. The technique processes an entire image is inefficient to process the whole image. Therefore, for partitioning the regions, image segmentation is utilized.

Infomax boost clustering is a machine learning ensemble technique that provides strong clustering results by combing the weak hypothesis. A weak hypothesis is a base clustering technique that provides slightly accurate results. On the contrary, a boost clustering technique provides well-correlated results with the true output results. For enhancing the accuracy and reducing the time, the proposed technique is applied ensemble clustering technique.

The ensemble technique uses mutual informative k means clustering technique is a weak hypothesis. Clustering is the method of grouping similar pixels into dissimilar clusters. Initialize the 'k' number of clusters $R_1, R_2, \ldots R_k$ and also centroid $s_1, s_2, s_3 \ldots s_k$. Then the mutual dependence between the cluster centroid and the pixels in the input image is measured. The mutual dependence is the probabilistic measure that groups the pixels into different clusters. The probabilities of mutual dependence between the clusters are computed as follows,

$$md\,(b_i, s_k) = p\,(b_i, s_k)\,log_2\left(\frac{p\,(b_i, s_k)}{p\,(b_i)p\,(s_k)}\right) \tag{6.4}$$

From Eq. (6.4), $md\,(b_i, s_k)$ indicates a mutual dependence between pixels (b_i) and cluster centroid s_k, $p\,(b_i, s_k)$represents the joint probability distribution, $p\,(b_i)$ and $p\,(s_k)$ symbolizes a marginal probability. By using (6.4), the mutual dependence between the pixels and cluster centroid is computed. Then the gradient ascent function is used for finding the maximum dependence between the pixels and cluster centroid.

$$D = \arg\max md\,(b_i, s_k) \tag{6.5}$$

Where, D indicates a gradient ascent function, arg*max* represents the argument of maximum function for grouping similar pixels as stated in (6.5) . Weak hypothesis results did not improve the clustering performance but it has some errors. So, the weak hypothesis results are boosted to obtain accurate results. The weak hypotheses are summed to obtain the final strong clustering results.

$$W = \sum_{t=1}^{n} g_i\,(b_i) \tag{6.6}$$

In (6.6), W denotes strong clustering results, and $g_i\,(b_i)$ symbolizes a weak hypothesis output. After that, a similar weight is assigned w t {\displaystyle w_{t}} to each weak cluster.

$$W = \sum_{t=1}^{n} g_i\,(b_i)_*\beta \tag{6.7}$$

In (6.7), β indicates the weight of the weak hypotheses. The weight is a random integer. Followed by, the training error is estimated based on actual and predicted error.

$$\varphi_E = (\varphi_a - \varphi_p)^2 \tag{6.8}$$

In (6.8), φ_E indicates a training error, φ_a denotes an actual error, φ_p represents a predicted error. Based on the error, weights get updated. Incorrectly grouped patterns gain a higher weight. If the weak hypotheses are correctly grouped, then the weight is minimized. As a result, strong clustering results are obtained. Based on the clustering results, the different segments of the regions are obtained.

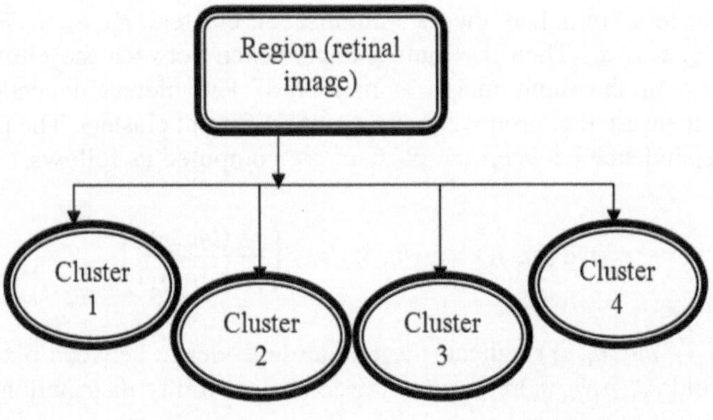

FIGURE 6.2 Division of segmented regions.

By using the clustering concept, the image segmentation is depicted in Figure 6.2. The clustering concept is used to cluster similar pixels and achieve the segmented region of the image. Next, select the segmenting the region of significant element the input fundus images to find the disease. This helps to eliminate the segmented region.

6.2.3 Clinical Feature Extraction

After the segmentation, the feature extraction process is performed to identify the glaucoma disease. The clinical features of the proposed technique such as cup to disk ratio (CDR), neuro-retinal rim (NRR), blood vessel ratio (BVR) are extracted from the segmented region.

The CDR is a major clinical feature that is defined as the ratio of the area of optic disc and optic cup,

$$CDR = \frac{ASOC}{ASOD} \tag{6.9}$$

In (6.9), '*ASOC*' indicates the area of the segmented optic cup and '*ASOD*' signifies the area of the segmented optic disk. The other clinical feature is a Neuroretinal rim (NRR), which is defined as an Optic cup that is segmented from the optic disk and gets a disk-shaped area.

$$NRR = NRR\_IQA + \frac{NRR\_SQA}{NRR\_NQA} + NRR\_TQA \tag{6.10}$$

In (6.10), '*NRR_IQA*' indicates theNRR in Inferior quadrant area and '*NRR_SQA*' point outs NRR in Superior Quadrant Area and '*NRR_NQA*'represents NRR in Nasal Quadrant Area and '*NRR_TQA*' is a Temporal Quadrant Area.

Finally, the last clinical features is a Blood Vessels Ratio (*BVR*) is measured as follows,

$$BVR = \frac{BVR\_IQA + BVR\_SQA}{BVR\_NQA + BVR\_TQA} \tag{6.11}$$

Where '*BVR_IQA*' designates the BVR in Inferior Quadrant Area and '*BVR_SQA*' indicates BVR in Superior Quadrant Area and '*BVR_NQA*' signifies BVR in Nasal Quadrant Area and '*BVR_TQA*' represents BVR in Temporal Quadrant Area in equation (6.11). Finally, the extracted features are matched with the testing value to obtain the final disease detection results.

$$Y = \begin{cases} CDR > CDR_t;\ \ NRR < 1;\ \arg\min\ BVR, \\ glaucoma\ \ impacted\ \ eye \\ \qquad otherwise,\ \ normal\ \ eye \end{cases} \tag{6.12}$$

Where Y denotes final output results in equation (6.12). When the CDR value is greater than the threshold (CDR_t), the NRR ratio is lesser than unity (i.e., 1), arg min *BVR* is minimal than the normal is said to be glaucoma impacted eye. Otherwise, it is said to be a normal one. As a result, the glaucoma disease from the given input fundus image is correctly identified. The algorithmic process of the NTKFIBC-IS technique is explained as follows,

Algorithm 6.1 is the step-by-step process of identifying glaucoma disease from the fundus images. Initially, the input image is preprocessed by applying the filtering technique to obtain the quality enhanced image. After that, the boosting ensemble clustering technique is applied for segmenting the input image. The ensemble technique constructs the multiple weak hypotheses to partition the input image into different regions. The clustering is performed based on mutual dependence between the centroid and pixels of the cluster. Finally, the ensemble technique combines all the weak hypotheses and creates a strong one for improving the clustering performance. Then a similar weight is assigned to each weak hypothesis that calculates the training error. The weight is then updated based on the training error. The weak hypothesis with minimum error is selected as the final result. Based on the clustering results, the segmented region of interest part of the fundus image is obtained. Different clinical features are then extracted and statistical analysis is performed. Based on the analysis, the glaucoma disease from the given input image is correctly identified, which reduces the false positive rate.

6.3 RESULTS AND DISCUSSION

In this section, the NTKFIBC-IS technique is executed in MATLAB with help of ACRIMA database. The result of the proposed NTKFIBC-IS technique is compared with conventional methods such as JointRCNN [1], LARKIFCM [2].

ALGORITHM 6.1 NONLINEAR TEAGER-KAISER FILTERATIVEINFOMAX BOOST CLUSTERING-BASED IMAGE SEGMENTATION

Input: HRF Image Database, input fundus images '$\delta_i = \delta_1, \delta_2, \ldots \delta_N$
Output: Increase disease detection accuracy
Begin
Collect fundus images $\delta_i = \delta_1, \delta_2, \ldots \delta_N$ from database
\\ **preprocessing**
  For each image δ_i
    Extract the number of pixels $b_1, b_2, \ldots b_n$
  Perform warped and interpolation of the pixels $V(i, j)$
  Normalize the pixels N_{ij}
    Remove noisy pixels by applying $F(x) = med\ \{N(b_{ij})\}$
  Obtain quality enhanced image
  End for
End
\\ **Segmentation**
  Construct 'n' number of weak hypotheses
    Initialize the 'k' number of clusters
    Initialize cluster centroid
For each centroid
For each pixel
      Measure the mutual dependence
      If arg max $md\ (b_i,\ s_k)$ **then**
        Assign pixels into a particular cluster
else
        Check another cluster centroid
End if
      End for
    End for
  Combine all the weak hypotheses $W = \sum_{t=1}^{n} g_i(b_i)$
  for eachweak hypotheses
  Initialize a weight 'β'
    Measure the training error φ_E
  Update the weight δ'
  Selectweak hypotheses with minimum error
  Obtain strong clustering results
  Obtain region of interest part of fundus images
  End for
\\ **feature extraction**
  Extracts clinical features using (4), (5), and (6)
    If ($CDR > CDR_t$; $NRR < 1$; arg min BVR) **then**
      Image is affected by the glaucoma

else
Image is said to be normal
End if
End

6.3.1 Quantitative Analysis

MSE is measured on the dissimilar among noisy images and quality improved images. The PSNR and MSE is formulated as follows in (6.13) and (6.14),

$$MSE = (\delta_i - \delta_{qe})^2 \quad (6.13)$$

$$PSNR = 10 * \log_{10}\left[\frac{Q^2}{MSE}\right] \quad (6.14)$$

The experimental result of PSNR versus different sizes of the images is shown in figure I. The number of image sizes is collected in the ACRIMA database. The ten dissimilar outcomes are observed for both proposed and existing methods in figure I.NTKFIBC-IS technique obtains the outcome of higher PSNR when compared to two conventional methods. To evaluate the PSNR, 21.3*KB* of the image is considered. By applying the NTKFIBC-IS technique, the MSE value is 0.25, and the PSNR value is 54.15*dB*. Similarly, the MSR ofJointRCNN [1] LARKIFCM [2] 0.36 and 0.64 and PSNR is 52.56*dB*and 50.06 *dB* respectively. The enhanced values of PSNR and minimal MSE demonstrate the outcome of the NTKFIBC-IS technique. Followed by, evaluate the ten diverse outcomes for both proposed and existing methods. The outcomes of the NTKFIBC-IS technique are discussed than the other two state-of-art methods. The overall observed results show the PSNR is improved by 4% and 8% using NTKFIBC-IS technique than the two existing methods Table 6.1.

By applying three dissimilar methods, the result of PSNR is illustrated in Figure 6.3. The horizontal and vertical axis corresponds to the various image sizes and PSNR respectively. With various input image sizes, the graph is increased nonlinearly. The Nonlinear Teager-Kaiser filtering technique is used for eliminating the noise artifacts in the input image. This is followed by elimination of the noisy pixels in the retinal image. Therefore, the quality of the image is higher and the MSE is less.

The experimental result of disease detection accuracy with respect to the different number of retinal images is described in Table 6.2. The number of retinal images in the range of 10 to 100 images is considered. For the experimental purpose, the ten dissimilar outcomes are measured. From the results, the accuracy of the NTKFIBC-IS technique is considerably improved. In the first iteration, 10 retinal images are considered. The NTKFIBC-IS accurately detects 8 images as normal or glaucoma and the percentages are 80%.

By applying the [1,2], 70% and 60% of accuracy are observed. The result of the NTKFIBC-IS technique is to provide a better outcome of the accuracy and

TABLE 6.1
Comparison of Peak Signal to Noise Ratio

Image size (KB)	Peak signal to noise ratio (dB)		
	NTKFIBC-IS	JointRCNN	LARKIFCM
21.3	54.15	52.56	50.06
15.4	52.56	50.06	49.04
16.5	54.15	51.22	48.13
19.8	56.08	54.15	52.56
23.2	52.56	50.06	49.04
26.9	51.22	50.28	48.13
20.4	50.06	48.13	47.30
17.9	51.22	49.04	48.13
25.1	52.56	50.06	49.04
24.6	54.15	52.56	50.06

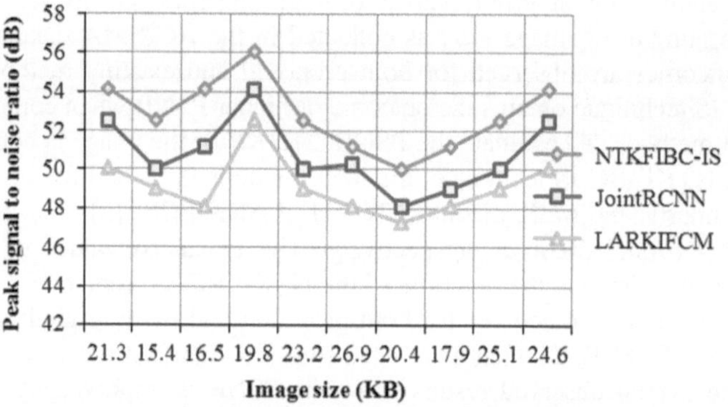

FIGURE 6.3 Graphical representation of the peak signal to noise ratio.

compared to two existing methods. Then, the different counts of the input images are used to perform the nine runs. Followed by, compares the performance of the proposed technique with the other existing methods. The comparison outcomes indicate that the disease detection accuracy is found to be improved by 6%, and 11% than the existing state-of-the-art methods.

The performance result of disease detection accuracy according to the 100 eye retinal images is demonstrated in Figure 6.4. Then, the different input images are employed to observe the accuracy of different outcomes. The NTKFIBC-IS technique is improved disease detection accuracy based on the three methods. This is due to the implementation of Infomax Boost Clustering Based Segmentation and feature extraction in the NTKFIBC-IS technique. Then, the input image is separated into dissimilar segments, by using the ensemble clustering technique. Next, choose the region of the important part of the image, therefore, eliminating the clinical

TABLE 6.2
Comparison of Disease Detection Accuracy

Number of images	Disease detection accuracy (%)		
	NTKFIBC-IS	JointRCNN	LARKIFCM
10	80	70	60
20	85	80	75
30	90	87	83
40	93	88	85
50	92	86	84
60	93	90	87
70	91	87	83
80	94	90	88
90	92	88	86
100	90	86	84

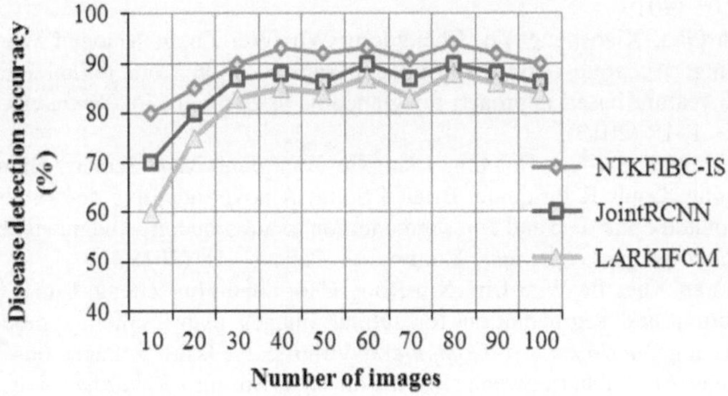

FIGURE 6.4 Graphical representation of the disease detection accuracy.

features. The input image is identified as glaucoma disease or normal in an accurate manner depending on the feature value.

6.4 CONCLUSION

Automatic screening systems named NTKFIBC-IS technique are introduced to enhance the accuracy for early identification and glaucoma. Initially, the nonlinear filtering technique is performed to remove the noises and improve the image contrast. The ensemble clustering-based segmentation process is then performed for eradicating the significant part of the region with improved detection performance. The segmented region of the image removes the dissimilar clinical features. Then, it is verified by using the predefined threshold value. This helps to exactly identify the normal or glaucomatous retinal images. The image database is utilized to perform the experimental estimation. Then the analysis of quantitative and qualitative results is conducted by using the NTKFIBC-IS technique and other methods. The results confirm that the NTKFIBC-IS technique improves disease detection accuracy and minimizes the disease detection time than the existing methods.

REFERENCES

[1] Jiang, Yuming, Duan, Lixin, Cheng, Jun, Gu, Zaiwang, Xia, Hu, Fu, Huazhu, Li, Changsheng, Liu, Jiang: JointRCNN: A region-based convolutional neural network for optic disc and cup segmentation. In: *IEEE Transactions on Biomedical Engineering*, Volume 67, Issue 2, Pages 335–343 (2020).

[2] Niharika Thakur, Mamta Juneja: Optic disc and optic cup segmentation from retinal images using hybrid approach. In: *Expert Systems with Applications, Elsevier*, Volume 127, Pages 308–322 (2019).

[3] Jyotika Pruthi, Kavita Khanna, Shaveta Arora: Optic cup segmentation from retinal fundus images using Glowworm Swarm Optimization for glaucoma detection. In: *Biomedical Signal Processing and Control*, Volume 60, Pages 1–12 (2020).

[4] László Varga, Attila Kovács, Tamás Grósz, Géza Thury, Flóra Hadarits, Rózsa Dégi, József Dombi: Automatic segmentation of hyperreflective foci in OCT images. In: *Computer Methods and Programs in Biomedicine*, Volume 178, Pages 91–103 (2019).

[5] Yuan Gao, Xiaosheng Yu, Chengdong Wu, Wei Zhou, Xiaonan Wang, Yaoming Zhuang: Accurate optic disc and cup segmentation from retinal images using a multi-feature based approach for glaucoma assessment. In: *Symmetry*, Volume 11, Pages 1–18 (2019).

[6] Muhammad Salman Haleem, Liangxiu Han, Jano van Hemert, Baihua Li, Alan Fleming, Louis R Pasquale, Brian J Song: A novel adaptive deformable model for automated optic disc and cup segmentation to aid glaucoma diagnosis. In: *Journal of Medical Systems, Springer*, Volume 42, Pages 1–18 (2018).

[7] Lan-Yan Xue, Jia-Wen Lin, Xin-Rong Cao, Shao-Hua Zheng, Lun Yu: Optic disk detection and segmentation for retinal images using saliency model based on clustering. In: *Journal of Computers*, Volume 29, Issue 5, Pages 66–79 (2018).

[8] Dhimas Arief Dharmawana, Boon Poh Nga, Susanto Rahardja: A new optic disc segmentation method using a modified Dolph-Chebyshev matched filter. In: *Biomedical Signal Processing and Control, Elsevier*, Volume 59, Pages 1–10 (2020).

[9] Fan Guo, Weiqing Li, Jin Tang, Beiji Zou, Zhun Fan: Automated glaucoma screening method based on image segmentation and feature extraction. In: *Medical & Biological Engineering & Computing*, Springer, Pages 1–20 (2020).

[10] Aneeqa Ramzan, M Usman Akram, Arslan Shaukat, Sajid Gul Khawaja, Ubaid Ullah Yasin, Wasi Haider Butt: Automated glaucoma detection using retinal layers segmentation and optic cup-to-disc ratio in optical coherence tomography images. In: *IET Image Processing* Volume 13, Issue 3, Pages 409–420 (2019).

[11] Yidong Chai, Hongyan Liu, Jie Xu: A new convolutional neural network model for peripapillary atrophy area segmentation from retinal fundus images. In: *Applied Soft Computing, Elsevier*, Volume 86, Pages 1–11 (2020).

[12] Zhe Xie, Tonghui Ling, Yuanyuan Yang, Rong Shu, Brent J Liu: Optic disc and cup image segmentation utilizing contour-based transformation and sequence labeling networks. In: *Journal of Medical Systems, Springer*, Volume 44, Page 1 (2020).

7 IoT-Based Deep Neural Network Approach for Heart Rate and SpO_2 Prediction

Madhusudan G. Lanjewar
School of Physical and Applied Sciences, Goa University, Taleigao Plateau, Goa, India

Rajesh K. Parate
Department of Electronics, S. K. Porwal College, Kamptee, India

Rupesh D. Wakodikar
Department of Electronics, N. H. College, Bramhapuri, India

Anil J. Thusoo
Govt. Secondary School, Kupwara, India

CONTENTS

7.1 Introduction ... 122
 7.1.1 Related Work ... 123
 7.1.2 Motivations ... 124
7.2 Materials and Methods ... 124
 7.2.1 Complete DNN-based System ... 124
 7.2.2 Principal Component Analysis (PCA) ... 125
 7.2.3 DNN Model ... 126
 7.2.4 Cloud Computing ... 126
7.3 Results ... 127
 7.3.1 DNN Model Accuracy Performance ... 128
 7.3.2 System Validation ... 129
  7.3.2.1 Bland-Altman Analysis ... 129
  7.3.2.2 R^2 (Coefficient of Determination) Regression Score Function ... 134
 7.3.3 Performance Analysis Criteria ... 134
7.4 Discussion ... 137

DOI: 10.1201/9781003217497-7

7.5 Conclusion 139
References 139

7.1 INTRODUCTION

Nowadays, innovations in the biomedical field have greatly influenced the life of human beings. Continuous monitoring of biomedical parameters like temperature, heart rate, and SpO_2 is important to understand the health status and provide mental satisfaction to patients [1]. In practice, doctors have to observe basic biomedical parameters for patients in the hospital. Such patients need a transportable, easy-to-use, cost-effective, and reliable device that ought to be ready to provide information about their health condition [2]. The advanced electronic sensors having low power consumption make them suitable to use to sense the biomedical parameters [3]. The parameters measured using such sensors show some error as compared with commercially available devices. So it's essential to scale back the error and improve the accuracy using suitable machine learning (ML) tools.

Measurement of HR and pulse oximetry are crucial factors to check the condition of the human cardiovascular system. HR is measured in 30 seconds by placing the thumb above the pulsation and usually counting pulses. HR was calculated by multiplying the measured value by two. This method is simple, but it is time-consuming, inaccurate, and can give errors when the rate is high [4]. Different techniques used to measure the HR include electrocardiography (ECG), phototherapy, oscillometry, and phonocardiography. ECG is one of the most common and precise HR measurement methods, but ECG is not economical [5]. HR in a healthy adult in rest is about 75(±15) beats per minute (bpm) or higher for women. Athletes generally have lower HR than those who are less active. At approximately 120 bpm, babies have far greater HR, while older children have HR at approximately 90 bpm. HR is very different in terms of fitness, age, and genetics between individuals [6]. On the other hand, the percentage of oxygen saturated blood (SpO_2) contributes to the efficacy of a patient's respiratory system. Pulse oximetry is the technique by which SpO_2 is determined. In the beginning, arterial blood gas measurements were the common method used to measure SpO_2. An Arterial Blood gas is a blood test involving a thin needle and syringe to puncture an artery and a small volume of blood to draw [7]. This method was invasive, costly, difficult, painful, and potentially risky. Pulse Oximeter was introduced, which is a non-invasive method based on the measurement of the absorption by using light sensors of red and infrared light, which goes through the patient's finger or ear lobe. The normal acceptable range for patients is 95% to 100%, whereas hypoxic-driven patients expect values to be between 88% and 92%. Oximetry of optical pulses was adopted as a standard patient monitoring technique for HR measurement because of its non-invasive nature, high precision, and reasonable costs [8]. SpO_2 extracting, especially during the current worldwide COVID-19 pandemic, is frequently vital to maintaining patients' health because of its prime function in the diagnosis of airborne conditions and patient monitoring. Pulse oximetry depends on direct contact, usually fingertip, which restricts and may become uneasy [9].

Artificial Neural Networks (ANNs), DNN, and deep learning (DL) are leading machine-learning (ML) tools in several biomedical areas like analysis, fault diagnosis, prediction, or classifications [10]. The applications of DL in biomedical areas cover the majority of fields like natural phenomena, prediction of demographic information, or disease epidemics. Due to development in DL and ML, there is exponential growth in the number of papers published in recent years [10]. There are many applications of DL models in the biomedical field, such as i) computer-aided diagnosis ML application to help the physicians for early diagnosis; ii) The medical care of patients with better-personalized therapies; and iii) analyzing the spread of disease and social behaviors [11]. ANN is a biological neural network like the brain and was introduced in the 1960s [11,12]. The advancements of technologies in the biomedical field are providing helpful information to understand human health and diseases [13]. ML is nothing but artificial intelligence (AI) field that develops statistical techniques to provide the power to find out the unknown thing [14]. The main focus of this research is on the automatic diagnosis of different diseases through the use of DL and ML, such as cardiac activity [15], diabetes retinopathia [16], and sleep apnoea [17].

7.1.1 Related Work

In recent years many researchers developed efficient HR and SpO_2 measurement devices. Naji et al. [18] proposed a SpO_2 measurement system using a digital camera based on a computer vision (CV) system. The authors used the concept of imaging photoplethysmography for measurement. It consists of a red and infrared light-emitting diode (LED) having different absorbance characteristics of oxygenated and deoxygenated hemoglobin. It uses a signal decomposition technique based on a complete Ensemble Empirical Mode Decomposition (EEMD) technique and Independent Component Analysis (ICA) technique to obtain the optical properties from these wavelengths and frequency channels. Bland-Altman test is used to test the validity of the designed system. Error analysis has been done on obtained data, and the sum of square error (SSE), mean absolute error (MAE), and root-mean-square error (RMSE) is determined. Yang et al. [19] demonstrated the photoplethysmography method for the measurement of SpO_2 and HR. They developed a portable watch that monitors SpO_2 and HR non-invasively. Elmoaget et al. [20] proposed a linear autoregressive model using historical SpO_2 data to predict critical de-saturation events. The authors use 20-second prediction intervals in which 88% to 94% of the important incidents were recorded with positive predictive values (PPVs) between 90% and 99%. Simultaneously they increase the prediction horizon to 60 seconds, and then 46% to 71% of the important incidents were detected with PPVs between 81% and 97%. In both cases, more than 97% of the non-important incidents were classified correctly. They investigated the comprehensive classification ability of the improved predictive models. The range of the developed models' area under ROC curves is from 0.86 to 0.98. Higoet al. [21] investigate the relationship between respiration and oxygen desaturation. Annapragada et al. [22] demonstrated DL model SWIFT (SpO_2 Waveform ICU Forecasting Technique) for the prediction of the SpO_2 signal for 5 minutes and 30 minutes. SWIFT model tested on novel data, and it is found that more than 80% and 60% of hypoxemic events in critically ill and COVID-19 patients, respectively. SWIFT also predicts SpO_2 waveforms with an average MSE below 0.0007. Inagaki et al. [23] proposed the system in which Thirty-one subjects with chronic thromboembolic pulmonary hypertension were respectively evaluated to examine the relationships between the changes in HR, HR acceleration time, the slope of HR acceleration, HR recovery. The change in SpO_2, SpO_2 reduction time, SpO_2recovery time, and the severity of pulmonary hemodynamic were assessed during the first-minute interval using right heart catheterization and echocardiography. Ajabe et al. [24] described the review on heart monitoring and heart disease prediction system. The detected heart information is transferred to the physician using the IoT, Bluetooth, GSM module, and cloud-based server. Sorte et al. [25] developed a healthcare monitoring system using the AD8232 ECG sensor module for remote monitoring of the patient. They developed an android based application for continuous monitoring of the ECG of a patient. The data extraction technique was used for the prediction of heart disease. It determines the amplitude of QRS and RR interval of an ECG wave. They predicted heart disease using data mining techniques, and remote transmission is done based on IoT technology. Similarly, Gajbhiye et al. [26] developed an android-based application for early detection of a heart attack. They designed the system in which HR and SpO_2 were displayed on the LCD module. Data transferred over the internet using ESP 8266 Wi-Fi module was observed on an Android-based application. Kalyan et al. [27], Ganesan et al. [28], Golande et al. [29], and Saadany et al. [30] developed IoT-based systems for heart disease prediction and monitoring. They built the system using Arduino and Raspberry pi-3. The AD8232 sensor module was used for the measurement of HR. Ublox NEO-6Mv2 module has been used to find patient location. They sent HR information to the cloud using a Wi-Fi module, and physicians access it from anywhere. Saranya et al. [31], Ahmed et al. [32], and Ani et al. [33] have implemented an IoT-based prediction and diagnosis of the healthcare system. They monitor various parameters such as HR, body temperature, and blood pressure. GPRS module is connected to Arduino microcontroller, and data was saved in the cloud. Doctors receive this data using a cloud server. Yahyaie et al. [34] described an IoT-based model for predicting heart attack. This model uses the ECG of the patient to analyze the heart condition. This model also sends the data of ECG patterns over the internet.

7.1.2 Motivations

The main purpose of designing a DNN-based system is to achieve an accurate measurement of HR and SpO_2. The main motivation of this work are i) design the system with sensors and raspberry pi ii) interfacing sensors with the raspberry Pi-4, iii) application of DNN in the biomedical area, iv) implementation of DNN model by using TensorFlow and Keras, iv) monitoring parameters on the cloud, v) uploading parameters to cloud to send the messages to the WhatsApp app and SMS. The main challenge for the proposed work is to find a suitable DNN model. It is observed that the using DNN model with TensorFlow and Keras achieved better accuracy.

7.2 MATERIALS AND METHODS

7.2.1 Complete DNN-based System

The proposed DNN-based system has been implemented on the Raspberry pi-4 board is shown in Figure 7.1. Raspberry pi has the features of the I2C interface to

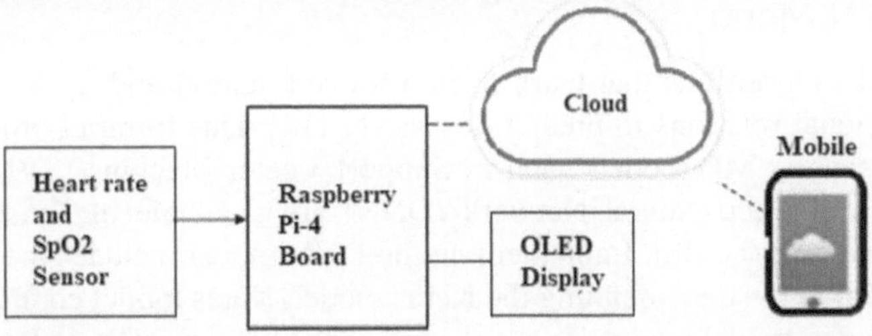

FIGURE 7.1 Complete block diagram of the proposed system with Raspberry pi-4.

attach the sensor. One sensor is used, which is compatible with the Raspberry pi is employed to detect the parameters like HR and SpO_2. Sensor interfaced with Raspberry pi through General Purpose Input/output (GPIO) pins. Sensor output is given to the PCA algorithm. PCA is usually transforming a large dataset into a smaller dataset by reducing the dimension [35]. The Performance of ML or DL can be improved using PCA [36]. The PCA data and corresponding output data are used to train the model. Now, the trained DNN model is prepared to predict the HR and SpO_2. Raspberry pi again reads the sensor data and passes it to the PCA algorithm. The PCA data unknown to the DNN model is given to the trained DNN model for prediction. The system sends the predicted values to the OLED display, to the cloud for future use, and sent to WhatsApp and SMS to the patient or concerned person's mobile number through the cloud.

7.2.2 Principal Component Analysis (PCA)

PCA has been used to reduce dimensionality in large datasets, typically reducing a large number of variables into a smaller one that still maintains most of the information. The PCA is also useful for data standardization to improve the performance of the model [37]. First, data standardization is employed to standardize the scope of the continuous starting variables so that each of them is equally involved in the analysis. It is essential for standardization before PCA operation because PCA is quite sensitive to variations in the initial variables. All the variables will be changed to the same scale when the standardization has been applied. The standardization is

$$z = \frac{value - mean}{Standered\ deviation} \tag{7.1}$$

The second stage is the calculation of the covariance matrix. This phase is to understand how the input data set variables differ from the median or, in other words, to see whether they are related. Because variables are sometimes highly connected, containing duplicated data. So we calculate the covariance matrix to identify these relationships. The final step is to calculate the eigenvectors and eigenvalues of the covariance matrix to identify the principal components.

7.2.3 DNN Model

ANNs are ML algorithms that learn from a trained dataset and try to find out the hidden functional relations to predict or classify [14]. Due to rapid progress in the field of AI, several ML models such as Support Vector Machine (SVM), Logistic Regression, and Deep Neural Network (DNN) are available in TensorFlow and Keras DL frameworks [38]. Implementing the DNN model includes the subsequent steps like loading the data, defining the Keras model, Keras model compiling, fitting the Keras model, model evaluations, and predictions. The NumPy or Pandas library is employed to load the dataset or initialize the dataset in the program. In the proposed work, the sequential model is employed and adds layers one at a time until the accuracy of the DNN model is above 99%. The Dense layers are defined and specify the number of nodes with an activation function. To compile the model first, choose a loss function to optimize the model like mean squared error or cross-entropy loss function, and also select optimizers like SGD or Adam. Select any performance metrics to test the performance of the model. DNN model fitting includes training the model with inputs and outputs, the number of epochs, and the batch size. In the training process of the DNN model, the training code will run for a fixed number of epochs (iterations) and also set the batch size that is considered before the model weights are updated in each epoch. The training process applies to the selected optimization algorithm to return the calculated errors by using the loss function and updates the model using the back propagation algorithm. Evaluating the model requires that to settle on a dataset that is not utilized during the training process to induce an unbiased estimate of the model performance while applying new data for prediction. The last step of the model is predicting unknown data. The architecture of the proposed system is shown in Figure 7.2.

7.2.4 Cloud Computing

Cloud computing is a broad word for any services offered via the Internet. These services are classified into three major categories: Platform as a Service (PaaS), Infrastructure as a Service (IaaS), and Software as a Service (SaaS). A private or public cloud may be available. A public cloud sells services on the Internet to anybody. A private cloud is a private network or data center that provides a small number of users with specific access and permission settings with hosting services. Cloud computing aimed to provide quick, scalable access to IT services and computer resources. Cloud infrastructure includes the hardware and software components necessary for a cloud computing architecture to be properly implemented. Cloud computing can also be seen as utility or on-demand computing. Cloud computing is that services such as storage and processing are delivered on-demand. In this work, two clouds were used. The ThinkSpeak cloud is used for data storage further analysis, and the Twilio cloud sends WhatsApp messages and the SMS of parameters to the authorized individual [39]. Cloud computing functions by allowing customer devices to access data from remote servers, databases, and computers via the internet. There are various examples like Microsoft Docs, Email, Calendar, Skype, Microsoft Office 365, WhatsApp, Zoom, and AWS Lambda.

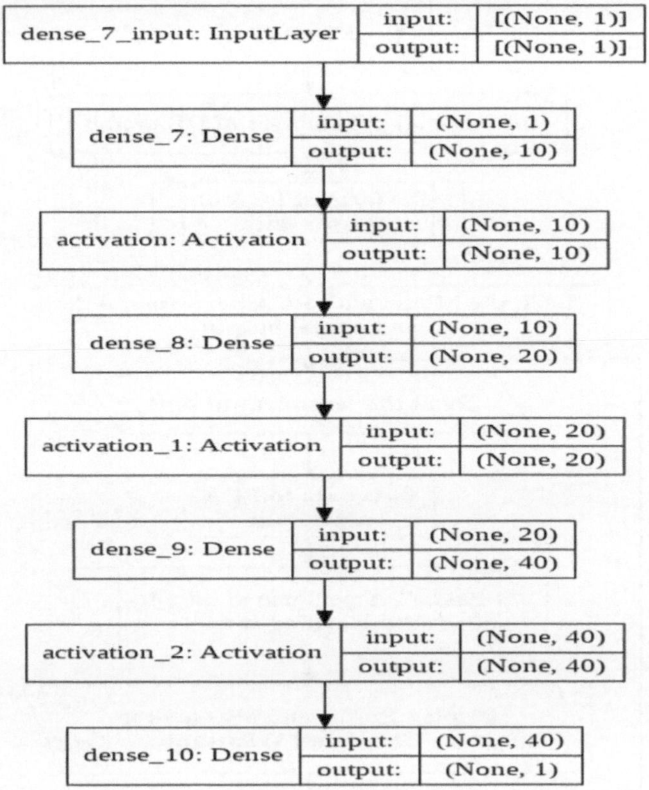

FIGURE 7.2 DNN model diagram for HR and SpO_2.

Cloud computing's key advantages are self-service, elasticity, pay per use, the resilience of workload, migration flexibility, wide network access, multi-tenancy, and resource pooling. Cloud computing offers many compelling advantages like cost reduction, mobility, and catastrophe recovery for companies and end-users. The flowchart of the complete DNN-based prediction system is shown in Figure 7.3.

7.3 RESULTS

There are 40 subjects with different age group that were used for the present work. Table 7.1 depicts the details of the 20 subjects out of 40. The 40 subject datasets were split into training and validation datasets with 80:20 ratios. The DNN model was trained with 30 and validated with 10 subjects. In the proposed DNN-based system, 40 subjects were used for checking the accuracy of the system. The sensor data was applied to the PCA algorithm. Among the 40 subjects recorded data, 30 PCA performed data are used for training the model, and 10 for system validation.

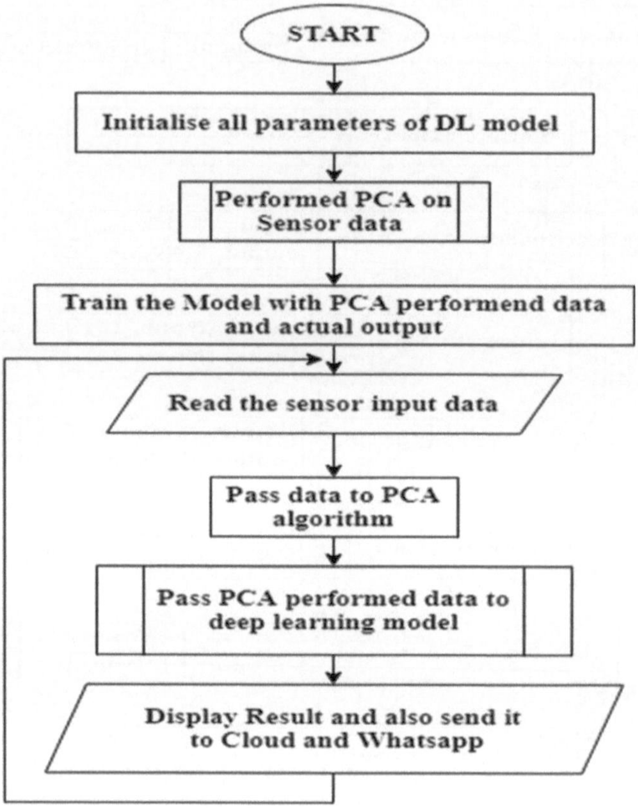

FIGURE 7.3 Flowchart of DL system.

7.3.1 DNN Model Accuracy Performance

In the present work, the DNN model is defined with Sequential API to predict the values of HR and SpO_2 parameters. DNN model has three hidden layers with ten nodes in the first layer, twenty within the second layer, forty in the third layer, and one in the output layer for HR and SpO_2. The activation function 'Relu' is employed in the first and 'sigmoid' in the second and third hidden layers. The mean square error loss function and SGD optimizer were used to compile the model. 30×1 matrix of PCA performed values, and a 10×1 matrix of expected output values was used to train the model. In the training process, display the accuracy of the model using the inbuilt Keras metrics accuracy function. The accuracy (Y-axis) and the number of epochs (X-axis) of the DNN model are shown in Figure 7.4. Figure 7.4a shows accuracy vs. epochs in the DNN-based prediction model for HR and Figure 7.4b for SpO_2.

It can be seen that from Figure 7.4a and 7.4b, the accuracy of the DNN model reaches above 100% after 400 epochs for HR and 200 epochs for SpO_2. In the present work, ThingSpeak and Twilio cloud were used for IoT applications. The real-time monitoring system assembles data from sensors using the IoT on

TABLE 7.1
Subjects Details

Subjects	Gender (Male = M, Female = F)	Age (Years)
1	M	32
2	F	23
3	F	27
4	F	35
5	M	46
6	M	27
7	M	53
8	F	41
9	F	28
10	F	61
11	M	21
12	M	21
13	M	19
14	F	19
15	F	19
16	M	21
17	M	20
18	M	20
19	F	20
20	M	19

the ThingSpeak cloud [40]. The DNN model predicted data uploaded to ThingSpeak cloud in the 5-minute interval, but interval time can modify as per requirement. Figure 7.5 shows the parameters like a) HR and b) SpO_2 on the ThinkSpeak Cloud.

The predicted results of the HR and SpO_2 values are tabulated in Table 7.2. The predicted values of HR and SpO_2 with the DNN model are almost near to the actual values.

7.3.2 System Validation

In the present work, Bland-Altman analysis and R2 (coefficient of determination) regression score function is applied to check the agreement in the predicted and actual (reference) values of HR and SpO_2.

7.3.2.1 Bland-Altman Analysis

The Bland-Altman analysis is the scatter plot and is used to compare the predicted and actual values graphically [41]. It is a plot between the differences of predicted values and actual health parameters values and the corresponding mean of

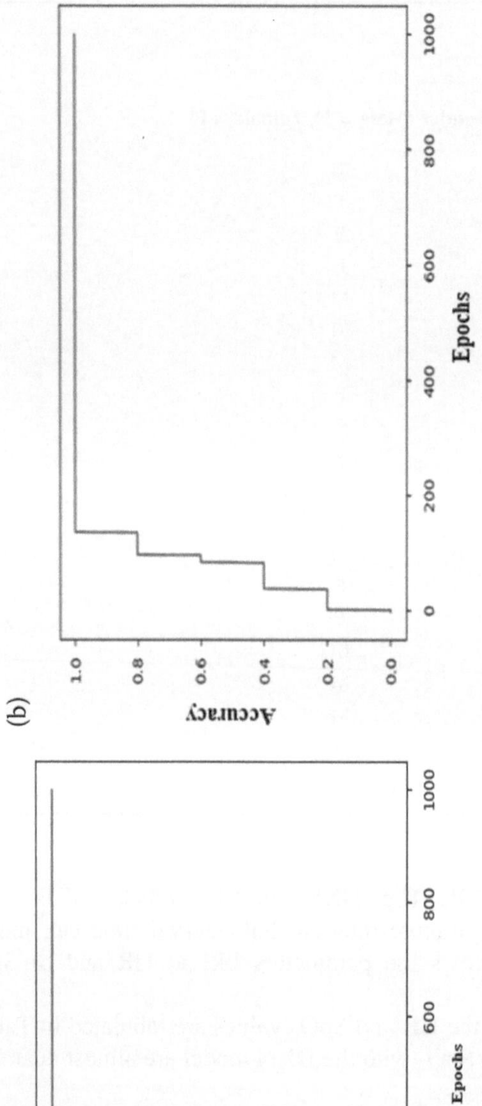

FIGURE 7.4 Accuracy vs. number of epochs of DNN-based prediction model a) for HR and b) for SpO_2.

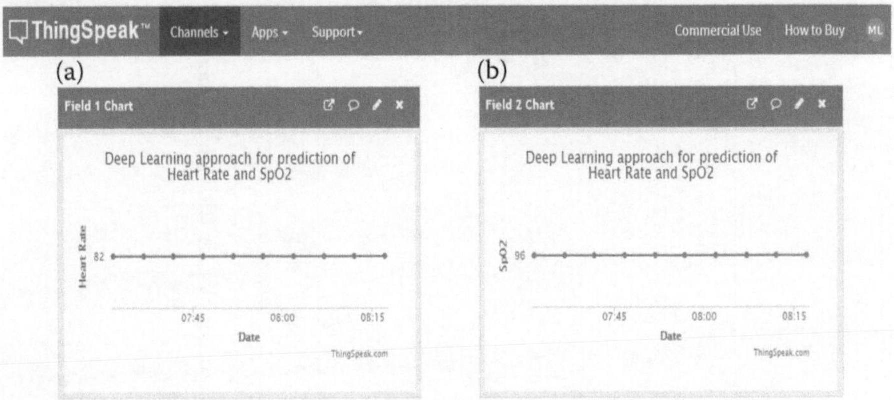

FIGURE 7.5 Health parameters a) SpO_2 and b) HR on the ThinkSpeak cloud.

TABLE 7.2
Estimated Result Without and With DNN Model

Actual HR	Predicted HR without DNN	Predicted HR with DNN	Actual SpO_2	Predicted SpO_2 without DNN	Predicted SpO_2 with DNN
76	76	76	98	97	97
75	76	75	96	95	96
73	73	73	96	96	96
78	76	77	96	97	96
74	75	74	96	95	96
89	88	89	97	96	97
71	69	71	94	94	94
90	91	90	96	96	96
87	86	87	96	95	96
75	75	75	95	94	95

parameters. The difference of actual and predicted values of health parameters is on the Y-axis and the corresponding means on the X-axis. Figure 7.6a shows the Bland-Altman scatter plot for HR without the DNN model, and Figure 7.6b shows the Bland-Altman scatter plot for HR with the DNN model.

Figure 7.7a shows the Bland-Altman scatter plot for SpO_2 without the DNN model, and Figure 7.7b shows with the DNN model. In the Bland-Altman scatter plot, three horizontal lines are drawn, shown in Figures 7.6 and 7.7. The first solid line at the mean of difference and the other two dotted lines at the boundaries of agreement. The boundaries can be defined from the mean of difference by multiplying Standard Deviation (SD) with ±1.96 in the Bland-Altman analysis scatter plot. The SD is defined as

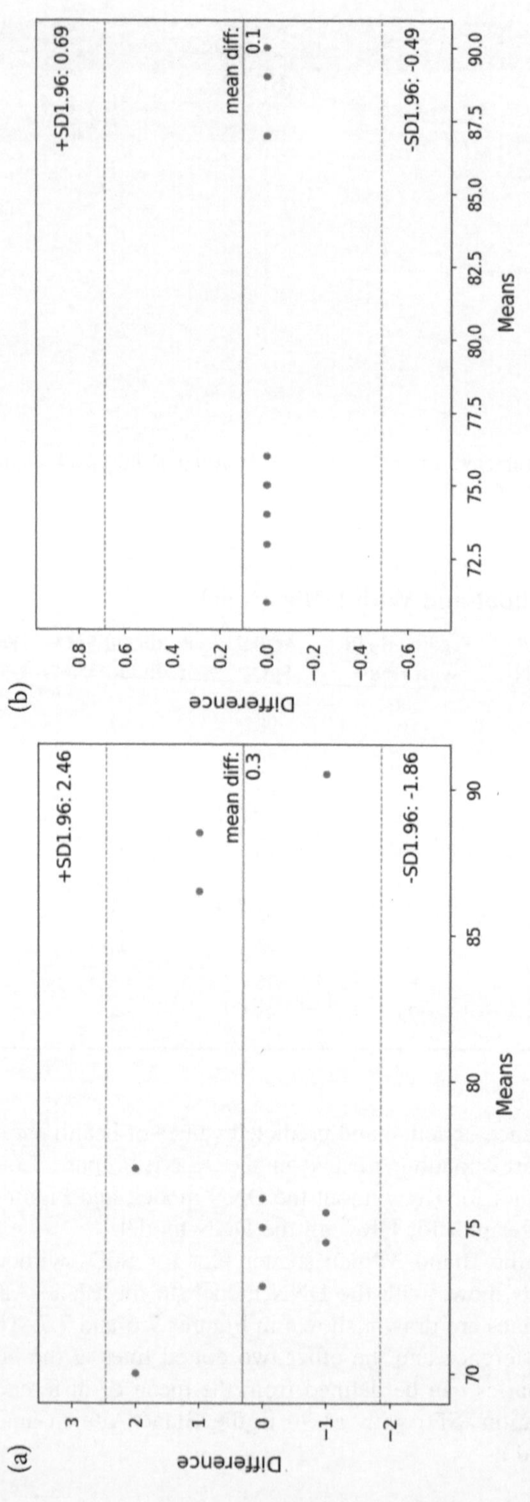

FIGURE 7.6 a) Bland-Altman analysis scatter plot for HR without DL model and b) Bland-Altman analysis scatter plot for HR with DL model.

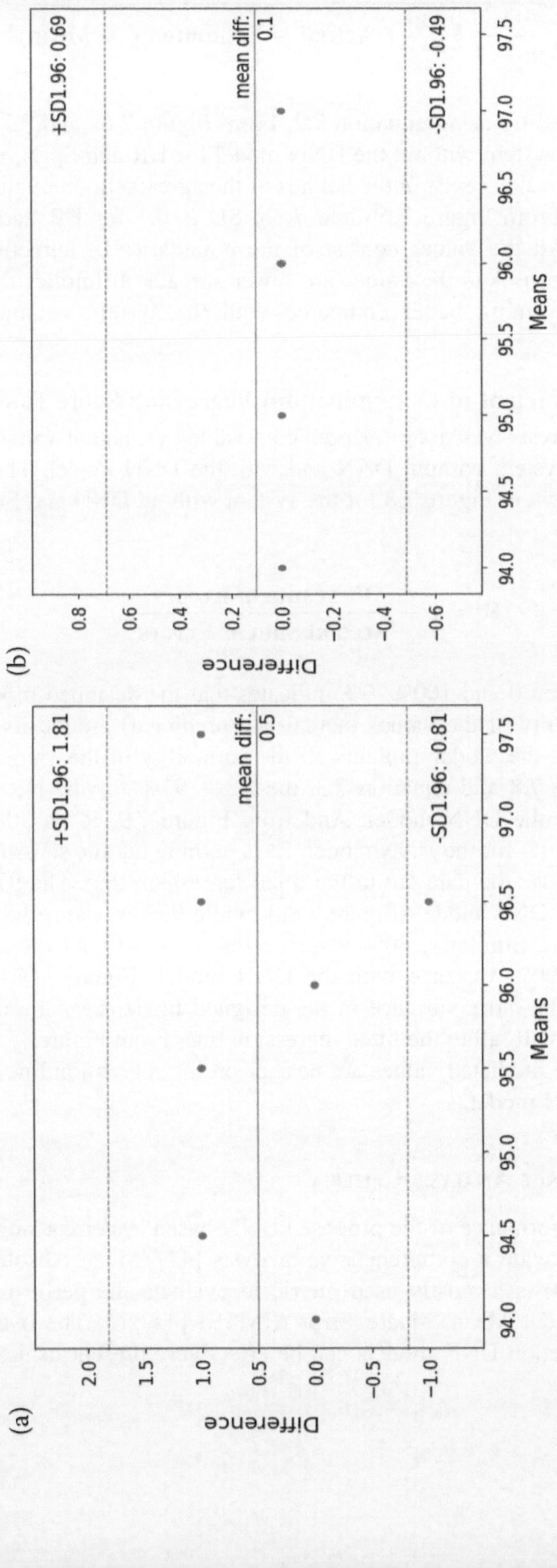

FIGURE 7.7 Bland-Altman analysis scatter plot a) for SpO_2 without DNN model and b) for SpO_2 with DNN model.

$$\mathbf{SD} = \sqrt{\frac{\mathbf{1}}{\mathbf{n-1}} \sum_{\mathbf{K=1}}^{\mathbf{n=10}} ((\mathbf{Actual} - \mathbf{Estimated})_{\mathbf{k}} - \mathbf{Mean})^{\mathbf{2}}} \tag{7.2}$$

The SD is calculated by using equation 7.2. From Figure 7.6a and 7.7a, the SD is 0.3 and 0.5 for the system without the DNN model for HR and SpO_2, respectively. The majority of the values exist in the bounds of the agreement, but values are more adjoin (deviated). From Figure 7.6b and 7.7b, SD is 0.1 for HR and SpO_2 with the DNN model. All the values consist of the boundaries of agreement and are very near to the mean. And the values are fewer spreads. It implies that a system with DNN is performing better compared with the system without the DNN model.

7.3.2.2 R^2 (Coefficient of Determination) Regression Score Function

The regression analysis was done for predicted values vs. actual values of the HR and SpO_2 for the system without DNN and with the DNN model. The regression analysis plot is shown in Figure 7.8 for the system without DNN and Figure 7.9 for the DNN model.

$$\mathbf{R^2 = 1 - \frac{First\ sum\ of\ Errors}{Second\ Sum\ of\ Errors}} \tag{7.3}$$

R^2 is always between 0 and 100%. 0% indicates that the designed model explains none of the variability of the values (actual and predicted) around its mean. And 100% indicates that the model explains all the variability of the values around its mean. From Figure 7.8 and equation 7.3, the R2 is 97% for the HR without the DNN and 99% for the DNN model. And from Figure 7.9, R^2 is 30% for SpO_2 without DNN and 90% for the DNN model. R^2 is nothing but the statistical measure of checking how close the data are to the fitted regression line. The 97% variance for HR without the DNN model (Figure 7.8a), while 99% variance with the DNN model (Figure 7.8b). Similarly, 30% variance for SpO_2 without the DNN model (Figure 7.9a) and 90% variance with the DNN model (Figure 7.9b). In the regression analysis, the more variance in the designed model near the actual or reference data points will fall to the fitted regression line. From Figures 7.8 and 7.9, it is observed that the predicted values are near or on the regression line for HR and SpO_2 with the DNN model.

7.3.3 Performance Analysis Criteria

To evaluate the performance of the proposed DNN-based system, a single metric is not sufficient to provide a comprehensive analysis [42]. Mean Absolute Relative Difference (MARD) is a mostly used metric to evaluate the performance of the system, just like Root Mean Square Error (RMSE) [42–46]. The overall performance of the prediction DNN models can be effectively present using RMSE and MARD [42].

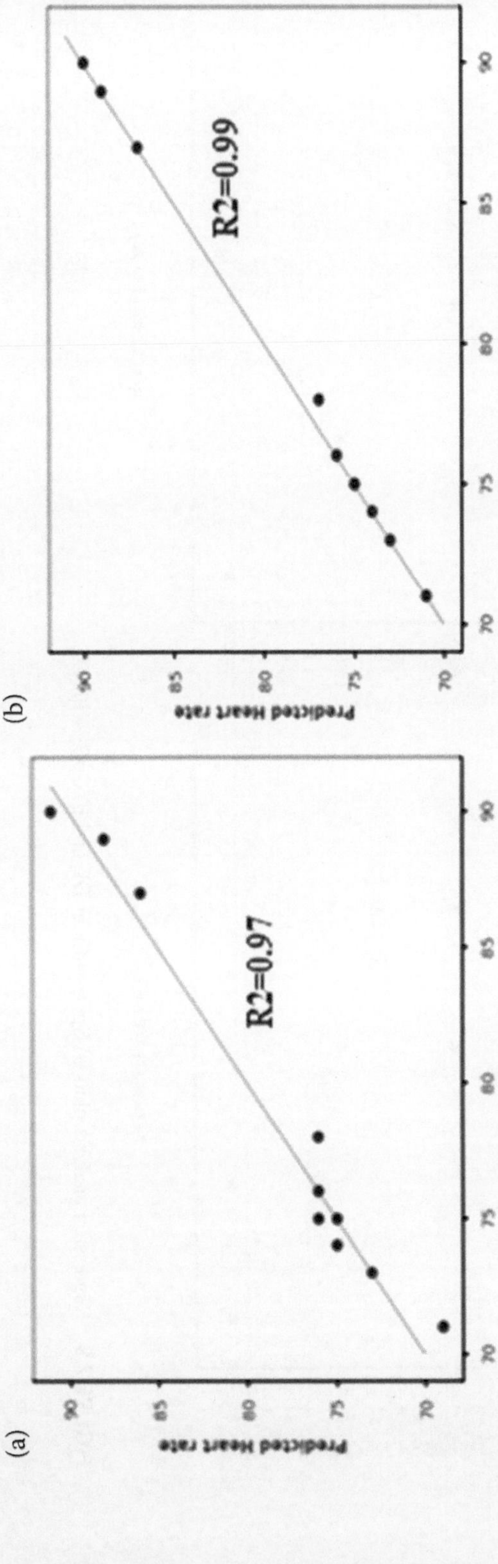

FIGURE 7.8 Regression analysis plots a) HR without DL b) HR with DL.

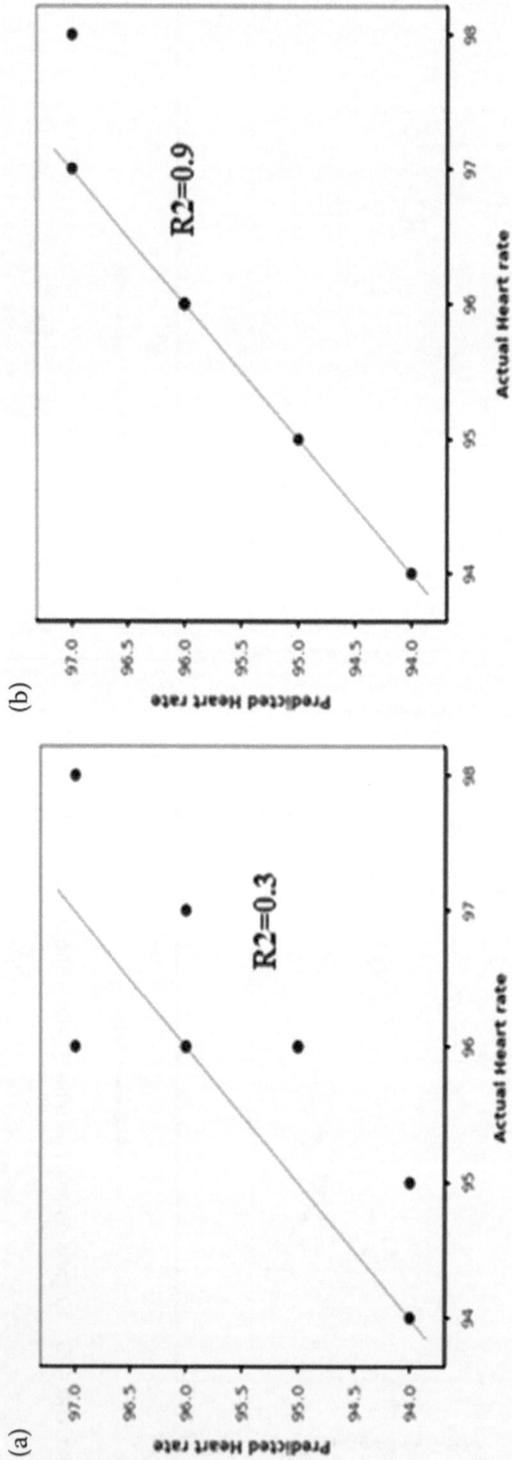

FIGURE 7.9 Regression analysis plots a) SpO_2 without DL and b) SpO_2 with DL.

The Root Mean Square Error (RMSE): It is defined as follows:

$$\textbf{RMSE} = \frac{1}{n}\sqrt{\sum_{k=1}^{n} (\textbf{Actual}_k - \textbf{Estimated}_k)^2} \quad (7.4)$$

Mean Absolute Relative Difference (MARD): it is defined as follows:

$$\textbf{MARD} = \frac{1}{n}\sum_{k=1}^{n}\left|\frac{(\textbf{Actual} - \textbf{Estimated})_k}{(\textbf{Actual})_k}\right| * \textbf{100\%} \quad (7.5)$$

Accuracy: it is defined as follows:

$$\textbf{Accuracy} = \left(1 - \frac{\sum \textbf{abs(Actual - Estimated)/Actual}}{\textbf{No of Subjects}}\right) * \textbf{100} \quad (7.6)$$

The accuracy of the proposed system is calculated by using equation 7.6. The accuracy for HR and SpO_2 without using the DNN model is 88.55 % and 92.73%, respectively. The accuracy for HR and SpO_2 using the DNN model is 98.72% and 98.98%, respectively. The RMSE for HR and SpO_2 without using the DNN model is 1.14 and 0.84, respectively, and the RMSE for the system with the DNN model is 0.32 and 0.35, respectively. Table 7.3 depicts the RMSE and MARD values with and without DNN, and it can be seen that the errors performance improved with the proposed DNN model.

The accuracy of the system with the DNN model is higher for HR and SpO_2 than the system without the DNN model. Results are excellent for both the DNN model and provide very accurate predictions. For both DNN models, the R2 is equal to 90% and 99%, so models report very high performance.

7.4 DISCUSSION

In the health sector, any parameters are vital for preventing and controlling the disease. If we measured the health parameters accurately and then it sends to the cloud. The measured data is available on the cloud, which can access by doctors from anywhere. This will help monitor the patient's health status on mobile from

TABLE 7.3
Performance Analysis of HR and SpO_2 With and Without DNN Model

Parameters	RMSE without DNN	RMSE with DNN	MARD without DNN	MARD with DNN	Accuracy without DNN	Accuracy with DNN	R^2 without DNN	R^2 with DNN
HR	1.14	0.32	1.1	0.1	88.55	98.72	97%	99%
SpO_2	0.84	0.35	0.7	0.1	92.73	98.98	30%	90%

anywhere. In the literature, various computational approaches for measuring parameters have been proposed earlier.

Nashif et al. [47] and Momin et al. [48] proposed a cloud-based heart disease prediction system. Authors use ML techniques to detect heart disease. The analysis of the received parameter will be performed by a Java-based open access data mining platform called WEKA. This algorithm uses two mostly used open-access databases. The 10 fold cross-validation technique was applied to analyze heart performance and achieved 97.53% accuracy. Arduino module sent this data to the cloud and also sent it to the doctor through SMS. The doctor can observe data stored over a cloud to analyze the patient's health in real-time. This system sent data to the cloud every 10 seconds interval.

Jahangir et al. [49] developed the system that monitors heartbeat using pulse sensor and body temperature using temperature sensor LM 35. The output of these sensors was applied to the Arduino microcontroller. Bluetooth chip will send this data to the android application. The doctor can analyze this data on his smartphone using the android application.

Patil et al. [50] have implemented a similar technique using AVR 328 micro-controller. It sends the data provided by the sensor to the Wi-Fi module. This work uses a temperature sensor, heartbeat sensor, ECG sensor. Also, the buzzer connected with the microcontroller alert caretaker in an emergency of the patient.

Islam et al. [1] presented an IoT-based health monitoring system. They designed a My-signal shield technique, which was low-power with a long-range wireless network. Body temperature sensor, HR sensor, SpO_2, and ECG sensor interfaced with My-signal shield for the acquisition of biomedical parameters. Physiological data and statistical analysis methods have been used to study the performances and effectiveness of the sensors and wireless platform devices. They used a wireless system with LoRa for transmission of the acquired parameter from My-signal shield to PC or Laptop.

Sethuraman et al. [51] designed IoT based HR and heart attack detection system. They developed a system using Node MCU ESP 8266, a pulse sensor, Adafruit with GPS technology, and the Blynk app. The real-time information was available on physicians', doctors', or nurses' mobile and monitor. GPS technology was used to monitor the live location of a patient anywhere in the world. The system provides security and privacy to patient data.

Malokar et al. [52] proposed methods for health care monitoring in which physicians were able to monitor patient conditions continuously on their mobile. The patient history was stored on the webserver so that physicians can access it anywhere in an emergency condition. They designed the whole system using the Rasberry-pi board.

Tastan et al. [53] developed an Android-based application that can monitor body temperature, HR, and heart rate variability (HRV) applicable for a patient suffering from cardiovascular disease. The system sends email and Twitter notifications regarding patient location to physicians and family members. Also, alert them when any one of the parameters goes below or above the predetermined value.

Many researchers are working on designing any biomedical system with high accuracy. In the present work, a DNN model was implemented using Python programming on Raspberry pi to improve the accuracy of the designed system. The designed system without DNN gives 89% and 93% accuracy for HR and SpO_2, respectively, but using the same hardware and sensors, a DNN model is implemented, and accuracy improves up to 99% for both the parameters. The predicted values of HR and SpO_2 are then uploaded to the ThinkSpeak cloud for further processing or future use. The predicted values are uploaded to the Twilio cloud to send WhatsApp messages and SMS to the concerned person. The R^2 value and accuracy of the system are compared with Jeyanthi et al. [54] and found that the prediction accuracy of both parameters is good compared with ANN, Fuzzy logic, and linear regression.

7.5 CONCLUSION

The main purpose of any measurement system is to measure the parameters accurately. There are so many other monitoring systems are available to monitor health parameters. First designed the HR and SpO_2 monitoring system with sensors and interfaced with a raspberry pi-4 board. But the designed system accuracy was less. The DNN model is implemented to improve the accuracy and achieve remarkable accuracy with the same sensors and hardware for both parameters. In this paper, DNN models were implemented successfully on Raspberry pi-4 by using a Python programming language. The present work is mainly focused on the implementation of the DNN model to improve the system performance. This system will help the patient to monitor HR and SpO_2 parameters. All recorded data are also available on the cloud to access doctors. The system will also send an alert message to the concerned person if the parameter values go beyond the critical values. This DNN-based system can be used for COVID-19 patients to monitor HR and SpO_2. In future work, authors will be implementing DL or ML models for all health parameters, including glucose and hemoglobin. DL model can train with more data set to improve accuracy further and compare it with the present work.

Conflict of Interest The authors declare that they have no conflict of interest.

REFERENCES

[1] M.S. Islam, M.T. Islam, A.F. Almutairi, G.K. Beng, N. Misran and N. Amin, “Monitoring of the Human Body Signal through the Internet of Things (IoT) Based LoRa Wireless Network System”, *Applied Sciences*, 9,1884 (2019).

[2] T. Landolsi, A.R. Al-Ali and Y.M. Al-Assaf, “Wireless Stand-alone Portable Patient Monitoring and Logging System”, *Journal of Communication*, 2(4) 65–70 (2007).

[3] S. Sali and C. Parvathi, “Integrated Wireless Health Monitoring System for Elderly People”, *International Journal of Innovative Research in Computer and Communication Engineering*, 5(4) 480–490 (2017).

[4] E. Jahan, T. Barrua and U. Salma, “An Overview on Heart Rate Monitoring and Pulse Oximeter System”, *International Journal of Latest Research in Science and Technology*, 3(5) 148–152 (2014).

[5] E. Dogo, F. Sado and S. Adah, “Design of a Simple and Low-Cost Microcontroller Based Medicare Device for Heart Beat Monitoring”, *African Journal of Computing and ICT*, 6(5)121–128 (2013).

[6] S. Das, "The Development of a Microcontroller Based Low Cost Heart Rate Counter for Health Care Systems", *International Journal of Engineering Trends and Technology*, 4(2) 207–211 (2013).
[7] K. Ajith, B. George, B. Aravind and K. Martin, "Integration of Low Cost SpO2 Sensor in Wearable Monitor", *ARPN Journal of Engineering and Applied Sciences*, 10(17) 7553–7558 (2015).
[8] D. Kaur, S. Kumar and S. Sharma, "Online Graphical Display of Blood Oxygen Saturation and Pulse Rate", *International Journal of Scientific and Engineering Research*, 2(6) 1–5 (2011).
[9] S. Alharbi, S. Hu, D. Mulvaney, L. Barrett, L. Yan, P. Blanos, Y. Elsahar, and S. Adema, "Oxygen Saturation Measurements from Green and Orange Illuminations of Multi-wavelength Optoelectronic Patch Sensors", *Sensors*, 19 118 (2019).
[10] W. Alvarado-Díaz, B. Meneses-Claudio and A. Roman-Gonzalez, "Implementation of a Brain-machine Interface for Controlling a Wheelchair", Proceeding CHILEAN Conference on Electrical, Electronics Engineering, Information and Communication Technologies (CHILECON), Pucon 1–6 (2017).
[11] S. Min, B. Lee and S. Yoon, "Deep Learning in Bioinformatics", *Brief Bioinform*, 18(5) 851–869 (2017).
[12] D.H. Hubel and T.N. Wiesel, "Receptive Fields, Binocular Interaction and Functional Architecture in the Cat's visual Cortex", *The Journal of Physiology*, 160 106–154 (1962).
[13] C. Cao, F. Liu, H. Tan, D. Song, W. Shu, W. Li, Y. Zhou, X. Bo and Z. Xie, "Deep Learning and Its Applications in Biomedicine", *Genomics, Proteomics & Bioinformatics*, 16(1) 17–32 (2018).
[14] C. Decaro, G.B. Montanari, R. Molinari, A. Gilberti, D. Bagnoli, M. Bianconi and G. Bellanca, "Machine Learning Approach for Prediction of Hematic Parameters in Hemodialysis Patients", *IEEE Journal of Translational Engineering in Health and Medicine*, 7 1–8 (2019).
[15] F. Beritelli, G. Capizzi, G.L. Sciuto, C. Napoli and F. Scaglione, "Automatic Heart Activity Diagnosis based on Gram Polynomials and Probabilistic Neural Networks", *Biomedical Engineering Letters*, 8(1) 77–85 (2018).
[16] F. Romany Mansour, "Deep Learning based Automatic Computer-aided Diagnosis System for Diabetic Retinopathy", *Biomedical Engineering Letters*, 8(1) 41–57 (2018).
[17] D. Dey, S. Chaudhuri, and S. Munshi, "Obstructive Sleep Apnoea Detection using Convolutional Neural Network based Deep Learning Framework", *Biomedical Engineering Letters*, 8(1) 95–100 (2018).
[18] A. Al-Naji, G.A. Khalid, J.F. Mahdi, and J.. Chahl, "Non-Contact SpO2 Prediction System Based on a Digital Camera", *Applied Sciences*, 11 4255(2021).
[19] D. Yang, J. Zhu and P. Zhu, "SpO2 and Heart rate Measurement with Wearable Watch based on PPG", 2015 IET International Conference on Biomedical Image and Signal Processing (ICBIS), 1–5 (2015).
[20] H. Elmoaqet, D.M. Tilbury and S.K. Ramachandran, "Evaluating Predictions of Critical Oxygen Desaturation Events", *Physiological Measurement*, 35(4) 639–655 (2014).
[21] R. Higo, N. Tayama, T. Watanabe and T. Nito., "Pulse Oximetry Monitoring for the Evaluation of Swallowing Function", *Eur Arch Otorhinolaryngol*, 260(3) 124–127 (2003).
[22] A.V. Annapragada, J.L. Greenstein, S.N. Bose, B.D. Winters, S.V. Sarma and R.L. Winslow, "SWIFT: A Deep Learning Approach to Prediction of Hypoxemic Events in Critically-Ill Patients Using SpO2 Waveform Prediction", (2021).

[23] T. Inagaki, J. Terada, M. Yahaba, N. Kawata, T. Jujo, K. Nagashima, S. Sakao, N. Tanabe and K. Tatsumi, "Heart Rate and Oxygen Saturation Change Patterns during 6-min Walk Test in Subjects with Chronic Thromboembolic Pulmonary Hypertension", *Respiratory Care*, 63(5) 573–583 (2018).

[24] D. Ajabe, N. Mahamuni, S. Lande and R. Kazi, "Heart Monitoring and Heart disease Prediction System: Survey", *International Journal of Advance Scientific Research and Engineering Trends*, 5(4) 29–43 (2020).

[25] P. Sorte, A. Golande, A. Yermalkar, V. Suryawanshi, U. Wanjare and S. Satpute, "Smart Hospital for Heart Disease Prediction Using IOT", *International Journal of Innovative Technology and Exploring Engineering*, 8(9) 321–326 (2019).

[26] S. Gajbhiye, B. Vyas, A. Janbandhu, S. Shrikhande, K.. Nagpure and M. Agashe, "Heart Attack Early Prediction Using IoT", *IOSR Journal of Engineering*", 50–54, (2019).

[27] P. Kalyan and G. Sharma, "IoT Based Heart Function Monitoring and Heart Disease Prediction System", *International Journal for Science and Advance Research in Technology*, 3(12) (2017).

[28] M. Ganesan and N. Sivakumar, "IoT Based Heart Disease Prediction and Diagnosis Model for Healthcare using Machine Learning Models", Proceeding of International Conference on Systems Computation Automation and Networking, (2019).

[29] A. Golande, P. Sorte, V. Suryawanshi, A. Yermalkar, U. Yermalkar and S. Satpute "Smart Hospital for Heart Disease Prediction Using IoT", *International Journal on Informatics Visualization*, 3(2) 198–202 (2019).

[30] Y. El Saadany, "A Wireless Early Prediction System of Cardiac Arrest ThroughIoT", *Proceeding of IEEE 41st Annual Computer Software and Applications Conference (COMPSAC)*, 690–695 (2017).

[31] E. Saranya and T. Maheswaran, "IOT Based Disease Prediction and Diagnosis System for Healthcare", *International Journal of Engineering Research and Development*, 7(2) (2019).

[32] F. Ahmed, "An Internet of Things (IoT) Application for Predicting the Quantity of Future Heart Attack Patients", *International Journal of Computers and Applications*, 164(6) 36–40 (2017).

[33] R. Ani, S. Krishna, N. Anju, M. SonaAslam and O.S. Deepa, "IoT Based Patient Monitoring and Diagnostic Prediction Tool using Ensemble Classifier", Proceedings of International Conference on Advances in Computing, Communications and Informatics (ICACCI), 1588–1593 (2017).

[34] M. Yahyaie, M.J. Tarokh and M.A. Mahmoodyar, "Use of Internet of Things to Provide a New Model for Remote Heart Attack Prediction", *Telemedicine and eHealth*, 25(6) 499–510 (2019).

[35] S. Mishra, U. Sarkar, S. Taraphder, S. Datta, D. Swain, R. Saikhom, S. Panda and M. Laishram, "Principal Component Analysis", *International Journal of Livestock Research*, 7(5) 60–78 (2017).

[36] T. Howley, M. Madden, M. O'Connell and A. Ryder, "The Effect of Principal Component Analysis on Machine Learning Accuracy with High Dimensional Spectral Data", Proceedings of AI-2005, 25th International Conference on Innovative Techniques and Applications of Artificial Intelligence, (2005).

[37] Z. Jaadi, "A Step by step Explanation of Principle Component Analysys (PCA)", (2021).

[38] Y.H. Chang and C. Chung, "Classification of Breast Cancer Malignancy Using Machine Learning Mechanisms in TensorFlow and Keras", *Proceedings of International Conference on Biomedical and Health Informatics*, (2019).

[39] W. Chai, "Cloud Computing". https://searchcloudcomputing.techtarget.com/definition/cloud-computing.

[40] D. Parida, A. Behera, J.K. Naik, S. Pattanaik and R.S. Nanda, "Real-time Environment Monitoring System using ESP8266 and Thing Speak on Internet of Things Platform", 2019 International Conference on Intelligent Computing and Control Systems (ICCS), Madurai, India, 225–229 (2019).
[41] J. Parab, M. Sequeira, M. Lanjewar, C. Pinto and G. Naik, "Backpropagation Neural Network-Based Machine Learning Model for Prediction of Blood Urea and Glucose in CKD Patients," *IEEE Journal of Translational Engineering in Health and Medicine*, 9, 1–8 (2021), Art no. 4900608, doi: 10.1109/JTEHM.2021.3079714.
[42] T. Zhu, K. Li and J. Chen, "Dilated Recurrent Neural Networks for Glucose Forecasting in Type 1 Diabetes", *Journal of Healthcare Informatics Research*, 4 308–324 (2020).
[43] D.A. Finan, J Francis, III Doyle, C.C. Palerm, W.C. Bevier, H.C. Zisser, L. Jovanovic and D.E. Seborg, "Experimental Evaluation of a Recursive Model Identification Technique for Type 1 Diabetes", *Journal of Diabetes Science and Technology*, 3(5) 1192–1202 (2009).
[44] C. Perez-Gand, A. Facchinetti, G. Sparacino, C. Cobelli, E. Gomez, M. Rigla, A. de Leiva and M. Hernando, "Artificial Neural Network Algorithm for Online Glucose Prediction from Continuous Glucose Monitoring", *Diabetes Technology & Therapeutics*, 12(1) 81–88 (2010).
[45] E.I. Georga, V.C. Protopappas, D. Ardigo, M. Marina, I. Zavaroni, D. Polyzos, D.I. Fotiadis and III Doyle, "Multivariate Prediction of Subcutaneous Glucose Concentration in Type 1 Diabetes Patients based on Support Vector Regression", *IEEE Journal of Biomedical and Health Informatics*, 17(1) 71–81 (2013).
[46] K. Li, J. Daniels, C. Liu, P. Herrero and P. Georgiou, "Convolutional Recurrent Neural Networks for Blood Glucose Prediction", *IEEE Journal of Biomedical and Health Informatics* (2019).
[47] S. Nashif, R. Raihan, R. Islam and M.H. Imam, "Heart Disease Detection by Using Machine Learning Algorithms and a Real - Time Cardiovascular Health Monitoring System", *World Journal of Engineering and Technology*, 6 854–873 (2018).
[48] M.A. Momin, N.S. Bhagat, S.B.. Chavhate, A.V. Dhiwar and N.S. Devekar, "Smart Body Monitoring system using IoT and Machine Learning", *International Journal of Advanced Research in Electrical, Electronics and Instrumentation Engineering*, 8(5) 1501–1506 (2019).
[49] A.K.M. JahangirAlamMajumder, Y.A. ElSaadany, Y. Roger and D.R. Ucci, "An Energy Efficient Wearable S mart IoT System to Predict Cardiac Arrest", *Hindawi Advances in Human-Computer Interaction*, 1–21 (2019).
[50] A. B. ChavanPatil, "An IoT Based Health Care and Patient Monitoring System to Predict Medical Treatment using Data Mining Techniques: Survey", *International Journal of Advanced Research in Computer and Communication Engineering*, 6(3) 24–26 (2017).
[51] T.V. Sethuraman, K. Rathore, G. Amritha and G. Kanimozhi, "IoT based System for Heart Rate Monitoring and Heart Attack Detection", *International Journal of Engineering and Advanced Technology*, 8(5) 1459–1464 (2019).
[52] S.N. Malokar and S.D. Mali, "An IOT Based Health Care Monitoring System-A Review", *International Journal of Innovative Research in Computer and Communication Engineering*, 5(6) 11583–11589 (2017).
[53] M. Taştan, "IoT Based Wearable Smart Health Monitoring System", *Celal Bayar University Journal of Science*, 14(3) 343–350 (2018).
[54] R. Jeyanthi, "An ANN based SpO2 Measurement for Clinical Management System", 1st International Conference on Power Engineering Computing and Control (PECCON-2017), VIT university, Chennai, Tamil Nadu, India, 117, 393–400 (2017).

8 An Intelligent System for Diagnosis and Prediction of Breast Cancer Malignant Features using Machine Learning Algorithms

Ritu Aggarwal
Maharishi Markandeshwar Institute of Computer Technology and Business Management, Mullana, Ambala, Haryana, India

CONTENTS

8.1 Introduction 143
8.2 Machine Learning Technologies 144
8.2.1 Naïve Bayes 144
8.2.2 K-Nearest Neighbor 145
8.2.3 Random Forest 145
8.2.4 Support Vector Machine 145
8.3 Related Work 145
8.4 Proposed Methodology 147
8.4.1 Experimental Results and Discussions 148
8.4.1.1 Efficiency 149
8.5 Conclusion 150
References 150

8.1 INTRODUCTION

In women, breast cancer (BC) is the main reason for mortality as well as the second most dangerous cancer after lung cancer. In other words, the cancer is vicious and is characterized by a malignant cyst. It is characterized by anomalous enlargement of cells and tissues in the body. It is a malignant disease that is responsible for many deaths across the world [1]. The researchers conducted studies on BC to detect it in the early stages, which helps in easy diagnosis of the disease and management and

DOI: 10.1201/9781003217497-8

treatment. Cancer progression rate is higher than the rate of curing. There is development of lump/mass on the breast. It can be detected by bioscopy and mammography. There are different types of cancers, such as BC, colorectum cancer, tracheal cancer, bronchus cancer, lung cancer, cervix uteri cancer, and ovarian cancer, out of which BC is the second most occurring cancer among women, which can lead to early death. Different types of detection algorithms are used to diagnose BC. There are some hidden layers and tissues where the activation functions can be applied. Some of the cytological characteristics in FNA could detect BC. There are two types of cancer—malignant and non-malignant [2]. The learning techniques are supervised to construct a best performance model. It is used in the field of medical and bio-medical sciences in data science field through machine learning with same techniques. With the help of imaging techniques and computer-aided microscopic images, data could be collected to perceive breast cancer. Different imaging and data removal techniques have been developed to detect breast cancer. Feature extraction is best method to detect the cancerous tumors [3]. Segmentation of images is achieved by extracting various properties, such as unevenness, uncouthness, declination, and consistency. Various techniques, such as texture analysis based on transformation, are used to transform particular image into newer one by measuring the intensity of pixels by using the properties of spatial frequency. With the help of images, the pixels easily verified the level of lumps near the breast. One technique of machine learning which gives better results in cases of BC is SVM.

The rest of the chapter is organized as follows: Section 8.2 discusses various machine learning technologies that are used in the diagnosis and prediction of breast cancer, literature analysis is done in Section 8.3, and Section 8.4 consists of proposed methodology along with experimentation and results. Finally, the chapter is concluded in Section 8.5.

8.2 MACHINE LEARNING TECHNOLOGIES

ML technologies are basically used to train computers by inputting facts, i.e., they are called supervised learning that further help in making decisions. ML tools evaluate various kinds of algorithms that could facilitate identification of pattern and prediction [2]. In ML we consider and implement the different phases, data collection, and selecting the model, and trained the test model. ML algorithms can be indentified as dissimilar kind of diseases. The logistic regression classifier could be analyzed BC by using different datasets that define BC to be malignant tumor or benign. The Wisconsin Database is used. There are numerous applications of ML, namely, biomedical sciences, recognition of objects, network security, data mining, social media, etc. Usage levels of ML techniques vary in cancer detection.

8.2.1 Naïve Bayes

Naïve Bayes algorithm is used to estimate the predictor densities within each class. It is a very powerful algorithm for predictive modeling. Naïve used the wrapper algorithm in the feature selection stage and the classification stage in breast cancer detection. It stores 683 data from UCI knowledge repository and namely 444 benign cancers and 239 malignant cancers with a type of attributes using Naïve Bayes algorithm. Naïve Bayes is a probability among the each class membership. It is based on the maximum probability obtained for that particular class for given tuple. It is also known as Bayes theorem.

8.2.2 K-Nearest Neighbor

It is used for detection of BC with malignant and benign tumors. It is use to envisage to determine a patient having a disease or not. It uses the Wisconsin dataset to detect BC. It is used as a supervised machine learning algorithm that solves both regression and classification problems on their datasets. It is also called k-nearest neighbor and is used to predict the tissues near the breast or developing of lumps/mass near the nipple area. It basically detects the growing tissues of cancer in the breast [4]. An algorithm training is given to computer in some particular field and then a new data set is given to it. Categorization of test data point depends upon the nearest training data points instead of assuming the dimensions of data set. KNN applies classification technique by classifying the objects based on the feature space where the K-closest training examples are used [5]. The output of classification problem is discrete in nature, i.e., either 1 or 0. In this, there is a predictor and a label. KNN works on data sets and envisages whether the patient is having cancer (malignant tumor) or not (benign tumor).

8.2.3 Random Forest

RF algorithm is used where the model quality and regularization point is highest. By using RF algorithm the biasness is removed and overcome the problem of DT. By using random samples RF algorithm basically is used in predictions used for learned patterns. It is used for the classification and regression. RF is based on unsupervised ML method. The RF is an ensemble classifier that uses a group of individual classifier to detect breast cancer by using different feature sets in supervised classification problem.

8.2.4 Support Vector Machine

This algorithm is used for classification and to extract patterns from large datasets. SVM includes single or hybrid models, such as standard SVM, proximal support vector machine, Newton SVM Lagrangian SVM linear programming SVM, and smooth SVM. SVM works by hyper plane that distinctly classifies the data points [1] where main focus is to chose hyper plane that has the highest margin, i.e., maximum distance between data points and both classes [6,7].

8.3 RELATED WORK

Dhahri et al. [8] solved the problem of automatic detection of breast cancer using a machine learning algorithm. This algorithm works in three phases. In the first phase, evolutionary algorithm based on genetic programming is used to attain the similar results to determine intended configuration. In the second phase, accuracy level is improved by using combining feature selection method. In the final phase, ML supervised classifier is designed automatically.

Abdel-Ilah et al.[1] used ML tools in classification of BC, and ANN to distinguish between different activation functions. They designed a neural network for a particular application that gives a high level of accuracy by altering the total number of hidden layers, total number of neurons that are present in hidden layers, and type of activation functions being used.

Y. Khourdifi and M. Bahaj [4] detected BC using digital/digitized to pathology images in the field of medical pathology. Here a network is designed by changing the network parameters and an encoder is used for compressing the data without affecting the original features of images. Images consisting of various wavelengths are also obtained by spectral imaging technique.

Shravya et al. [6] used advanced predictive models to achieve the valid disease outcomes using supervised ML methods. Supervised ML techniques on predictive models are used for predicting the appropriate disease and its accuracy level. It is analyzed by different techniques that are preprocessing, feature selection, and dimensionality reduction technique, which can provide conducive tools for interpretation in the detection of BC.

Chtihrakkannan et al. [5] diagnosed breast cancer by using the DNN algorithms by using classification methods. This paper basically focused on the prediction of breast cancer at an initial stage by using deep neural network based on artificial neural network. By using Python as a tool, training and computational time have been decreased to a great extent.

Ganggayah et al. [9] in their paper analyzed BC using some prognostic factors through ML techniques. Six variables were recognized. With the help of these variables results may vary according to different datasets and life style of cancer patients. These variables affect the living rate of patients suffering from breast cancer, which can be practiced in clinics.

Shen et al. [10,11] in their paper used screening mammograms classification with the imaging techniques using deep learning model. A whole image classifier is designed, which can further be used for more datasets, which is deficient in ROI annotations even in uneven distribution of pixels intensity.

Tapak et al. [12] in their paper used different models of SVM and LDA to predict survival rate in BC. For detection of BC, six ML and two classical techniques were used for predicting the survival rate and generated level of BC in patients.

Turkki et al. [13] used CNN methods to detect tumor tissues by using ML techniques. With the help of prognostication factors, they reduced the risk that formed in a group of cancer patients by using clinic pathological variables used during mammograms of tissue images and provide the results. These tissue images could be identified to a large extent to describe the image lines using the technique of morphology.

Sharma et al. [14] detected BC by making a comparison between different algorithms. ML using Wisconsin Diagnosis Breast Cancer dataset. This paper compared the most popular ML algorithms like KNN, RF, and NB for achieving high accuracy.

TABLE 8.1
Classification Groups for Benign and Malignant Samples

Groups Classification Samples	Healthy Samples	Unhealthy Samples
1	400	150
	Σ550	

Dabeer et al. [15] identified micro calcification clusters at a very early stage and classify them as benign or malignant cancer cells with very high accuracy, which helped to determine true positive and true negative results.

Singh and Choudhary et al. [16] presented different applications of CNN in the field of mammogram analysis for detection of BC.

Tahmooresi et al. [17] studied the different cancer applications by using ML techniques SVN and CNN. With the help of SVN and CNN, they achieved higher accuracy in breast cancer detection.

8.4 PROPOSED METHODOLOGY

WBCD is a breast cancer database that is collected from the UCI. There are various scalar observations having different elements. The number of samples taken is 550 in which there are two types of datasets, benign and malignant samples. 150 samples in the dataset were malignant and others were found to be benign in this research. In the original UCI datasets there are 11 attributes with their sample id numbers. In this research, the concept of FNA was used to diagnosis lesions and lumps in breast. From value 1 to 9 the cytological characteristics were used to describe benign and malignant features, as shown in Table 8.1.

Different cytological characteristics of breast cancer are given in Table 8.2. With the cytological characteristics of breast cancer, the value is assigned according to their characteristics that shows if the value is closest to 1 it is benign and the value

TABLE 8.2
Different Number of SVM With Different Accuracies of Testing Outputs in Second Group

Index	SVM	Number of Correct Results	Number of Incorrect Results	Accuracy %
1	21	98	2	98
2	22	98	2	98
3	23	96	4	96
4	24	97	3	97
5	25	97	4	96

TABLE 8.3
Hidden Layers With Different Accuracies of Testing Outputs in First Group

Index	Number of Hidden Layers	Number of Correct Results	Number of Incorrect Results	Accuracy %
1	1	96	5	96
2	2	95	4	95
3	3	97	3	97

TABLE 8.4
Cytological Characteristics

Sr. No	Cytological Characteristics	Values Assigned
1	Clump thickness	1–10 with 1 being the closest to benign and 10 the most malignant.
2	Regularity of cell size	
3	Equality of cell shape marginal adhesion	
4	Distinct epithelial cell size	
5	Bare nuclei	
6	Bland chromatin	
7	Normal nucleoli	
8	Mitoses	

is 10 it is most malignant. The middle range value gives symptoms of breast cancer but is considered less as shown in Table 8.4. Table 8.2 gives the accuracy obtained which varies from 98 to 96% for different number of SVM. Table 8.3 gives the accuracy obtained for the various values of hidden layers 1, 2 and 3.

8.4.1 Experimental Results and Discussions

The WBCD dataset is used for detecting BC by the defined range 1–10 for each cytological characteristic. Those are experimented according to the attributes mentioned in table. In this chapter, the classifiers used some libraries from Jupyter notebook ML environment with Python 3.7. It is the collection of different ML techniques for classification, regression, and association rule. ML techniques are applied to solve real problems. Performance in terms of accuracy in breast cancer classification by using fixed recursive elimination method is shown in Table 8.5. Using RFE algorithms the most relevant feature of datasets using BC is found with the help of their feature ranks. In this section, results are analyzed with the help of classifiers and then evaluated. The classification approach across 10-fold cross-validation is used for evaluation. The predictive models are used to test and train the data. Before application,

TABLE 8.5
RFE Algorithms

S. No	Attributes	Feature Ranks based on RFE in				
1	clump_thickness	6	4	5	4	4
2	size_uniformity	2	7	8	2	7
3	shape_uniformity	3	2	2	6	2
4	marginal_adhesion	5	1	1	8	8
5	epithelial_size	9	8	6	8	8
6	bare_nucleoli	2	2	6	1	1
7	bland_chromatin	5	5	5	3	3
8	normal_nucleoli	6	3	6	7	5
9	mitoses	9	6	9	5	2

preprocessing is performed for analyzing and visualizing data. The outcomes are measured in terms of their effectiveness and efficiency as shown in Figure 8.1.

In this section, to build the model we estimated the efficiency of all classifiers in requisites of time, classified instances , and accuracy incorrectly (Table 8.6).

8.4.1.1 Efficiency

The results are based on the confusion matrix that is used by TPR, false value by which the different performance evaluation metrics are used, such as True Positive (TP), False Positive (FP), Precision, Recall F1 score, and Target Value by the class that predicts benign and malignant (Table 8.7).

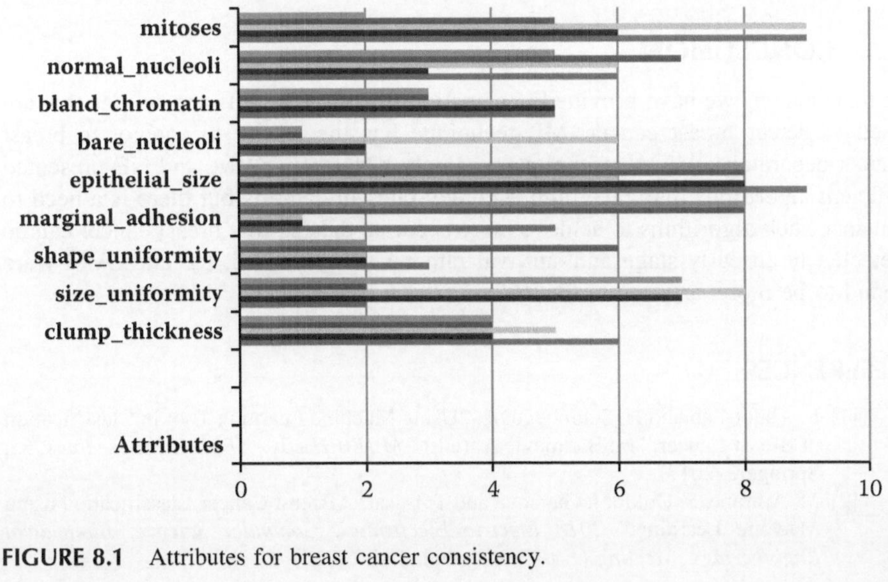

FIGURE 8.1 Attributes for breast cancer consistency.

TABLE 8.6
Results Using Classifiers

RF	SVM	NB	KNN
0.09	0.068	0.08	0.03
689	679	690	667
40	38	25	46
98.11	96.2	92.7	94.29

TABLE 8.7
Evaluation Metrics

TP	FP	Precision	Recall	F1 Score	Class
0.92	0.02	0.97	0.92	0.98	Benign
RF					
0.94	0.03	0.91	0.93	0.94	Malignant
	0.03	0.93	0.96	0.97	Benign
SVM					
0.94	0.03	0.94	0.93	0.92	Malignant
	0.04	0.95	0.94	0.96	Benign
NB	0.05	0.89	0.93	0.94	Malignant
0.98	0.091	0.93	0.96	0.98	Benign
KNN	0.03	0.94	0.91	0.95	Malignant

8.5 CONCLUSION

In this chapter, we have provided explanation for different ML approaches that are used to detect breast cancer. ML technique has the ability to categorize breast cancer accurately. All ML techniques, namely KNN, RF, SVM, and NB presented efficient algorithms that gave high accuracy rates in datasets but there is a need to enhance such algorithms to achieve more accurate data so that breast cancer can be detected in an early stage and survival rate can be increased. RF and SVM were found to be more accurate in the detection of breast cancer.

REFERENCES

[1] L. Abdel-Ilah and H. Šahinbegović, "Using Machine Learning Tool in Classification of Breast Cancer," In: Badnjevic A. (ed.) *CMBEBIH 2017. IFMBE Proceedings*, 62, Springer, (2017).

[2] M. Amrane, S. Oukid, I. Gagaoua and T. Ensarİ, "Breast Cancer Classification using Machine Learning," *2018 Electric Electronics, Computer Science, Biomedical Engineerings' Meeting (EBBT)*, Istanbul, 1–4, (2018).

[3] T. Klonisch, E. Wiechec, S. Hombach-Klonisch, S.R. Ande, S. Wesselborg, K. Schulze-Osthoff and M. Los, "Cancer Stem Cell Markers in Common Cancers–therapeutic Implications," *Trends in Molecular Medicine*, 14(10), 450–460, (2008).
[4] Y. Khourdifi and M. Bahaj, "Applying Best Machine Learning Algorithms for Breast Cancer Prediction and Classification," 2018 International Conference on Electronics, Control, Optimization and Computer Science (ICECOCS), Kenitra, 1–5, (2018).
[5] R. Chtihrakkannan, P. Kavitha, T. Mangayarkarasi and R. Karthikeyan, "Breast Cancer Detection using Machine Learning," *International Journal of Innovative Technology and Exploring Engineering*, 8(11), September 2019, 3123–3126, (2019).
[6] Ch. Shravya, K. Pravalika and S. Subhani, "Prediction of Breast Cancer Using Supervised Machine Learning Techniques," 8(6), April 2019, (2019).
[7] E. Halim, P.P. Halim and M. Hebrard, "Artificial Intelligent Models for Breast Cancer Early Detection," 2018 International Conference on Information Management and Technology (ICIMTech), Jakarta, 517–521, (2018).
[8] H. Dhahri, E. Al Maghayreh, A. Mahmood, W. Elkilani and M. Faisal Nagi, "Automated Breast Cancer Diagnosis Based on Machine Learning Algorithms," *Hindawi Journal of Healthcare Engineering* Volume 2019, Article ID 4253641, 11 pages, (2019).
[9] M.D. Ganggayah, N.A. Taib, Y.C. Har, et al., "Predicting Factors for Survival of Breast Cancer Patients using Machine Learning Techniques," *BMC Medical Informatics and Decision Making* 19, 48, (2019).
[10] L. Shen, L.R. Margolies, J.H. Rothstein, et al., "Deep Learning to Improve Breast Cancer Detection on Screening Mammography," *Scientific Reports* 9, 12495, (2019).
[11] R. Sangeetha and K.S. Murthy, "A Novel Approach for Detection of Breast Cancer at an Early Stage Using Digital Image Processing Techniques," 2017 International Conference on Inventive Systems and Control (ICISC), Coimbatore, 1–4, (2017).
[12] L. Tapak, N.S. Khorram, P. Amini, B. Alafchi, O. Hamidi and J. Poorolajal, "Prediction of Survival and Metastasis in Breast Cancer Patients using Machine Learning Classifiers," *Clinical Epidemiology and Global Health*, 7(3), September 2019, 293–299, (2018).
[13] R. Turkki, D. Byckhov, M. Lundin, et al., "Breast Cancer Outcome Prediction with Tumour Tissue Images and Machine Learning," *Breast Cancer Research and Treatment* 177, 41–52, (2019).
[14] S. Sharma, A. Aggarwal and T. Choudhury, "Breast Cancer Detection Using Machine Learning Algorithms," 2018 International Conference on Computational Techniques, Electronics and Mechanical Systems (CTEMS), Belgaum, India, 114–118, (2018).
[15] S. Dabeer, M.M. Khan and S. Islam, "Cancer Diagnosis in Histopathological Image: CNN based approach," *Informatics in Medicine Unlocked*, 16, (2019), 100231.
[16] O.V. Singh and P. Choudhary, "A Study on Convolution Neural Network for Breast Cancer Detection," 2019 Second International Conference on Advanced Computational and Communication Paradigms (ICACCP), Gangtok, India, 1–7, (2019).
[17] M. Tahmooresi, A. Afshar, B. Bashari Rad, K.B. Nowshath and M.A. Bamiah, "Early Detection of Breast Cancer Using Machine Learning Techniques," *Journal of Telecommunication, Electronic and Computer Engineering*, 10(3-2), 21–26, (2018).

9 Medical Image Classification with Artificial and Deep Convolutional Neural Networks: A Comparative Study

Amen Bidani and Mohamed Salah Gouider
SMART Lab, ISG, University of Tunis, Tunis, Tunisia

Carlos M Travieso-Gonzalez
IDeTIC, Universidad de Las Palmas de Gran Canaria, Las Palmas, Spain

CONTENTS

9.1 Introduction 154
9.2 Machine and Deep Learning Methods 155
9.2.1 Machine Learning Techniques 155
9.2.1.1 Supervised Learning 155
9.2.1.2 Unsupervised Learning 156
9.2.1.3 Semi-Supervised Learning 156
9.2.1.4 Reinforcement Learning 156
9.2.1.5 Deep Learning 156
9.2.2 Deep Learning Techniques 156
9.2.2.1 DL Definitions 156
9.2.2.2 DL Class 157
9.2.2.3 Deep Architectures 157
9.3 Comprehensive Study 158
9.3.1 Concept of Brain MRI Data 158
9.3.2 Image Classification for Medical Disease Diagnosis 158
9.3.3 Medical Image Classification for Machine and Deep Learning 159
9.4 Comparative Study 161
9.5 Artificial and Convolutional Deep Neural Networks based on Medical Image Classification for Alzheimer Disease 162

DOI: 10.1201/9781003217497-9

9.5.1 Brain MRI Datasets 162
9.5.2 MRI Data Pre-processing 164
9.5.3 Features Extraction and Selection from Brain MRI Datasets 164
9.5.4 Classification Methods 164
9.5.5 Proposed Machine-Deep Model 167
9.6 Discussion and Conclusion 167
References 168

9.1 INTRODUCTION

Nowadays, Artificial Intelligence (AI) applications like Machine Learning (ML) and Deep Learning (DL) play a significant role in medical image classification, which is an important research issue in the medical disease diagnosis and neuroscience fields. Many works of researchers and computer scientists have applied AI applications in ML and DL in medical science, healthcare [Wang W. et al. (2020)], Medicine [A. Nogales et al. (2021), Chaddad, A. (2021)], Radiology [Hosny A et al. (2018)], Neurology [Ganapathy K et al. (2018)], and bioinformatics domains were described in recent years. Accordingly, AI is a major branch of Computer science which is used successfully of creating intelligent applications and machines for many medical and clinical decision goals when ML and DL are subsets of AI. In addition, ML suggests training algorithms to solve tasks individually using pattern recognition and DL purposes trust on neural networks with artificial neurons models after a human brain. These networks have multiple hidden layers and can improve more visions than linear techniques. These DL techniques are usually used to reconstruct medical images and improve their quality. The ways of using AI in healthcare and medical science are based on programming and Letting Learning algorithms from large volumes of data with supervised, unsupervised and deep techniques. AI is integrated into numerous technologies that people use every day when early AI applications of AI comprised many intelligent machines and programs. [Emanuel EJ. et al. (2019), Matheny M. et al. (2019); Signaevsky M. et al. (2019); Valliani, A.AA et al. (2019)]. A large amount of data in healthcare is generated by Artificial Intelligence (AI) applications, which mostly is due to the advent of accurate classification ML and DL models. Specifically, in the brain care domain, several novel AI approaches have achieved better results and opened new perspectives in terms of Medical diseases diagnosis, detection, classification, and prediction tasks. AI techniques have received growing interest in the field of brain imaging and computational neurosciences. Segato present a systematic and careful review that contains an overview of different AI techniques used in brain diseases and a review of important clinical applications in healthcare domain. It is based on search in main databases, such as PubMed, Scopus, and Web of Science was accomplished via the main keywords of AI and brain diseases. Additional references were combined by cross-referencing from key articles. 155 studies out of 2696 were identified, which actually made use of AI algorithms for different purposes such as diagnosis and treatment. Brain MRI images data are one of the commonly used data types. The possibility of AI focus to help clinicians and computers sciences to increase decision-making ability in neuroscience applications. However, major medical research problems need to be addressed for better use of AI applications in the brain. To this aim, it is significant in both data processing and building effective AI algorithms.

Hence this chapter book, we present a comprehensive and comparative study on medical image classification and analyzes the improvement in Machine and Deep Learning techniques, such as ANN and DCNN models. To develop the performance of Neural Networks in medical diagnosis applications, image pre-processing and learning algorithms are crucial steps in feature extraction from brain MRI databases. After this previous overview of medical diagnosis of ND with AI applications in neuroscience domain, we make the main essential parts of this issue in the rest of this chapter in the following sections. In the first part, we study a comprehensive literature of the medical image classification using ML and DL techniques from Brain MRI datasets that are used in this work. In the second part, related works of ANN and DCNN models and a comparative study between those models for medical image classification are presented. In the third part, we propose a new deep model entitled to ANN-DCNN model combining the ANN and CNN models from those brain datasets. In the fourth part, we discuss by the recent visions and future ways to develop better performance of those learning models in medical diagnosis applications.

9.2 MACHINE AND DEEP LEARNING METHODS

This section is subdivided into two important subsections: (9.2.1) Machine Learning methods and (9.2.2) Deep Learning methods.

9.2.1 Machine Learning Techniques

Machine Learning (ML) techniques are a set of rules and procedures of AI in which a computer algorithm is developed to analyze and make predictions from data that is fed into the system. Machine learning applications are more used in recent years, such as personalized news feeds and traffic prediction maps. *Neural Networks* are ML approaches modelled like the brain in which algorithms process signals via interconnected nodes called artificial neurons. Mimicking biological nervous systems, Artificial Neural Networks (ANN) have been used successfully to recognize and predict patterns of neural signals elaborated in the functions of the brain. ML techniques are devised in different groups, Supervised Learning, Unsupervised Learning and Reinforcement Learning, and Deep Learning.

9.2.1.1 Supervised Learning

This type is a branch of ML techniques that a function is concluded based on labeled training data. The algorithm prepares a function which can be used for mapping future unknown inputs. The training data is made of a set of training examples, each data is a pair (x; y) where x is an input "vector" and y is the output "value". Supervised learning algorithms devised in two main categories: Regression Algorithms (Linear, Polynomial, Logistic; Regression) and Classification Algorithms (Decision Tree, ANN, SVM, CNN, RNN,).

9.2.1.2 Unsupervised Learning

This type is the branch of ML techniques in which a function/pattern is inferred based on unlabeled training data. The training data consists of only inputs and no known outputs. Thus, unsupervised learning algorithms aim to make sense of the training data by finding relations and patterns within it. Unsupervised learning algorithms can be divided into 3 main categories: Clustering (k-Means algorithm), Dimensionality Reduction, and Anomaly Detection.

9.2.1.3 Semi-Supervised Learning

This type is a branch of ML technique in which a function/pattern is inferred based on partially labeled training data. It associates fundamentals from supervised and unsupervised learning. The goal of this type of technique is to try to make use of both the labeled and unlabeled data to get better learning models. To be able to make use of the unlabeled training data, some assumptions as in the following need to be made to have some structure to the data distribution (Smoothness Assumption, Cluster Assumption, Manifold Assumption, Self-training, Low-density Separation Models).

9.2.1.4 Reinforcement Learning

This type is a branch of ML technique that the action is to take the role to maximize a cumulative reward metric. This is often done using a trial-and-error sort of way in an attempt to discover the actions with the highest rewards. These two features, which are the trial-and-error and delayed reward, are the two most distinguishing characteristics of reinforcement learning: Dynamic Programming, Monte Carlo techniques.

9.2.1.5 Deep Learning

This type is one of the special classes of supervised ML techniques then considered a special case of. In literature, DL algorithms can be believed of as a large-scale neural networks. However, due to the fact that deep learning is also able to perform automatic unsupervised feature extraction, also commonly referred to as feature learning, it cannot be classified as a traditional neural network. Moreover, this type of ML technique tries to model abstractions using databases using a graph with multiple processing layers which contain units that apply linear and non-linear transformations on the data to extract as much useful information as possible.

9.2.2 Deep Learning Techniques

Deep Learning (DL) techniques are a form of ML techniques that use many layers of computation to practice what is defined as a Deep Neural Network, capable of learning from large volumes of complex and unstructured data.

9.2.2.1 DL Definitions

The term of Deep Learning (DL) is used in various definitions can be recognized in the literature. "Deep learning is a set of learning methods attempting to model data with complex architectures relating different non-linear transformations. The elementary bricks of DL are the Neural Networks that are combined to form the DNNs". Deng and Yu (2014) defined the DL technique as "A class of ML techniques based on representations" that exploit many layers of non-linear information processing for transformation, pattern analysis, classification, for supervised or unsupervised feature extraction step.

9.2.2.2 DL Class

- ***Deep networks for supervised learning*** are also named discriminative deep networks until they are proposed to directly give discriminative power for pattern classification tasks. They present in direct or indirect structures a target label data that are always obtainable. These techniques of supervised learning focus to characterize the later distributions of classes trained on visible data.
- ***Deep networks for unsupervised learning*** are proposed to capture a high association of visible data for pattern analysis. They submit to deep networks category when any information about target class labels is obtainable. These unsupervised features or representation learning focus to describe joint statistical distributions of visible data and their associated classes when it is used in generative mode with obtainable treated as components of this data.
- ***Hybrid Deep Networks*** are proposed to give the discrimination that is helped with generative or unsupervised deep networks category. They aim to be able when discriminative criteria for them. These supervised learning techniques focus to estimate the parameters of the deep generative or unsupervised deep networks in the first class beyond then they can also be estimated by better optimization of the deep networks in the second class.

9.2.2.3 Deep Architectures

- ***Deep Neural Networks (DNNs)*** are similar to multi-layers perceptron MLP networks but with more hidden layers. The number of layers is increased and allowed a network of neurons to detect small variations in the learning model, favoring over-learning or over-fitting.
- ***Deep Convolutional Neural Networks (DCNNs)*** are composed of many layers of hierarchy with some layers for feature representations and other types of CNNs for classification. Two altering types of layers called the convolutional and sub-sampling layers. These techniques are prone to get attentive in local optima of a non-convex objective function that often leads to lowly performance and cannot take advantage of unlabeled data.
- ***Deep Belief Networks (DBNs)*** are operated in the first unsupervised phase followed by supervised conventional training. Unsupervised phases aim to learn data distributions without using label information and it aims to facilitate the supervised learning phase that achieves a local search for fine-tuning. These techniques integrate both the unsupervised pre-training phase and the supervised fine-tuning phase to build these learning models.

9.3 COMPREHENSIVE STUDY

This section is based on comprehensive literature that is subdivided into four subsections: (9.3.1) Concept of Brain MRI data, (9.3.2) Image Classification for Medical disease diagnosis, and (9.3.3) Medical Image Classification for ML and DL techniques.

9.3.1 Concept of Brain MRI Data

Magnetic Resonance Imaging (MRI) is the most common imaging practice used to detect neurodegenerative diseases and abnormal tumors in the parts of the brain. Usually, MRI images are analyzed manually by radiologists to detect abnormal brain conditions, however, the huge volume of image dataset is difficult to extract and analyse in a short time. (AbdulAzeem, Y., et al. (2021); Lundervold A. S. and Lundervold A. (2019); Işik A.H. et al. (2021); Kunapuli and Bhallamudi (2021)).

Segato A. et al. (2020) present the different types of MRI data in literature that are reported in the following:

- *Magnetic Resonance Imaging (MRI)* uses a robust magnet and radio-frequency waves to offer clear and full images of internal organs and tissues.
- *MRI Diffusion Tensor Imaging (MRI-DTI)* is a MRI sequence that allows the dimension of the restricted diffusion of water in tissue in order to produce neural tract images in its place of using these data specially for the purpose of conveying contrast or colors to pixels in a cross-sectional image.
- *MRI Diffusion Weighted Imaging (MRI-DWI)* measures the power of molecular motions of diffusion inside a tissue structure or frontiers of white and gray matter brain tissues and brain lesions that have their own diffusion size and can be limited by the diseases.
- *MRI Fluid-Attenuated Inversion Recovery (MRI-FLAIR)* is an MRI sequence to null fluids with an inversion recovery set.
- *MRI T1-Weighted Image (MRI-T1WI)* is one of the principal pulse sequences in MRI when it establishes some modifications in the T1 relaxation times of tissues.
- *MRI T2-Weighted Image (MRI-T2WI)* is one of the basic pulse sequences in MRI when the sequence increase attractions some modifications in the T2 relaxation time of tissues.

9.3.2 Image Classification for Medical Disease Diagnosis

Researchers are more focused towards AI in medical disease diagnosis at the merger of healthcare and medical science. (Anwar, S.M. et al. (2018); Razzak M.I. et al. (2018); Valliani Ranti and Oermann (2019)). Over the past few years, AI in medical diagnosis has shown massive potential in changing the medical standards cares while reducing the life-threatening pressures. It aims with clinical decision

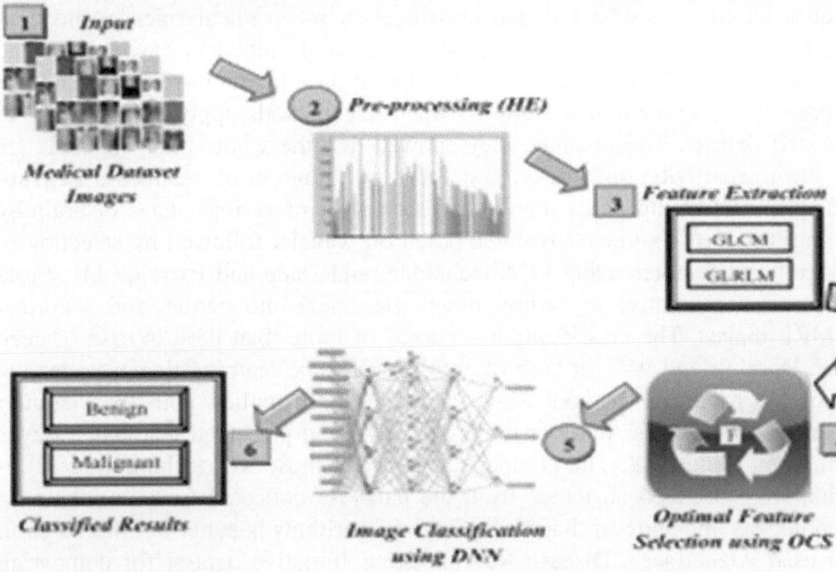

FIGURE 9.1 The general process of medical image classification.

support, robotics, management, and organization. AI is rich in data analytics, image processing, medical image classification, neural networks, and ML and DL algorithms and insights adapting to the needs of the patients. It can be used to diagnose disease in medical imaging provide radiologists with the help in management of diseases. (Fan, Z et al. 2020; Ashraf et al., (2020); Kunapuli and Bhallamudi (2021); Mirbabaie et al. (2021)). Therefore, ML and DL techniques designed to diagnose diseases are trained on huge medical data of normal and abnormal cases like patient's history, symptoms, laboratory things, scans, and images when predicting diseases by efficient and more accurate results. Medical imaging is a way in AI to read images and extract patterns from huge medical image data. In medical diagnosis, clinicians use sources of medical images that are MRI, CT scan, X-ray, ultrasound, and other techniques to decide the presence of one disease. Figure 9.1

9.3.3 Medical Image Classification for Machine and Deep Learning

In this section, we present related works of recent articles based on neurodegenerative disorders detection and classification using Machine and Deep Learning from brain image datasets. *Medical image classification* is an essential task in medical science and image analysis. Although ML and DL techniques have shown proven advantages over traditional methods that presented in these recent research articles: Farid, A. et al. (2020), Termine et al. (2021), Nogales A. et al (2021), Agrawal R.K. and Juneja A. (2019), Lundervold A. S. and Lundervold A. (2019), Jyotiyana M. et al. (2021), Balne S. and Elumalai A. (2021), Işik A.H. et al. (2021).

Although other articles are presented, different comparative studies focused on comparing from 2011 to 2021 over Medical Image Classification for ML and DL techniques based on medical image classification for medical science and neurology, such as ANN, DCNN, and SVM. For Neural Networks based ANN and DCNN, we selected 11 comparison studies based on a literature review. Cuingnet et al. presented a comparative study between ten methods applying MRI images from ADNI dataset. To conclude, they showed that the whole brain methods are taking great sensitivity, specificity, and accuracy. Singh et al. realized a new approach for investigating brain abnormalities on MRI of various states of brain by extracting the most significant features based on wavelet followed by selection of most significant features using PCA technique, and Deep and Extreme ML-based classification comparative to various others classifiers into normal and abnormal brain MRI images. The classification accuracy of more than 93% in case of deep machine learning and 94% in case of extreme machine learning demonstrates the utility of the proposed method. Shree and Sheshadri applied both the classifier "J48" and "Naïve Bayes" in order to diagnose AD and presented that Naïve Bayes performed outshines J48. The comparison between those ML techniques of classification were used 24 attributes from the database collected from various neuropsychologists and showed that Naïve Bayes algorithms is better in all. Fan et al. (2020) used Alzheimer's Disease Neuroimaging Initiative dataset for comparing various techniques of feature selection using ML technique for dementia for anatomical brain MRI. It is shown that age removal recovers the regular accuracy with all the classifiers when SVM and Logistic Regression are used as classifiers and after applying feature selection techniques for brain diseases. Bansal et al. compared between four ML models such as Naïve Bayes, Random Forest, Multilayer Perceptron, and J48. They applied the feature selection that decreases the set of attribute to 4 and indicated the overall greater accuracy. They used CFS Subset Eval for the attribute decrease. They concluded that J48 is favored because it has been considered the best among all the models to detect dementia disease. Zhang et al., (2018) proposed a hybrid new approach named CDHVF algorithm (Combined Deep and Handcrafted Visual Feature) that uses features learned by per-trained Deep Convolutional Neural Networks (DCNNs) and three fine-tuned and two handcrafted descriptors in a combined approach. They estimated the CDHVF algorithm on the Image CLEF 2016 Subfigure Classification dataset and it realized an accuracy of 85.47% that is higher than the better performance of other purely visual approaches listed in the challenge leader board. Experimental results specify that handcrafted features complement the image representation learned by DCNNs on small training datasets and develop accuracy in certain medical image classification problems. Alebiosu and Muhammad (2019) presented a research paper about image classification by using DL via TensorFlow framework. It has three aims that are related directly with conclusions because it can decide whether all aims are effectively achieved or not. It can be finished that all results that have been achieved, showed quite impressive outcomes. The deep neural network (DNN) develops the key agenda for this research, particularly in image classification technology. DNN technique was studied in more details starting from assembling, training model and to classify images into categories. Termine et al. (2021) introduced generally, the need of effective ML applications treatments for neurodegenerative diseases. They discussed how ML can aid early diagnosis and interpretation of medical images as well as the discovery and development of new therapies. A unifying theme of the different applications of machine learning is the integration of multiple high-dimensional sources of data, which all provide a different view of the disease, and the automated derivation of actionable insights. Sharma A.K. et al. (2021) presented a paper that aims to provide an introduction of deep learning in the medical sector for image processing. First, the process of image processing neural network has been discussed and then a review of ML algorithms about CNN, learning with CNN, RNN, Boltzmann machine is presented. The application of neural networks in medical image analysis has also been discussed, such as detection, segmentation, registration, and localization, etc. They concluded by adding some opinions about challenges and future directions of AI, ML, and DL techniques that has also been presented by the advantages in terms of accuracy. Although the ML techniques are able to offer great knowledge and information about MIA because it has so effective and accurate methods that are able to interact with image detection. Ajagbe et al. (2021) presented a study that was designed the improvements of AD Image classification with DCNN concerning CNN and transfer learning (Visual Geometry Group (VGG) 16 and VGG19) using MRI and extend the evaluation metrics since limitations and capacity of algorithms cannot be revealed by few metrics. The objectives of this research are to classify AD images into four known classes by neurologists and results of the finding are subjected to many evaluation metrics. This research used computer algorithms majorly DCNN and transfer learning to classify AD. This study has proven that computer algorithms are capable of classifying AD into four classes known to medical experts. Jyotiyana et al. (2021) Deep Learning (DL) is an emerging field that attracts researchers, especially in the field of engineering and medical sciences. DL gives us many solutions to date, that is why it is still an active field of interest and will for many years. They provided a brief introduction of DL architectures and the applications and the role of DL in the ND prediction such as Alzheimer's, Parkinson's, Huntington's disease, MCI, and other dementia when they also discussed other brain disorders and how DL is important, nowadays, in the medical science field for providing better, accurate, and fast treatment for the patient.

9.4 COMPARATIVE STUDY

This section proposes a comparative study of medical image classification for neurodegenerative disorders with Machine and Deep Learning techniques. *The neurodegeneration* is a common cause of cognitive impairment in the elderly persons when it is placing a considerable pressure on a gradually aging society. Neurodegenerative diseases, such as Dementia, Alzheimer's, and Parkinson's disease, are a large group of neurological disorders with heterogeneous clinical symptoms that affect a specific subset of neurons in specific functional anatomic systems. These disorders present an essential issue in medical science and image processing, which causes the change on the level of the brain and nerve organs by difficulties as memory, concentration, daily comportments, and psychological situation. Neurodegenerative disease detection and classification among massive data is applicable in medical image processing. As shown in Figure 9.2, we present the

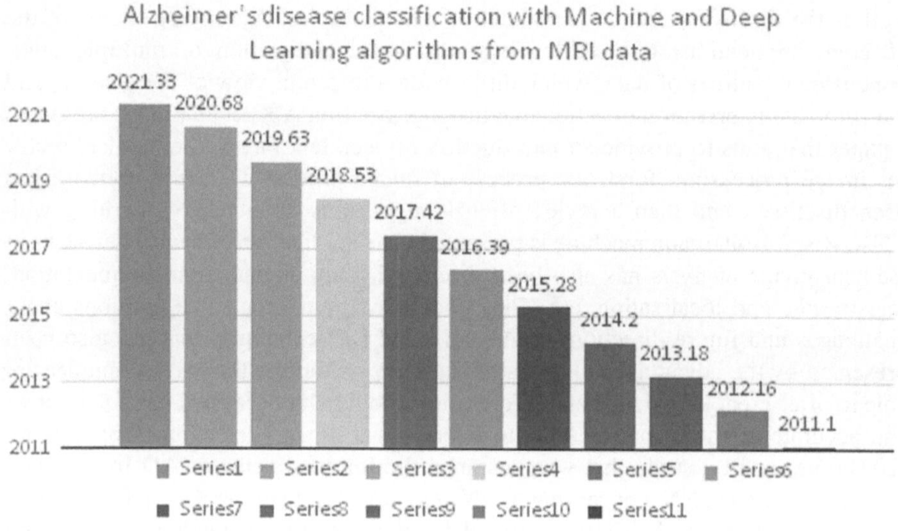

FIGURE 9.2 Machine and deep learning methods for Alzheimer's disease classification in recent ten years.

number of publications for Machine and Deep Learning in the recent five years. Also, as shown in Table 9.1 and Table 9.2, we propose a comparison between the medical image classification based on the different ML and DL techniques in order to detect and classify the ND using brain MRI datasets.

9.5 ARTIFICIAL AND CONVOLUTIONAL DEEP NEURAL NETWORKS BASED ON MEDICAL IMAGE CLASSIFICATION FOR ALZHEIMER DISEASE

This section proposes a new Machine and Deep model based on medical image classification using artificial and convolutional deep neural networks for Alzheimer's disease, which is subdivided into four subsections: (9.5.1) brain MRI datasets, (9.5.2) MRI data pre-processing, (9.5.3) features extraction and selection from Brain MRI datasets, and (9.5.4) classification methods.

9.5.1 Brain MRI Datasets

The brain MRI images, relative of OASIS dataset, are processed by using three major phases, namely image processing, feature extraction and selection, and classification, and each of these phases will be discussed. Based on Figure 9.3, it is mainly the image classification framework where artificial and deep convolutional neural networks are applied. In this chapter, we used OASIS open-access Brain datasets. These datasets investigate during preparation from Neuroimaging Informatics Analysis Center (NIAC) at Washington University School of Medicine. We create four classes based on CDR score, such as No Dementia (CDR-0), Very Mild Dementia (CDR-0.5), Mild-Dementia (CDR-1), and Moderate AD (CDR-2).

TABLE 9.1
Medical Image Classification with Machine Learning for Medical Science and Alzheimer's Disease

Papers	Machine Learning Methods	Brain Datasets	Performance
Maruyama T., et al., (2018)	Support Vector Machine (SVM), Artificial Neural Network (ANN), and Convolution Neural Network (CNN).	Low-quality medical images	CNN is more accurate than conventional ML methods that utilize the manual feature extraction.
Shahbaz, M., et al., (2019)	Decision Tree, KNN, Naive Bayes, GLM, Rule Indection, Deep Leanrning, Confusion Matrix	Brain MRI dataADNI dataset	88,24%
Fan, Z., et al., (2020)	SVM model	Brain MRI data	The accuracy of classification and prediction is the best.
Kotturu P. K. and Kumar A., (2020)	Random Forest, Naïve BayesMulti Correlation Method	Brain data	Early diagnose of AD is dealt with different ML models and that proposed work was explained clearly.
Uysal G, Ozturk M (2020)	Machine Learning techniques	MRI dataADNI dataset	The better performance of the computer-aided diagnosis of AD
Lanka P, et al., (2020)	Supervised machine learning for diagnostic classification	large-scale neuroimaging datasets	They combined feature importance scores obtained from all classifiers to infer the discriminative ability of connectivity features.
Zhang F, et al., (2019)	Extreme Machine Learning Method	ADNI dataset	
Ferreira et al. (2017)	SVM model-based AD classification	Brain MRI data	rCBF-SPECT still has a role to play in AD diagnosis.
Donnelly-Kehoe PA, et al., (2018)	Multi Classifier System (MCS)	Brain MRI data	The proposed MCS showed a better performance than state-of-the-art classifier.
Tan et al. (2018)	Instance Transfer Learning algorithm (ITL) based on wrapper mode	Brain MRI data	It is helpful for the small sample problems of AD. and heuristics to the relevant researchers
Zhou T., et al., (2019)	Latent Representation Learning for Alzheimer's Disease Diagnosis With	ADNI dataset MRI, PET and Genetic Data	The experimental results verify the effectiveness of our proposed method.

(Continued)

TABLE 9.1 (Continued)
Medical Image Classification with Machine Learning for Medical Science and Alzheimer's Disease

Papers	Machine Learning Methods	Brain Datasets	Performance
Castellazzi G, et al. (2020)	Machine Learning algorithms	Brain fMRI data	High discriminant power to classify AD and VD profiles. With rate 77,33%
Binny Naik et al., (2020)	SVM model	Brain MRI data	It is presenting the optimal multimodal paradigm for the classification of AD.
Mehmood A, et al., (2021)	Transfer Learning algorithm	Brain MRI data	highest rates of the classification accuracy on AD vs NC is 98.73%, also distinguish between EMCI vs LMCI patients testing accuracy 83.72%, whereas remaining classes accuracy is more than 80%.

We have 382 images achieved from the OASIS dataset when AD patients have aged in the range of 20 to 96 years.

9.5.2 MRI Data Pre-processing

Image pre-processing is the major part to extract efficient and accurate results for those algorithms based on the ANN and CNN models. The OASIS dataset image size is 256 × 256 but the proposed CNN model requires an image size of 224 × 224.

9.5.3 Features Extraction and Selection from Brain MRI Datasets

The feature extraction and selection is one of the significant steps that can regulate the accuracy of brain MRI images classification in which the results will help detect the disease.

9.5.4 Classification Methods

- *Artificial Neural Networks (ANN)* are computational systems that "learn" to perform tasks by considering examples, generally without being programmed with any task-specific rules. As shown in Figure 9.3, it contains of four data inputs of four types of different NDs.
- *Convolutional neural networks (CNN)* are models proposed by the development of biotechnology. Neurons are like local filtering of the entire input space, and they are well-organized together to achieve an understanding of the image in the entire field of view. The convolution process is configured with as it produces Deep convolution neural networks.

TABLE 9.2
Medical Image Classification with Deep Learning for Medical Science and Alzheimer's Disease

Papers	Deep Learning Methods	Brain Datasets	Performance
Chen M. et al., (2021)	CNN	Brain MRI data	it shows that the proposed scheme is superior to other approaches, which effectively solves the intrinsic labor-intensive problem during artificial image labeling
Mohsen H., et al., (2018)	DNN	Brain MRI data	The classifier was combined with the discrete wavelet transform (DWT) the powerful feature extraction tool and principal components analysis (PCA) and the evaluation of the performance was quite good over all the performance measures.
Zhang Xia Xie Fulham and Feng (2018)	Synergic Deep Learning	Brain MRI data	results indicate that handcrafted features complement the image representation learned by DCNNs on small training datasets and improve accuracy in certain medical image classification problems.
Talo M., et al., (2019)	Deep Transfer Learning	Brain MRI data	The proposed model achieved 5-fold classification accuracy of 100% on 613 MR images. Our developed system is ready to test on huge database and can assist the radiologists in their daily screening of MR images.
Alebiosu and Muhammad (2019)	Deep Pre-Trained Neural Networks	Medical X-ray images	AlexNet + SVM produced a total classification accuracy of 84.27% and as a fine-tuned network produced a total of 86.47% which is the highest among the four techniques across all the 116 image classes.
Basaia et al. (2019)	Deep Learning Algorithm	Brain MRI data	High levels of accuracy were demonstrated in all the classifications, with the highest rates demenstrated in the AD vs HC classification tests using both the ADNI dataset only (99%) and the combined ADNI + non-ADNI dataset (98%). CNNs discriminated c-MCI from s-MCI patients with an accuracy up to 75% and no difference between ADNI and non-ADNI images.

(*Continued*)

TABLE 9.2 (Continued)
Medical Image Classification with Deep Learning for Medical Science and Alzheimer's Disease

Papers	Deep Learning Methods	Brain Datasets	Performance
Alaeddine, H., and Jihene, M. (2020)	Deep Convolutional Neural Network	ImageNet database	an analysis of different characteristics of existing topologies is detailed in order to extract the various strategies used to obtain better performance
Ajagbe S. A., et al., (2021)	Deep Convolutional Neural Network	Brain MRI data	VGG-19 was the best in three, CNN was the best in two and VGG-16 was the best in one. Conclusively, this study has proven that computer algorithms are capable of classifying AD into four classes known to medical experts.
AbdulAzeem, Y., et al., (2021)	Convolutional Neural Network	Brain MRI dataADNI Dataset	Proposed framework achieved 97.5% classification accuracy
Işik A.H., et al., (2021)	Convolutional Neural Network	OASIS datasetSectional MR Brain Medical Image Data	80% accuracy rate was obtained. The model's loss rate fell to 0.3 s.
Nemoto, K., et al., (2021)	Residual neural network (ResNet) type of convolutional neural network	Brain MRI data	Results confirmed that the DL method with gray matter images can detect fine differences between DLB and AD that may be underestimated by the conventional method.
(So et al. 2019)	deep learning multi-layer perceptron (MLP) model	ADNI dataset	We obtained the highest accuracy of 85% in the AD-NC
Tufail, A. B., et al., (2020)	Deep Neural Networks	SMRI data	The transfer learning approaches exceed the performance of non-transfer learning-based approaches demonstrating the effectiveness of these approaches for the binary AD classification task.
Marzban EN et al., (2020)	Deep Convolution Neural Network	diffusion tensor images	The results were competitive among the existing literature, which paves the way for improving medications that could slow down the progress of the AD or prevent it.

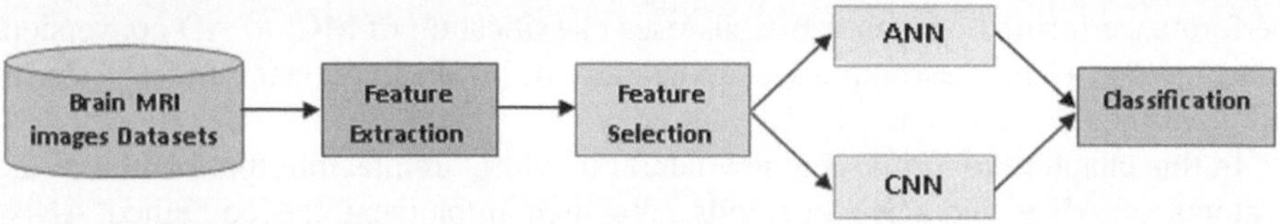

FIGURE 9.3 Overview of the proposed model using ANN-DCNN for classifying brain MRI images.

9.5.5 Proposed Machine-Deep Model

In this chapter, we propose a deep model named ANN-DCNN model to address this issue by using multiple DCNN simultaneously and enabling them to mutually learn from each other. For the proposed model, the training and testing on medical images go through the preprocessing steps. MRI images during the process of their forming compression and rotation. To overcome this issue for the improvement of MRI scans, image enhancement approaches were applied for the upgrade of the distribution of pixels over an extensive range of intensities, linear contrast stretching was applied on the images. The accuracy of this new deep model demonstrate 91% when it focus on the classification of four class; Normal, Mild demented, Very Mild demented, Alzheimer's patient. Figure 9.4

9.6 Discussion and Conclusion

The performance comparison by DL approaches needs huge amounts of data to achieve the desired levels of performance accuracy. In currently partial neuroimaging data, the hybrid methods that combine traditional ML methods for diagnostic classification with DL approaches for feature extraction generated better performance and can be a good alternative to handle the brain image data. Though hybrid approaches have produced relatively good results, they do not take full advantage of DL approaches, which automatically extracts features from large amounts of neuroimaging data. The most DL techniques in medical science and image classification studies is the CNN, which specializes in extracting characteristics from images. Recently, CNN models using MRI images showed better

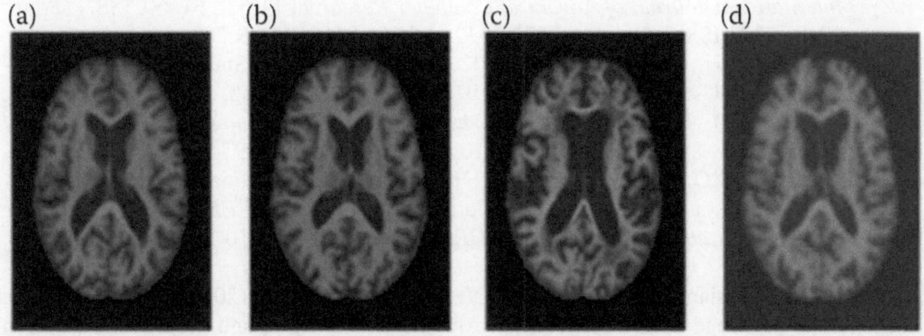

FIGURE 9.4 The brain MRI images presented for Alzheimer's disease stages.

performance for neurodegenerative diseases classification of MCI to AD conversion. Machine and Deep Learning applications may occur an important part between all different medical data science and neurology.

In this chapter, we propose a new neural network architecture that combines the features of ANN and CNN methods. We then implement the combined ANN-DCNN framework from MRI scans for medical image classification. Our proposed model preserves the extraction information of image features and can learn structured information of image features. Compared with the previous existing methods, our proposed technique achieved the highest performance in terms of classification based on the MRI datasets. We hope that this segmentation-free, highly accurate medical image classification method can be used to develop medical-aided diagnostic systems for brain-related diseases in the future research works. In this chapter book, we based on a related works of the image classification applications and analyzes the improvement of Machine and Deep Learning techniques. First, we studied a comprehensive literature of the medical image classification using ML and DL techniques from brain MRI data as ADNI datasets, which are used in this work. Second, a related works of ANN and DCNN models and a comparative study between those models for medical image classification are presented. Third, we propose a new Machine-Deep model combining the ANN and DCNN models from these brain datasets. Fourth, we discuss the recent visions and future ways to develop better performance of these learning models in medical diagnosis applications.

REFERENCES

[1] AbdulAzeem, Y., Bahgat, W.M., and Badawy, M. A. (2021). CNN Based Framework for Classification of Alzheimer's Disease. *Neural Computing and Applications* 33, 10415–10428. doi: 10.1007/s00521-021-05799-w.

[2] Agrawal, R.K., and Juneja, A. (2019). Deep Learning Models for Medical Image Analysis: Challenges and Future Directions. In: Madria S., Fournier-Viger P., Chaudhary S., Reddy P. (eds) *Big Data Analytics. BDA 2019. Lecture Notes in Computer Science*, 11932. Springer, Cham. doi: 10.1007/978-3-030-37188-3_2.

[3] Ajagbe, S.A., Amuda, K.A., Oladipupo, M.A., Oluwaseyi, F.A.F.E., and Okesola, K.I. (2021). Multi-classification of Alzheimer Disease on Magnetic Resonance Images (MRI) using Deep Convolutional Neural Network (DCNN) Approaches. *International Journal of Advanced Computer Research*, 11(53), 51–60. ISSN (Print): 2249- 7277 ISSN (Online): 2277-7970. doi:10.19101/IJACR.2021.1152001.

[4] Alaeddine, H., and Jihene, M. (2020). A Comparative Study of Popular CNN Topologies Used for Imagenet Classification. In A. Suresh, R. Udendhran, & S. Vimal (Eds), *Deep Neural Networks for Multimodal Imaging and Biomedical Applications*, 89–103. IGI Global. 10.4018/978-1-7998-3591-2.ch007.

[5] Alebiosu, D.O., and Muhammad, F.P. (2019). Medical Image Classification: A Comparison of Deep Pre-trained Neural Networks. *2019 IEEE Student Conference on Research and Development (SCOReD)*, 306–310, doi: 10.1109/SCORED.2019.8896277.

[6] Altaf, F., Islam, S.M.S., Akhtar, N., and Janjua, N.K. (2019). Going Deep in Medical Image Analysis: Concepts, Methods, Challenges, and Future Directions. In *IEEE Access*, 7, 99540–99572, doi: 10.1109/ACCESS.2019.2929365.

[7] Anwar, S.M., Majid, M., Qayyum, A. et al. (2018). Medical Image Analysis using Convolutional Neural Networks: A Review. *Journal of Medical Systems*, 42, 226. doi: 10.1007/s10916-018-1088-1.

[8] Ashraf, R. et al. (2020). Deep Convolution Neural Network for Big Data Medical Image Classification," in *IEEE Access*, vol. 8, pp. 105659–105670, doi: 10.1109/ACCESS.2020.2998808.

[9] Balne, S., and Elumalai, A., Machine Learning and Deep Learning Algorithms used to Diagnosis of Alzheimer's: Review, *Materials Today: Proceedings*, 2021, ISSN 2214-7853, doi: 10.1016/j.matpr.2021.05.499.

[10] Basaia, S., Agosta, F., Wagner, L., Canu, E., Magnani, G., Santangelo, R., Filippi, M., and Alzheimer's Disease Neuroimaging Initiative (2019). Automated Classification of Alzheimer's Disease and Mild Cognitive Impairment Using a Single MRI and Deep Neural Networks. *NeuroImage: Clinical*, 21, 101645. doi: 10.1016/j.nicl.2018.101645.

[11] Bringas, S., Salomón, S., Duque, R., Lage, C., and Montaña, J.L. (2020). Alzheimer's Disease Stage Identification using Deep Learning Models. *Journal of Biomedical Informatics*, 109, 103514. doi: 10.1016/j.jbi.2020.103514.

[12] Castellazzi, G., Cuzzoni, M.G., Cotta Ramusino, M., Martinelli, D., Denaro, F., Ricciardi, A., Vitali, P., Anzalone, N., Bernini, S., Palesi, F., Sinforiani, E., Costa, A., Micieli, G., D'Angelo, E., Magenes, G., and Gandini Wheeler-Kingshott, C. (2020). A Machine Learning Approach for the Differential Diagnosis of Alzheimer and Vascular Dementia Fed by MRI Selected Features. *Frontiers in Neuroinformatics*, 14, 25. doi: 10.3389/fninf.2020.00025.

[13] Chaddad, A., Katib, Y., and Hassan, L. (2021). Future Artificial Intelligence Tools and Perspectives in Medicine. *Current Opinion in Urology*. Jul 1; 31(4), 371–377. doi: 10.1097/ MOU.0000000000000884. PMID: 33927099.

[14] Chen, M., Shi, X., Zhang, Y., Wu, D., and Guizani, M., (2021). Deep Features Learning for Medical Image Analysis with Convolutional Autoencoder Neural Network, in *IEEE Transactions on Big Data*, 7(4), 750–758. doi: 10.1109/TBDATA.2017.2717439.

[15] Deng, L. and Yu, D. (2014) Deep Learning: Methods and Applications. *Foundations and Trends in Signal Processing*, 7, 197–387.

[16] Donnelly-Kehoe, P.A., Pascariello, G.O., and Gómez, J.C. (2018). Looking for Alzheimer's Disease Morphometric Signatures using Machine Learning Techniques. *Journal of Neuroscience Methods*, 302, 24–34.

[17] Emanuel, E.J. and Wachter, R.M. (2019). Artificial Intelligence in Health Care: Will the Value Match the Hype? *JAMA*, 321(23), 2281–2282. doi: 10.1001/jama.2019.4914.

[18] Falahati, F., Westman, E., and Simmons, A. (2014). Multivariate Data Analysis and Machine Learning in Alzheimer's Disease with a Focus on Structural Magnetic Resonance Imaging. *Journal of Alzheimer's Disease*, 41(3), 685–708. doi: 10.3233/JAD-131928.

[19] Fan, Z., Xu, F., Qi, X. et al. (2020). Classification of Alzheimer's Disease based on Brain MRI and Machine Learning. *Neural Computing and Applications*, 32, 1927–1936. doi: 10.1007/s00521-019-04495-0.

[20] Farid, A.A., Selim, G., and Khater, H. (2020). Applying Artificial Intelligence Techniques for Prediction of Neurodegenerative Disorders: A Comparative Case-Study on Clinical Tests and Neuroimaging Tests with Alzheimer's Disease. *Preprints* 2020, 2020030299. doi: 10.20944/preprints202003.0299.v1.

[21] Feng, W., Halm-Lutterodt, N.V., Tang, H., Mecum, A., Mesregah, M.K., Ma, Y., Li, H., Zhang, F., Wu, Z., Yao, E., and Guo, X. (2020). Automated MRI-Based Deep Learning Model for Detection of Alzheimer's Disease Process. *International Journal of Neural Systems*, 30(6), 2050032. doi: 10.1142/S012906572050032X.

[22] Ferreira, L.K., Rondina, J.M., Kubo, R., Ono, C.R., Leite, C.C., Smid, J., Bottino, C., Nitrini, R., Busatto, G.F., Duran, F.L., and Buchpiguel, C.A. (2017). Support Vector Machine-based Classification of Neuroimages in Alzheimer's Disease: Direct Comparison of FDG-PET, rCBF-SPECT and MRI Data Acquired from the same Individuals. *Revista brasileira de psiquiatria (Sao Paulo, Brazil: 1999)*, 40(2), 181–191. doi: 10.15 90/1516-4446-2016-2083.

[23] Fotin, S.V., Yin, Y., Haldankar, H., Jeffrey, W., Hoffmeister, M.D., and Periaswamy, S. (2016). Detection of Soft Tissue Densities from Digital Breast Tomosynthesis: Comparison of Conventional and Deep Learning Approaches, Proceeding SPIE 9785, Medical Imaging 2016: Computer-Aided Diagnosis, 97850X (24 March 2016); doi: 10.1117/12.2217045.

[24] Ganapathy, K., Abdul, S.S., and Nursetyo, A.A. (2018). Artificial Intelligence in Neurosciences: A Clinician's Perspective. *Neurology India* 2018; 66, 934–939.

[25] Gao, J., Jiang, Q., Zhou, B., and Chen, D. (2019). Convolutional Neural Networks for Computer aided Detection or Diagnosis in Medical Image Analysis: An Overview. *Mathematical Biosciences and Engineering*. Jul 15; 16(6), 6536–6561. doi: 10.3934/mbe.2019326. PMID: 31698575.

[26] Gupta, A., & Kahali, B. (2020). Machine Learning-based Cognitive Impairment Classification with Optimal Combination of Neuropsychological Tests. *Alzheimer's & Dementia (New York, N. Y.)*, 6(1), e12049. doi: 10.1002/trc2.12049.

[27] Han-Qing, L., Xiao-Dong, L., Bo, K., Hua-Li, Z., Ji-Chao, F., and Jun-Ling, H. (2021). Comparative Study on Classification and Recognition of Medical Images Using Deep Learning Network [J]. *Computer Science*, 48(6A), 89–94.

[28] Hesamian, M.H., Jia, W., and He, X. (2019). Deep Learning Techniques for Medical Image Segmentation: Achievements and Challenges. *Journal of Digital Imaging* 32, 582–596. doi: 10.1007/s10278-019-00227-x.

[29] Hosny, A., Parmar, C., Quackenbush, J., Schwartz, L.H., and Aerts, H.J.W.L. (2018). Artificial Intelligence in Radiology. *Nature Reviews Cancer*. 18(8), 500–510. doi: 10.1038/s41568-018-0016-5.

[30] Işik, A.H., Ersoy, M., Köse, U., Türkçetin, A.Ö., and Çolak, R. (2021). Deep Learning Based Classification Method for Sectional MR Brain Medical Image Data. In: Hemanth J., Yigit T., Patrut B., Angelopoulou A. (Eds) *Trends in Data Engineering Methods for Intelligent Systems. ICAIAME 2020. Lecture Notes on Data Engineering and Communications Technologies*, 76. Springer, Cham. doi: 10.1007/978-3-030-79357-9_62.

[31] Jan, B., Farman, H., Khan, M., Imran, M., Islam, I.U., Ahmad, A., Ali, S., and Jeon, G. (2019). Deep Learning in Big Data Analytics: A Comparative Study, *Computers & Electrical Engineering*, 75, 275–287, ISSN 0045-7906, doi: 10.1016/j.compeleceng.2017.12.009.

[32] Jo, T., Nho, K., and Saykin, A.J. (2019). Deep Learning in Alzheimer's Disease: Diagnostic Classification and Prognostic Prediction Using Neuroimaging Data. *Frontiers in Aging Neuroscience*, 11, 220. doi: 10.3389/fnagi.2019.00220.

[33] Jyotiyana, M., and Kesswani, N. (2021). A Study on Deep Learning in Neurodegenerative Diseases and Other Brain Disorders. In: Rathore V.S., Dey N., Piuri V., Babo R., Polkowski Z., Tavares J.M.R.S. (Eds) *Rising Threats in Expert Applications and Solutions. Advances in Intelligent Systems and Computing*, 1187. Springer, Singapore. doi: 10.1007/978-981-15-6014-9_95.

[34] Ker, J., Wang, L., Rao, J., and Lim, T. (2018). "Deep Learning Applications in Medical Image Analysis," in *IEEE Access*, 6, 9375–9389, doi: 10.1109/ACCESS.2017.2788044.

[35] Khan, S., Islam, N., Jan, Z., Ud Din, I., and Rodrigues, J.J.P.C. (2019). A Novel Deep Learning based Framework for the Detection and Classification of Breast

Cancer using Transfer Learning, *Pattern Recognition Letters*, 125, 1–6, ISSN 0167-8655, doi: 10.1016/j.patrec.2019.03.022.

[36] Khatami, A., Khosravi, A., Nguyen, T., Lim, C.P., and Nahavandi, S. (2017). Medical Image Analysis using Wavelet Transform and Deep Belief Networks, *Expert Systems with Applications*, 86, 190–198, ISSN 0957-4174, doi: 10.1016/j.eswa.2017.05.073.

[37] Kotturu, P.K. and Kumar, A. (2020). Comparative Study on Machine Learning models for Early Diagnose of Alzheimer's Disease: Multi Correlation Method, *2020 5th International Conference on Communication and Electronics Systems (ICCES)*, 778–783, doi: 10.1109/ICCES48766.2020.9137872.

[38] Kunapuli, S.S., and Bhallamudi, P.C. (2021). A Review of Deep Learning Models for Medical Diagnosis, in *Machine Learning, Big Data, and IoT for Medical Informatics* (pp. 389–404), Elsevier.

[39] Lanka, P., Rangaprakash, D., Dretsch, M.N., Katz, J.S., Denney, T.S., and Deshpande, G. (2020). Supervised Machine Learning for Diagnostic Classification from Large-scale Neuroimaging Datasets. *Brain Imaging and Behavior*, 14(6), 2378–2416. doi: 10.1007/s11682-019-00191-8.

[40] Litjens, G., Kooi, T., Bejnordi, B.E., Setio, A.A.A., Ciompi, F., Ghafoorian, M., van der Laak, J.A.W.M., van Ginneken, B., and Sánchez, C.I. (2017). A Survey on Deep Learning in Medical Image Analysis, *Medical Image Analysis*, 42, 60–88, ISSN 1361-8415, doi: 10.1016/j.media.2017.07.005.

[41] Liu, X., Chen, K., Wu, T., Weidman, D., Lure, F., and Li, J. (2018). Use of Multimodality Imaging and Artificial Intelligence for Diagnosis and Prognosis of Early Stages of Alzheimer's Disease. *Translational Research: the Journal of Laboratory and Clinical Medicine*, 194, 56–67. doi: 10.1016/j.trsl.2018.01.001.

[42] Lundervold, A.S. and Lundervold, A. (2019). An Overview of Deep Learning in Medical Imaging Focusing on MRI, *Zeitschrift für Medizinische Physik*, 29(2), 102–127, ISSN 0939-3889, doi: 10.1016/j.zemedi.2018.11.002.

[43] Madusanka, N., Choi, H.K., So, J.H., and Choi, B.K. (2019). Alzheimer's Disease Classification Based on Multi-feature Fusion. *Current Medical Imaging Reviews*, 15(2), 161–169. doi: 10.2174/1573405614666181012102626.

[44] Maruyama, T., Hayashi, N., Sato, Y., Hyuga, S., Wakayama, Y., Watanabe, H., Ogura, A., and Ogura, T. (2018). Comparison of Medical Image Classification Accuracy among Three Machine Learning Methods. *Journal of X-Ray Science and Technology*, 26(6), 885–893. doi: 10.3233/xst-18386. PMID: 30223423.

[45] Marzban, E.N., Eldeib, A.M., Yassine, I.A., Kadah, Y.M., and Alzheimer's Disease Neurodegenerative Initiative. (2020). Alzheimer's Disease Diagnosis from Diffusion Tensor Images using Convolutional Neural Networks. *PloS one*, 15(3), e0230409. doi: 10.1371/journal.pone.0230409.

[46] Mateos-Pérez, J.M., Dadar, M., Lacalle-Aurioles, M., Iturria-Medina, Y., Zeighami, Y., and Evans, A.C. (2018). Structural Neuroimaging as Clinical Predictor: A Review of Machine Learning Applications. *NeuroImage: Clinical*, 20, 506–522. doi: 10.1016/j.nicl.2018.08.019.

[47] Mirbabaie, M., Stieglitz, S. and Frick, N.R.J. (2021). Artificial Intelligence in Disease Diagnostics: A Critical Review and Classification on the Current State of Research Guiding Future Direction. *Health and Technology*. 11, 693–731 doi: 10.1007/s12553-021-00555-5.

[48] Matheny, M., Israni, S.T., Ahmed, M., and Whicher, D. (Editors. 2019). *Artificial Intelligence in Health Care: The Hope, the Hype, the Promise, the Peril. NAM Special Publication*. Washington, DC: National Academy of Medicine.

[49] Mehmood, A., Yang, S., Feng, Z., Wang, M., Ahmad, A.S., Khan, R., Maqsood, M.,

and Yaqub, M. (2021). A Transfer Learning Approach for Early Diagnosis of Alzheimer's Disease on MRI Images. *Neuroscience*, 460, 43–52.

[50] Mirzaei, G., Adeli, A., and Adeli, H. (2016). Imaging and Machine Learning Techniques for Diagnosis of Alzheimer's Disease. *Reviews in the Neurosciences*, 27(8), 857–870. doi: 10.1515/revneuro-2016-0029.

[51] Mohsen, H., El-Dahshan, E.A., El-Horbaty, E.M. M. and Salem, A.B. (2018). Classification using Deep Learning Neural Networks for Brain Tumors, *Future Computing and Informatics Journal*, 3(1), 68–71, ISSN 2314-7288, doi: 10.1016/j.fcij.2017.12.001.

[52] Naik, B., Mehta, A., and Shah, M. (2020). Denouements of Machine Learning and Multimodal Diagnostic Classification of Alzheimer's Disease. *Visual Computing for Industry, Biomedicine, and Art*, 3(1), 26. doi: 10.1186/s42492-020-00062-w.

[53] Nemoto, K., Sakaguchi, H., Kasai, W., Hotta, M., Kamei, R., Noguchi, T., Minamimoto, R., Arai, T., and Asada, T. (2021). Differentiating Dementia with Lewy Bodies and Alzheimer's Disease by Deep Learning to Structural MRI. *Journal of Neuroimaging: Official Journal of the American Society of Neuroimaging*, 31(3), 579–587. doi: 10.1111/jon.12835.

[54] Nguyen, M., He, T., An, L., Alexander, D.C., Feng, J., Yeo, B., and Alzheimer's Disease Neuroimaging Initiative. (2020). Predicting Alzheimer's Disease Progression using Deep Recurrent Neural Networks. *NeuroImage*, 222, 117203. doi: 10.1016/j.neuroimage.2020.117203.

[55] Nogales, A., García-Tejedor, Á.J., Monge, D., Vara, J.S., and Antón, C. (2021). A Survey of Deep Learning Models in Medical Therapeutic Areas, *Artificial Intelligence in Medicine*, 112, 102020, ISSN 0933-3657, doi: 10.1016/j.artmed.2021.102020.

[56] Puente-Castro, A., Fernandez-Blanco, E., Pazos, A., and Munteanu, C.R. (2020). Automatic assessment of Alzheimer's Disease Diagnosis based on Deep Learning Techniques. *Computers in Biology and Medicine*, 120, 103764. doi: 10.1016/j.compbiomed.2020.103764.

[57] Ravishankar, H. et al. (2016). Understanding the Mechanisms of Deep Transfer Learning for Medical Images. In: Carneiro G. et al. (ed.) *Deep Learning and Data Labeling for Medical Applications*. DLMIA 2016, LABELS 2016. Lecture Notes in Computer Science, 10008. Springer, Cham. doi: 10.1007/978-3-319-46976-8_20.

[58] Razzak, M.I., Naz, S., and Zaib, A. (2018). Deep Learning for Medical Image Processing: Overview, Challenges and the Future. In: Dey N., Ashour A., and Borra S. (eds) *Classification in BioApps. Lecture Notes in Computational Vision and Biomechanics*, 26, Springer, Cham. doi: 10.1007/978-3-319-65981-7_12.

[59] Shahbaz, M., Ali, S., Guergachi, A., Niazi, A. and Umer, A. (2019). Classification of Alzheimer's Disease using Machine Learning Techniques. In *Proceedings of the 8th International Conference on Data Science, Technology and Applications (DATA 2019)*, 296–303. SCITEPRESS–Science and Technology Publications. ISBN: 978-989-758-377-3. doi: 10.5220/0007949902960303).

[60] Sharma, A.K., Nandal, A., Dhaka, A., Dixit, R. (2021). Medical Image Classification Techniques and Analysis Using Deep Learning Networks: A Review. In: Patgiri R., Biswas A., Roy P. (eds) *Health Informatics: A Computational Perspective in Healthcare. Studies in Computational Intelligence*, 932. Springer, Singapore. doi: 10.1007/978-981-15-9735-0_13.

[61] Signaevsky, M., Prastawa, M., Farrell, K. et al. (2019). Artificial Intelligence in Neuropathology: Deep Learning-based Assessment of Tauopathy. *Laboratory Investigation*, 99, 1019–1029 doi: 10.1038/s41374-019-0202-4.

[62] So, J.H., Madusanka, N., Choi, H.K., Choi, B.K., and Park, H.G. (2019). Deep Learning for Alzheimer's Disease Classification using Texture Features. *Current*

Medical Imaging Reviews, 15(7), 689–698. doi: 10.2174/1573405615666190404163233.
[63] Tai, A., Albuquerque, A., Carmona, N.E., Subramanieapillai, M., Cha, D.S., Sheko, M., Lee, Y., Mansur, R., and McIntyre, R.S. (2019). Machine Learning and Big Data: Implications for Disease Modeling and Therapeutic Discovery in Psychiatry. *Artificial Intelligence in Medicine*, 99, 101704. doi: 10.1016/j.artmed.2019.101704.
[64] Talo, M., Baloglu, U.B., Yıldırım, Ö., and Acharya, U.R., (2019). Application of Deep Transfer Learning for Automated Brain Abnormality Classification using MR Images, *Cognitive Systems Research*, 54, 176–188, ISSN 1389-0417, doi: 10.1016/j.cogsys.2018.12.007.
[65] Tan, X., Liu, Y., Li, Y., Wang, P., Zeng, X., Yan, F., and Li, X. (2018). Localized Instance Fusion of MRI Data of Alzheimer's Disease for Classification based on Instance Transfer Ensemble Learning. *Biomedical Engineering Online*, 17(1), 49. doi: 10.1186/s12938-018-0489-1.
[66] Termine, A., Fabrizio, C., Strafella, C., Caputo, V., Petrosini, L., Caltagirone, C., Giardina, E., and Cascella, R. (2021). Multi-Layer Picture of Neurodegenerative Diseases: Lessons from the Use of Big Data through Artificial Intelligence. *Journal of Personalized Medicine*, 11(4), 280. doi: 10.3390/jpm11040280.
[67] Tufail, A.B., Ma, Y.K., and Zhang, Q.N. (2020). Binary Classification of Alzheimer's Disease Using sMRI Imaging Modality and Deep Learning. *Journal of Digital Imaging*, 33(5), 1073–1090. doi: 10.1007/s10278-019-00265-5.
[68] Uysal, G. and Ozturk, M. (2020). Hippocampal Atrophy based Alzheimer's Disease Diagnosis via Machine Learning Methods. *Journal of Neuroscience Methods*, 337, 108669.
[69] Valliani, A.A.A., Ranti, D., and Oermann, E.K. (2019). Deep Learning and Neurology: A Systematic Review. *Neurology and Therapy*, 8, 351–365 doi: 10.1007/s40120-019-00153-8.
[70] Wang, W., et al. (2020). Medical Image Classification using Deep Learning. In: Chen Y.W. and Jain L. (Eds) *Deep Learning in Healthcare. Intelligent Systems Reference Library*, 171. Springer, Cham. doi: 10.1007/978-3-030-32606-7_3.
[71] Wei, B., Han, Z., He, X., and Yin, Y. (2017). Deep Learning Model Based Breast Cancer Histopathological Image Classification. *2017 IEEE 2nd International Conference on Cloud Computing and Big Data Analysis (ICCCBDA)*, 348–353, doi: 10.1109/ICCCBDA.2017.7951937.
[72] Yang, R. and Yu, Y. (2021). Artificial Convolutional Neural Network in Object Detection and Semantic Segmentation for Medical Imaging Analysis. *Frontiers in Oncology* 11, 638182. doi: 10.3389/fonc.2021.638182.
[73] Zhang, J., Xie, Y., Wu, Q., and Xia, Y. (2019) Medical Image Classification using Synergic Deep Learning. *Medical Image Analysis*, 54, 10–19, ISSN 1361–8415, doi: 10.1016/j.media.2019.02.010.
[74] Zhang, J., Xia, Y., Xie, Y., Fulham, M., and Feng, D.D. (2018). Classification of Medical Images in the Biomedical Literature by Jointly Using Deep and Handcrafted Visual Features. In *IEEE Journal of Biomedical and Health Informatics*, 22(5), 1521–1530, , doi: 10.1109/JBHI.2017.2775662.
[75] Zhang, F., Tian, S., Chen, S., Ma, Y., Li, X., and Guo, X. (2019). Voxel-Based Morphometry: Improving the Diagnosis of Alzheimer's Disease Based on an Extreme Learning Machine Method from the ADNI cohort. *Neuroscience*, 414, 273–279. doi: 10.1016/j.neuroscience.2019.05.014.
[76] Zhou, T., Liu, M., Thung, K.H., and Shen, D. (2019). Latent Representation Learning for Alzheimer's Disease Diagnosis With Incomplete Multi-Modality Neuroimaging and Genetic Data. *IEEE Transactions on Medical Imaging*, 38(10), 2411–2422. doi: 10.1109/TMI.2019.2913158.

10 Convolutional Neural Network for Classification of Skin Cancer Images

Giang Son Tran, Quoc Viet Kieu, and Thi Phuong Nghiem
ICTLab, University of Science and Technology of Hanoi, Vietnam Academy of Science and Technology, Hanoi, Vietnam

CONTENTS

10.1 Introduction ... 175
10.2 State-of-the-Art ... 177
10.3 Materials and Methods ... 178
10.3.1 Data Preprocessing and Augmentation ... 178
10.3.2 Data Augmentation ... 180
10.3.3 Classification Models ... 181
10.3.3.1 Convolutional Neural Network (CNN) ... 181
10.3.3.2 Transfer Learning and Pre-trained Models ... 185
10.3.3.3 Pre-trained Xception Model ... 185
10.3.3.4 Xception Model Fine-tuning ... 186
10.3.3.5 Evaluation Metrics ... 187
10.4 Experimental Results ... 189
10.4.1 Learning Performance ... 189
10.4.2 Classification Results ... 190
10.4.3 Comparative Study ... 191
10.5 Conclusion and Perspectives ... 192
References ... 193

10.1 INTRODUCTION

Skin cancer is a severe and popular cancer disease. It is the abnormal development of skill cells in the outermost layer of skin. If not early diagnosed and treated, these cells will multiply uncontrollably and become malignant tumors [1]. Skin cancer usually appears on sun-exposed parts of the skin such as the face, neck, or hands. In

DOI: 10.1201/9781003217497-10

these parts, the sun's unhealthy ultraviolet (UV) rays are absorbed into the skin and gradually cause skin damage [1]. Two general categories of skin cancer include (1) melanoma skin cancer and (2) nonmelanoma skin cancer. In the first case, melanoma, the deadliest type of skin cancer, presents a malignant skin lesion arising from melanocytes which are skin cells producing melanin pigment. In the second case, nonmelanoma skin cancer is usually diagnosed by clinical images and histopathology images such as cut lesions in rhombohedral or elliptical shapes by surgical methods; burning laser; or radioactivity, radiotherapy (X-rays, radium rays) [2].

It was reported by [2] that each day there are nearly 10,000 people having skin cancer in the United States, and two people die every hour. Moreover, the treatment cost of skin cancer is very high. For example, in the United States, around $8.1 billion is used each year for skin cancer treatment [2]. In 2021, more than 5,400 people worldwide are estimated to get death due to nonmelanoma skin cancer each month, in which around 7,180 people (64% men, 36% women) will die of melanoma [2]. With large numbers of deaths caused by skin cancer, early detection will save lives for many patients. The statistics show that if a melanoma patient is treated appropriately at an early stage, they can achieve up to a 99% 5-year survival rate [2]. Therefore, a patient's survival rate can be enhanced by early detection, and diagnosis of skin cancer can help enhance the survival rate of patients.

Dermoscopy images are widely used by dermatologists to examine suspicious skin lesions [3]. To do so, the doctor usually looks at the dermoscopic images of skin lesions to determine if there exists cancer and, if so, which type of cancer the lesion may represent. Nevertheless, one problem that arises is that to analyze these million images of skin cancer is a massive workload for dermatologists due to the high variance of size, shape, texture, location between the healthy skin and the damaged skin.

Thanks to advances in machine learning technologies, computers are used to automate the detection process of malignant skin lesions [4]. Using computer methods to classify skin cancer, we can ease the workload of dermatologists during the clinical stages [5–7]. As a result, the time and treatment cost of skin cancer can be reduced. The general pipeline for skin lesion detection includes data preprocessing, feature extraction, image classification, and disease diagnosis. The classification of skin lesion images is essential to support the subsequent step of disease diagnosis in the general pipeline.

In this chapter, the main goal is to develop an automatic system to aid dermatologists in skin cancer examination and diagnosis. Specifically, we propose an automatic system using deep learning techniques to categorize multiple classes of skin lesions. Our system utilizes data preprocessing and augmentation to enlarge data on skin cancer. After that, transfer learning is applied to fine-tune a pre-trained model for extracting and classifying the image features. The experiments conducted on the publicly available ISIC 2019 dataset are used to measure the effectiveness of our proposed system for skin lesion image classification.

10.2 STATE-OF-THE-ART

Traditional approaches usually use image processing techniques and conventional learning models to classify skin lesion images. For example, Murugan et al. [8] utilized the support vector machine (SVM) as a classifier to determine skin lesion images as benign or melanoma. With different experiments, the experiments show that SVM produced better classification results compared to several other methods. Farooq et al. [9] segmented cancerous areas in the skin lesions by combining active contours and watershed techniques. Later, SVM was used to classify the cancer moles. Finally, an additional classification artificial neural network is used to fine-tune the SVM results and check the indeterminate cases produced from SVM's output. However, these traditional methods highly depend on preprocessing and post-processing steps of images and the hand-crafted features of skin lesion images. These methods are difficult to achieve satisfactory results due to the high variability of size, shape, and texture between healthy skin and damaged skin.

Recently, deep neural networks have been popular in skin lesion image classification. Following this direction, one common approach is the use of transfer learning to fine-tune pre-trained models for this task. For example, Chaturvedi et al. [10] proposed an automated system in order to categorize multiple classes of skin cancer. The authors performed fine-tuning of deep learning networks to improve classification performance by (1) adding "ReLU" activation to dense layers, (2) putting dropout and softmax layers at the end of the network, and (3) adapting values of hyperparameters. The maximum performance for an individual network is 93.20% of accuracy, and for the ensemble model is 92.83%. Through extensive experiments, ResNeXt101 is recommended by the authors for skin cancer image's multi-class classification.

Dorj et al. [11] utilized a pre-trained deep network called AlexNet to extract features of skin cancer images from four types, including SCC, BCC, MEL, and actinic keratosis (AK). SVM classifier is then applied to classify the skin cancer images. From the experiments, the method obtains maximum performances for accuracy, sensitivity, and specificity are 95.1% for SCC, 98.9% for AK, and 94.17% for SCC, respectively. Similarly, the minimum performances are 91.8% accuracy for BCC, 96.9% sensitivity for SCC, and 90.74% specificity for MEL. It is noticed that this work gains very good sensitivity results for AK and SCC cancers.

Hosny et al. [12] fine-tuned a pre-trained deep learning model, namely AlexNet, to improve the classification performance of skin lesions. Specifically, the authors replaced the pre-trained AlexNet's last layer with a softmax activation function to categorize three types of skin lesions (MEL, common nevus, and atypical nevus). The method was evaluated on the PH2 public dataset and achieved 98.61% accuracy, 98.33% sensitivity, 98.93% specificity, and 97.73% precision. The results of this work are much higher than the existing methods. However, the trained and tested dataset was a small one compared to other datasets such as ISIC challenge datasets.

Although these methods have obtained satisfactory results, the classification performance of skin cancer in dermoscopic images still needs further improvement to meet the high variability in size, shape, texture, and location of skin lesions. This chapter aims to improve the skin lesions' multi-class classification by employing and fine-tuning pre-trained Xception, a deep learning network. A detailed description of the materials and methods to implement this objective is presented in the next section.

10.3 MATERIALS AND METHODS

We propose an automatic system using a deep neural network and transfer learning to classify multiple types of skin cancer images. Figure 10.1 demonstrates a visualization of our proposed method. From the figure, we perform data preprocessing to clean input data and data augmentation to enhance training samples. Some parts of the pre-trained Xception model are kept intact for extracting features of input images, while the remaining parts are fine-tuned for fitting with the problem of multi-class classification of skin lesions.

10.3.1 Data Preprocessing and Augmentation

An international organization named International Skin Imaging Collaboration (ISIC) aims to support researchers worldwide about skin cancer diagnosis. Through its challenges in 2017, 2018, 2019, and 2020, ISIC provides the largest publicly available datasets of skin lesions' dermoscopy images, which now become the benchmark datasets for scientists worldwide. All photos in ISIC datasets were collected from various skin microscopes, from different surgical sites and several hospitals.

In this chapter, we use the ISIC 2019 challenge dataset [13–15] to train and test our model. The dataset contains 25,331 images collected from three other datasets, namely HAM10000, BCN_20000, and MSK. The HAM10000 dataset contains 12,413 images of size 600x450 centered and cropped around the lesions, while BCN_20000 has 10,015 images of size 1024x1024. The pictures of BCN_20000 dataset is challenging since they are uncropped and skin lesions are in different locations, scale, and angle to spot out. The last one is MSK with 819 images of various sizes. Qualified dermatologists created the ground truth labels.

Table 10.1 demonstrates the detailed description of each class with the corresponding number of images, and Figure 10.2 shows image examples in ISIC 2019 challenge dataset. From the tables, it can be seen that ISIC 2019 challenge dataset is imbalanced. There are only 239 images in the smallest class (Dermatofibroma class) and up to 12,875 photos in the dataset's largest class (Melanocytic nevi class). The properties of skin lesion images in the ISIC 2019 dataset vary differently from irregular boundaries, thick hair, or dark edges.

Having 25,331 images from ISIC 2019 challenge dataset, we randomly get 2,534 images (10%) to form the test set. For the remaining 22,797 images (90%), since there exist cases where the same lesion of one person may have several images, we removed 15,959 duplicate images to clean data. After this step, we obtained 5,357 images without duplication. From this number of data, we get 1,072 photos (20%) for the validation set. The last 4,285 images (80%) were merged with 15,959 photos to create the training set of 20,244 images.

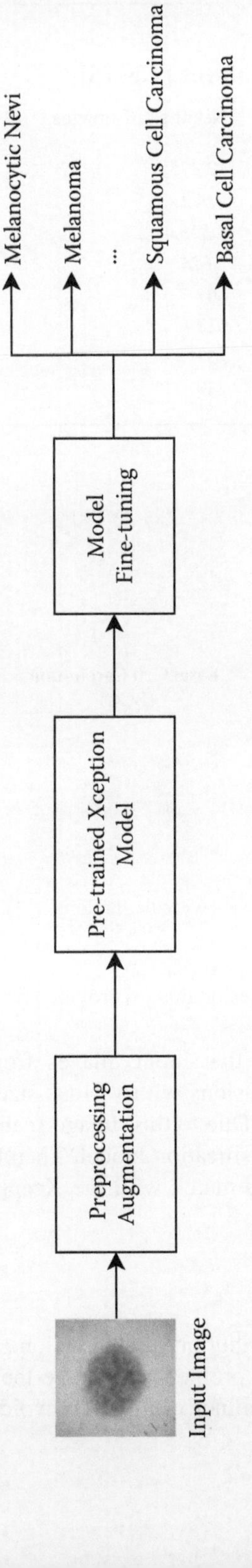

FIGURE 10.1 Our classification system of skin lesion images.

TABLE 10.1
Description of ISIC 2019 Challenge Dataset [13–15]

Class	Number of Images	Ratio (%)
Melanocytic nevi (NV)	12,875	50.83
Melanoma (MEL)	4,522	17.85
Basal Cell Carcinoma (BCC)	3,323	13.12
Benign keratosis-like lesions (BKL)	2,624	10.36
Actinic keratoses (AK)	867	3.42
Squamous Cell Carcinoma (SCC)	628	2.248
Vascular lesions (VASC)	253	1.00
Dermatofibroma (DF)	239	0.94

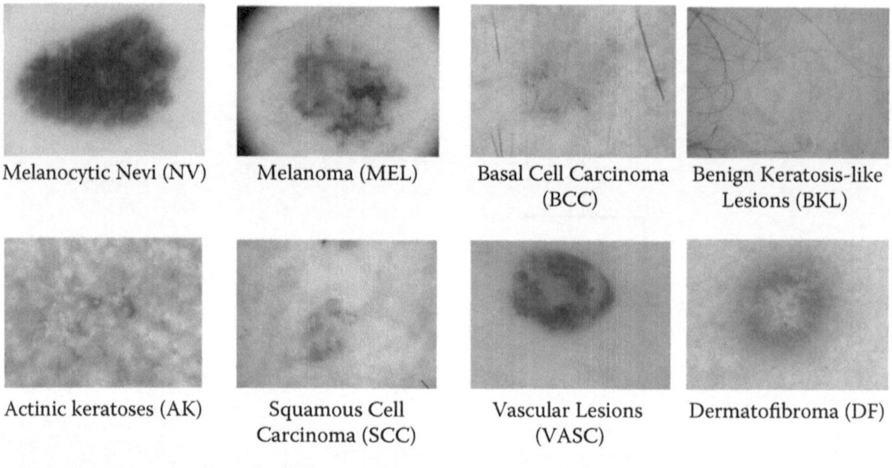

FIGURE 10.2 Examples of ISIC 2019s skin lesion images provided by the dataset [13–15].

For data preprocessing, it is noticed that input images from the ISIC 2019 challenge dataset have inconsistent dimensions with various sizes, while our classification model requires fixed input size. Due to this, image scaling is necessary to feed our input image data to train the classification model. Therefore, we scaled all images to the size of 299 × 299 pixels to match with the Xception model's input size.

10.3.2 Data Augmentation

As can be seen from Table 10.1, the distribution of skin lesion classes in the ISIC 2019 challenge is very imbalanced. This problem can make the model learn bias towards the major classes more than the minor classes. To avoid this problem, we

TABLE 10.2
Training Images After Augmentation

Class	Training Images After Augmentation	Ratio (%)
Melanocytic nevi (NV)	9128	13%
Melanoma (MEL)	9104	13%
Basal Cell Carcinoma (BCC)	9098	13%
Benign keratosis-like lesions (BKL)	9114	13%
Actinic keratoses (AK)	8960	13%
Squamous Cell Carcinoma (SCC)	7818	11%
Vascular lesions (VASC)	8358	12%
Dermatofibroma (DF)	8506	12%

apply different data augmentation techniques to increase more image samples from minor classes in order to be equal to the major classes. Another benefit of data augmentation is to have more samples for the training set, which is often required for deep learning models.

Having 20,244 images from ISIC 2019 challenge dataset, the following data augmentation methods are utilized:

- Random rotation from 0° to 180°
- Shift horizontally and vertically: 10%
- Zoom in the inputs: 10%
- Flip horizontally and vertically

After augmentation, we have 70,086 images for the training set, in which the ratio of images in each class is much more balanced compared to the original dataset. Table 10.2 shows a detailed description of images in each category in our training set.

Table 10.3 presents a description of our training and testing dataset for the experiments in this work. It is noticed that the test set contains only original images from the ISIC 2019 dataset, while the validation set consists of clean data with duplicate image removal and the training set contains both original and augmented image data.

10.3.3 Classification Models

10.3.3.1 Convolutional Neural Network (CNN)

CNN is an important building block of many intelligent systems with high accuracy [16]. Generally, a CNN consists of an input layer, several hidden layers for feature extraction, an optionally fully connected layer for classification, and an output layer (Figure 10.3). A CNN hidden layer is usually a convolutional layer followed by an activation function. Additionally, after the activation function, a pooling layer can

TABLE 10.3
Detail of Training and Testing Data in Our Experiments

	Training Set	Validation Set	Test Set
Number of images	70,086	1,072	2,534

be added in order to down-sample the input features but does not affect the image channels. The fundamental purpose of a CNN hidden layer is to extract spatial information of the image features automatically. A CNN network can contain as many as needed hidden layers for better accuracy performance. After the feature extraction step, a dense layer can be used to perform the classification of image features. This dense layer is usually followed by an activation function for generating probabilistic distribution of output values.

The **convolutional layer** is the most important hidden layer in a CNN. It applies convolutional products with many filters/kernels on the input image, then is followed by an activation function to break the linearity of the CNN network. It is the heavy part of a CNN that performs most computational tasks to learn the meaningful features. The output of a feature map j at the convolutional layer l is defined as follows [10]:

$$C_j^l = f\left(\sum_{i=1}^{N^{l-1}} C_i^{l-1} * w_{ij}^l + b_j^i\right) \tag{10.1}$$

Where l is the layer number, C_j^l is the output of activation function of feature map j, f is the activation function, w_{ij}^l are kernel weights from the feature map i at the previous layer to the feature map j at the current layer, N^{l-1} is the feature map number of the previous layer and b_j^i is the bias coefficient between the two feature maps i and j.

An **activation function** transforms a neuron's output from linear to non-linear. In our model, after each convolutional layer, we use ReLU activation function. At the end of the network, after the fully connected layer, we apply softmax activation function. ReLU is defined as follows:

$$relu(x) = \begin{cases} x & for\ x \geq 0, \\ 0 & for\ x < 0. \end{cases} \tag{10.2}$$

Where x is the vector output of convolutional layer before the activation function. $relu(x)$ is the ReLU activation function applied to x to transform its values from linear to non-linear. Softmax is defined as follows:

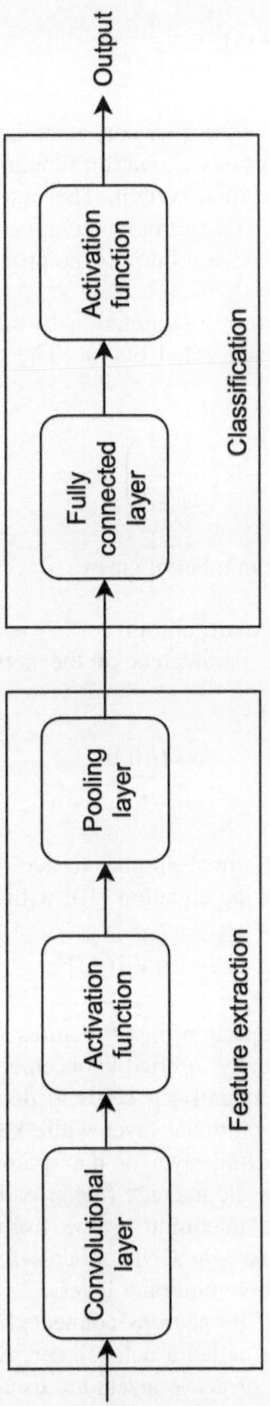

FIGURE 10.3 General architecture of a CNN.

$$softmax\,(x)_i = \frac{e^{x_i}}{\sum_{j=1}^{K} e^{x_j}} \tag{10.3}$$

Where x is the input vector (the same as the fully connected layer's output) and K is the desired number of classes. The softmax activation function converts the output values by dividing each value by the total weight. The output is a vector of the predicted probabilities of the classes. The softmax activation function is beneficial in multi-class classification problems since it outputs the probability of each image over the K classes.

We use the categorical cross-entropy loss function to measure the difference between the model's output and the expected output. The definition of the loss function E is as follows [10]:

$$E = -ln\left(\frac{e^{\partial_p}}{\sum_i^K e^{\partial_i}}\right) \tag{10.4}$$

Where i is the iteration index, K is the number of classes, ∂_p is the network score for the positive class, and.

To optimize the loss function E, Adam optimizer [17] is applied. Specifically, after each iteration, weight and bias parameters of the network are updated as follows [10]:

$$\partial_{i+1} = \partial_i - \frac{\alpha \nabla \mathrm{E}(\partial_i)}{\sqrt{\nu_i} + \varepsilon} \tag{10.5}$$

Where α is the learning rate, ε is a minimal number to avoid zero in the denominator, ν_i is calculated using the following equation [10] with γ is the decay rate:

$$\nu_i = \gamma\nu_{i-1} + (1 - \gamma)[\nabla \mathrm{E}(\partial_i)]^2 \tag{10.6}$$

A **pooling player** performs down-sampling of input features without impacting the channel number of the image. It is usually inserted between convolutional layers to reduce the spatial dimensions. Consequently, it helps to decrease the number of training parameters for the next convolutional layer while keeping the depth of a CNN model unchanged. Average pooling layer or max-pooling layer are usually used in a CNN. The former calculates the average (mean) value of all elements in the filter, while the latter takes the maximum value from all filter elements. Nowadays, max pooling is widely used in CNN models for performing down-sampling input features between the convolutional layers.

A **fully connected layer** has all of its neurons connected to all neurons in the previous layer. This layer can also be called a dense layer. After applying hidden layers for feature extraction, a couple of dense layers are usually added to perform feature classification. One layer gathers the feature layers, and another converts the data from 3-D or 2-D into 1-D, representing probability output for each class.

10.3.3.2 Transfer Learning and Pre-trained Models

Following the rapid development of deep learning models, various well-known classification models are pre-trained on different datasets, for instance, CIFAR-100 or ImageNet [18]. The model's source codes and weights are usually publicized to the public. We call such models *pre-trained models*. A new model reusing some (or all) parts of a pre-trained one to another task is called a *transferred model*.

Utilizing and adapting a pre-trained model for new tasks is called *transfer learning* [19]. This progress is becoming popular since training a new deep learning model is very costly and time-consuming since it requires a vast number of data samples and parameters to train. Using transfer learning, we can get a better model based on the modifications of pre-trained models without training it from scratch.

The main steps of using transfer learning in this work are as follows:

1. Pre-trained model selection: find pre-trained models (those trained on a large and diverse image dataset) such that the pre-learned features can fit with skin lesion ones. After doing a survey, we decided to choose a modern pre-trained classification model provided by Google called Xception for this work.
2. Fine-tune pre-trained model: the next step is to analyze the model architecture to perform its fine-tuning. We need to decide which part of the pre-trained Xception will be kept and which part will be re-trained to learn new features from a new dataset of skin lesions.

Using the pre-trained model is essential for researchers to follow in their predecessor's accomplishments, leveraging existing pre-trained models to create new models for more specific target tasks and more practical applications.

10.3.3.3 Pre-trained Xception Model

Proposed by Chollet, 2017 [20], Xception is an improved version of Inception, a very deep popular CNN model produced by Google for image classification. The name "Xception" is short for "Extreme Inception". The principle of Xception architecture is the use of depthwise separable convolution layers. In such an architecture, instead of using the regular convolution layer, the author divided it into two separated types: depthwise and pointwise convolutions. In the former layer, each channel is convolved with a filter of depth 1. In the latter layer, the output feature maps of the depthwise convolution are convolved with 1x1 filters, which have the depth representing the desired number of channels in the output image. Figure 10.4 illustrates the general architecture of Xception with three blocks, namely entry, middle, and exit flows.

The entry flow takes input tensors of size $299 \times 299 \times 3$ and performs two blocks of convolutional layers and ReLU. After that, it performs various depthwise separable convolutional layers, followed by 3×3 max-pooling layers. There are skip connections with 1×1 convolution where the "add" operator is used to merge two tensors. The shape of input and output in each flow is also presented. For example,

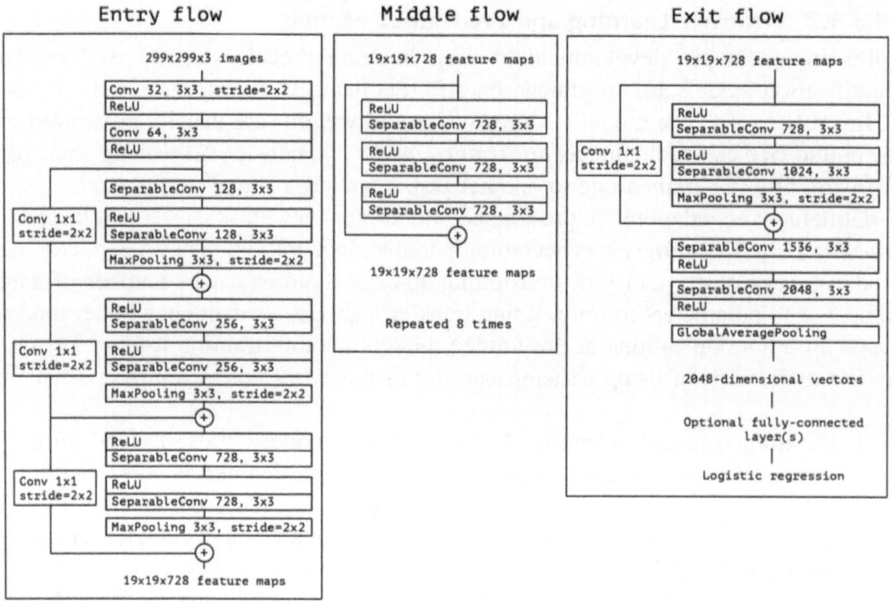

FIGURE 10.4 General architecture of Xception [20].

the dimension of the entry flow is 299 × 299 × 3, and the output size of feature maps is 19 × 19 × 728.

The middle flow takes feature maps of size 19 × 19 × 728 as input and performs eight modules of depthwise separable convolution layers, one after the other. All of these modules utilize a stride of 1 without any pooling layers. As a result, the spatial size of the tensor stays the same as passed from the entry flow's output. Besides, the channel depth is the same as the input's depth of 728 since the middle flow modules have 728 filters.

The exit flow contains two convolution modules. The first module uses max pooling and the skip connection, while the second one uses global average pooling without skip connection. Besides, fully connected layers can be optionally used before passing the output to the logistic regression layer.

In this work, we employ the pre-trained Xception model. This model has been previously pre-trained on the popular ImageNet dataset [21]. Xception is currently one of the latest and most accurate models for classification problems provided by Google. The network has a total of 71 layers with 22.9 million parameters.

10.3.3.4 Xception Model Fine-tuning

In order to make the pre-trained Xception model work efficiently with the problem of multiple classifications of skin cancer, we perform the model fine-tuning as follows:

1. The batch size for model training and validation is set to 20.
2. The last two layers of the pre-trained Xception model are removed.

3. We append a dense layer to Xception for 8-class classification.
4. Dropout ratio is set to 0.25 to prevent overfitting.
5. We use Adam optimizer, having a learning rate of 10^{-2}.
6. Replace Logistic Regression with softmax.
7. Categorical cross-entropy loss function is used to measure the model performance.
8. The weights of the first 36 pre-trained layers are reused for extracting features, while the last 35 layers are re-trained to learn new features and perform class prediction of skin lesion images. We choose to reuse 36 layers of the pre-trained Xception model since these layers represent basic features, for instance, lines or edges, that can be suitable for skin lesion properties.
9. The model is trained using a total of 30 epochs.

To facilitate the experiments, we use ModelCheckpoint callback to save checkpoints of the model during training. The learning rate is halved after two epochs when the metric has stopped improving.

To perform Xception model fine-tuning, we used Keras as the deep learning framework. Keras contains different pre-trained models on the ImageNet dataset. Additionally, it supports various deep learning libraries as backend, for instance, TensorFlow or Theano. We performed our experiments using Keras 2.2.1 with TensorFlow 1.14 on Python 3.7.3, running on Debian 10.

Regarding hardware infrastructure, our experiments are conducted on a server equipped with a GeForce RTX 2080 Ti GPU.

10.3.3.5 Evaluation Metrics

After training the model, it is crucial to measure its effectiveness to categorize skin lesions into multiple classes. A confusion matrix is used to show a model's classification performance in each class. In a confusion matrix, one dimension presents the values of each actual class, while another dimension provides the predicted values of each class. A cell value shows the number of instances in which the model guesses correctly or incorrectly to a given actual class. As a result, a confusion matrix is generally used to evaluate a given classification model's performance.

A binary classifier has only positive and negative values. Prediction output can be one of these four cases:

- True positive (TP): a positive case is correctly predicted as positive.
- True negative (TN): a negative case is correctly predicted as negative.
- False positive (FP): a negative case is incorrectly predicted as positive (Type I error).
- False negative (FN): a positive case is incorrectly predicted as negative (Type II error).

For a multi-class classifier, the number of classes K is not 2, and there are neither positive nor negative cases. However, it can be desirable to measure the effectiveness of the classifier on each class. To do this, for each class C_i, $i = 1 \ldots K$, we consider a binary classification in the test set: C_i as positive class while the rest

$\{C_j,\ j \neq i\}$ as negative class. As such, for each class C_i, we can calculate TP_i, TN_i, FP_i, and FN_i values based on the prediction output.

To measure the validity of a model, a set of more statistical metrics are used:

- **Accuracy** measures overall correct predictions:

$$Accuracy = \frac{\Sigma_0^{n-1}(TP_i + TN_i)}{\Sigma_0^{n-1}(TP_i + TN_i + FP_i + FN_i)}$$

- **Precision** measures the proportion of true positives among those classified as positives:

$$Precision = \frac{\Sigma_0^{n-1} TP_i}{\Sigma_0^{n-1}(TP_i + FP_i)}$$

- **Recall**, also called sensitivity, measures the proportion of predicted positives that are truly positive:

$$Recall = \frac{\Sigma_0^{n-1} TP_i}{\Sigma_0^{n-1}(TP_i + FN_i)}$$

- **Specificity** measures the proportion of predicted negatives that are truly negative:

$$Recall = \frac{\Sigma_0^{n-1} TN_i}{\Sigma_0^{n-1}(TN_i + FP_i)}$$

- **F1-score** is the precision's and recall's harmonic mean:

$$F1 = 2*\frac{Precision*Recall}{Precision + Recall}$$

F1-score is valid between half intervals (0,1]. F1-score indicates the quality of the classifier. In the best scenario, $F1 = 1$ when recall and precision are equal to 1.

- **Balanced Multi-class Accuracy (BMA)** is the mean recall of the confusion matrix:

$$BMA = \frac{1}{8}*\sum_{j=1}^{8} Recall_j$$

According to the ISIC 2019 challenge definition, BMA represents the diagnosis category score of the model. Hence, it is used to rank the participants of the challenge.

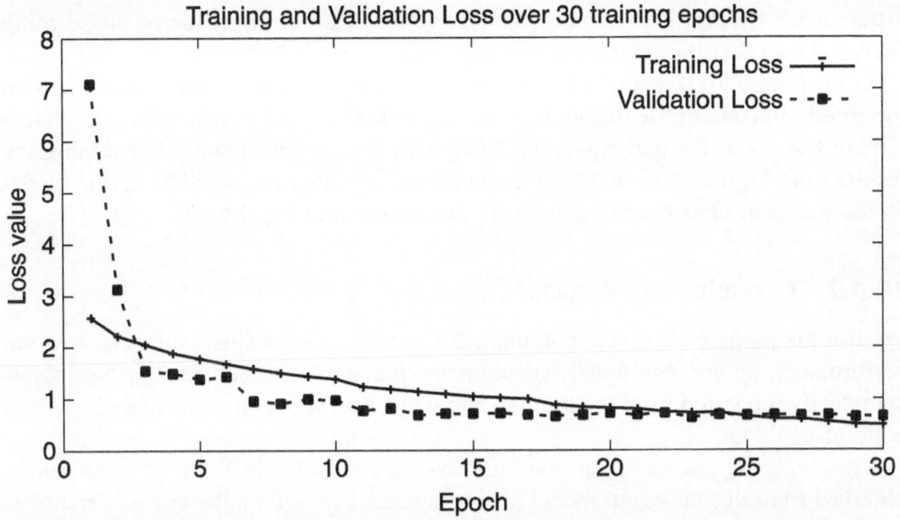

FIGURE 10.5 Learning curve of fine-tuned Xception model: training and validation loss.

10.4 EXPERIMENTAL RESULTS

10.4.1 LEARNING PERFORMANCE

Figure 10.5 and Figure 10.6 illustrate the learning performance of the fine-tuned Xception model during training. From Figure 10.5, it can be observed that the validation loss is very close to the training loss, leading to a good generalization ability. Specifically, from epoch 25 onward, our model converges since the

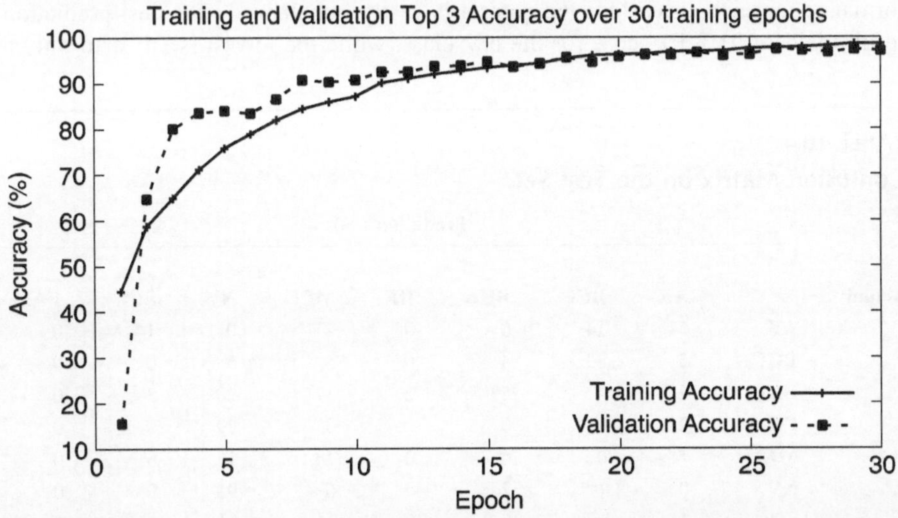

FIGURE 10.6 Learning curve of fine-tuned Xception model: training and validation accuracy.

difference between the two curves is negligible. Besides, the shape of the learning curves shows that the learning process is stable.

From Figure 10.6, it indicates that the validation accuracy nearly matches with the training accuracy. It means that the algorithm is confident in accurately classifying lesions to the corresponding categories during the training. Combining the results from Figures 10.4 and 10.5 demonstrates that the fine-tuned Xception model learns well and does overfit or underfit during the training process.

10.4.2 Classification Results

We use the prepared test set containing 2,534 images to evaluate the classification performance of our fine-tuned Xception model. It is noticed that this test set is completely separated from the training and validation sets so that the model is tested with unseen data.

The confusion matrix of our fine-tuned model is detailed in Table 10.4. As can be observed from this table, our model performs relatively well on the test set. The most successful predictions come from the NV class (the most popular one with the highest number of data samples), with 91% actual NV instances predicted as NV and the remaining 9% as BCC, BLK, or MEL. The following highest prediction results come with MEL class (the most dangerous type with the second-highest number of data samples), with 78% of samples being identified correctly. We perform data augmentation during the training process so that the number of samples is similar in each class. However, the test set is imbalanced because it is randomly extracted from the ISIC 2019 challenge dataset. Hence, in summary, although our model is trained on a balanced dataset, it can still predict an imbalanced dataset relatively well.

We summary the classification performance of our model for each class in Table 10.5. As depicted from this table, there is a clear difference between performance for each class since the dataset is vastly imbalanced. The best prediction result yields a 91% F1-score for the NV class, while the lowest is DF with only a

TABLE 10.4
Confusion Matrix on the Test Set

		Predicted (%)							
Actual		AK	BCC	BKL	DF	MEL	NV	SCC	VASC
	AK	51	14	0	0	21	0	14	0
	BCC	3	83	4	0	5	5	0	0
	BKL	2	4	53	2	17	20	2	0
	DF	0	0	0	71	0	29	0	0
	MEL	1	0	6	0	78	15	0	0
	NV	0	1	2	0	6	91	0	0
	SCC	11	6	0	0	11	11	61	0
	VASC	0	0	0	0	0	0	25	75

TABLE 10.5
Classification Result for Each Class

Class	Precision (%)	Recall (%)	F1-Score (%)
AK	47	57	52
BCC	80	78	79
BKL	72	54	62
DF	40	29	33
MEL	45	81	58
NV	93	89	91
SCC	62	44	52
VASC	75	75	75

33% F1-score. The performances are slightly better for AK and SCC classes than the DF class, yielding a 52% F1-score. These results show that the number of data samples in the test set has certain effects on the classification output.

From Table 10.5, it can also be seen that MEL class achieves much better recall than precision. This result can be explained as the similarity between MEL images and NV images in the test set. Figure 10.7 shows one example of similar images between MEL and NV classes. In general, all of the classes (except the DF class with the lowest number of samples in the test set) yield over 50% F1-score, which are acceptable results for multiple classifications of skin lesion images.

10.4.3 Comparative Study

This section compares our approach with the literature using the same ISIC 2019 dataset. Table 10.6 summarizes these result comparisons. From Table 10.6, our fine-tuned Xception model is a good classifier among other similar works on the same dataset. For example, our work obtains the best accuracy of 95.96% and the best BMA score of 64.3%. Regarding other performances such as precision, recall, and

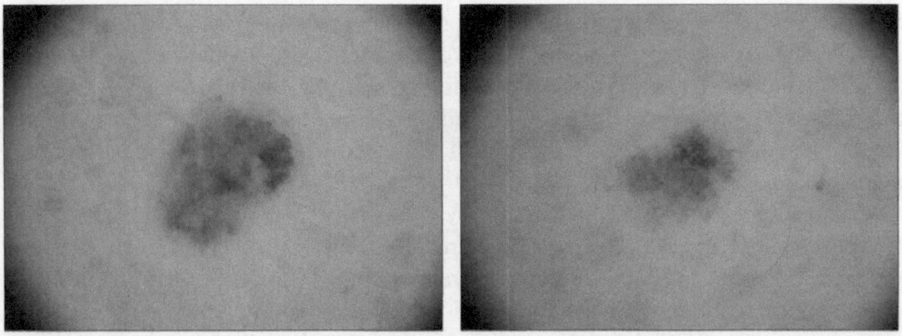

FIGURE 10.7 Example of the similarity between a MEL image (left) and an NV image (right).

TABLE 10.6
Performance Comparison With Other Works

Work	Method	Performance (%)				
		Accuracy	Precision	Recall	Specificity	BMA
Kassem et al., 2020 [22]	GoogleNet	94.92	80.36	79.8	97	–
Gessert et al., 2020 [21]ISIC 2019 Leaderboard rank 1	Multi-Res EfficientNets, SEN154 2	92.6	59.7	50.7	97.7	63.6
ISIC 2019 Leaderboard rank 2	EfficienetB3-B4-Seresnext101	91.7	50.7	60.7	95.2	60.7
ISIC 2019 Leaderboard rank 3	ResNet-152, DenseNet-201, SeResNext-101	92.4	58.4	54.0	96.3	59.3
ISIC 2019 Leaderboard rank 4	Ensemble 13 models	91.9	56.0	50.7	96.5	57.8
ISIC 2019 Leaderboard rank 5	Densenet-161	91.0	45.0	47.3	96.7	56.9
ISIC 2019 Leaderboard rank 6	Divide and conquer, Ensemble CNN networks	92.6	59.7	50.7	97.7	63.6
Ours	Xception	95.96	71.98	70.5	96.64	64.3

specificity, our model also gets quite good results compared to other works. It is also noticed that it is difficult to make a fair comparison since the test set of this work is randomly extracted from the ISIC 2019 dataset, thus different from other compared works in the literature.

10.5 CONCLUSION AND PERSPECTIVES

Skin cancer has raised attention in recent years, pressing needs to address this global general medical problem. This work presents a computer-aided diagnosis system capable of classifying eight different skin cancer types with reasonable accuracy by applying transfer learning and fine-tuning techniques to the pre-trained Xception model. We evaluate the model with dermoscopy images on a publicly available dataset named ISIC 2019.

Our method achieves 95.96% accuracy, 71.98% precision, 70.50% recall, 96.64 F1-score and 64.3% BMA score. These results show that our fine-tuned Xception model is a good classifier for the problem of multiple classifications of skin lesion images. This work can still go further if we have more data, especially for small classes like AK, SCC, VASC, and DF classes. Another direction is to continue improving the Xception model to deal with imbalanced dataset problems rather than just performing data augmentation to generate balanced classes.

REFERENCES

[1] Skin Cancer Foundation. Skin Cancer 101, Knowledge is Your Best Defense. Available online: https://www.skincancer.org/skin-cancer-information/. June 2021.

[2] Skin Cancer Foundation. Skin cancer facts & statistics. Available online: https://www.skincancer.org/skin-cancer-information/skin-cancer-facts/. June 2021.

[3] Vestergaard M. E., Macaskill P. H. P. M., Holt P. E., Menzies S. W. (2008). Dermoscopy compared with naked eye examination for the diagnosis of primary melanoma: a meta-analysis of studies performed in a clinical setting. *British Journal of Dermatology* 159(3):669–676. 10.1111/j.1365-2133.2008.08713.x.

[4] Lopez A. R., Giro-i-Nieto X., Burdick J., Marques O. (2017). Skin lesion classification from dermoscopic images using deep learning techniques. In: *IEEE 13th IASTED International Conference on Biomedical Engineering (BioMed'2017)*, pp 49–54. 10.2316/P.2017.852-053.

[5] Korotkov K., Garcia R. (2012). Computerized analysis of pigmented skin lesions: a review. *Artificial Intelligence in Medicine* 56(2):69–90. 10.1016/j.artmed.2012.08.002.

[6] Oliveira R. B., Papa J. P., Pereira A. S., Tavares J. M. R. (2018). Computational methods for pigmented skin lesion classification in images: review and future trends. *Neural Computing and Applications* 29(3):613–636. 10.1007/s00521-016-2482-6.

[7] Pathan S., Prabhu K. G., Siddalingaswamy P. C. (2018).Techniques and algorithms for computer aided diagnosis of pigmented skin lesions-a review. *Biomedical Signal Processing and Control* 39:237–262. 10.1016/j.bspc.2017.07.010.

[8] Murugan A., Nair S. A. H., Kumar K. S. (2019). Detection of skin cancer using SVM, random forest and kNN classifiers. *Journal of Medical Systems* 43(8):1–9

[9] Farooq M. A., Azhar M. A. M., Raza, R. H. (2016). Automatic lesion detection system (ALDS) for skin cancer classification using SVM and neural classifiers. *In 2016 IEEE 16th International Conference on Bioinformatics and Bioengineering (REF10_E)*, pp. 301–308. IEEE.

[10] Chaturvedi S. S., Tembhurne J. V., Diwan T. (2020). A multi-class skin Cancer classification using deep convolutional neural networks. *Multimedia Tools and Applications* 79(39), 28477–28498.

[11] Dorj U. O., Lee K. K., Choi J. Y. Lee M. (2018). The skin cancer classification using deep convolutional neural network. *Multimedia Tools and Applications* 77(8), 9909–9924.

[12] Hosny K. M., Kassem M. A., Foaud, M. M. (2018). Skin cancer classification using deep learning and transfer learning. In *2018 9th Cairo International Biomedical Engineering Conference (CIBEC)*, 90–93. IEEE.

[13] Tschandl P., Rosendahl C., Kittler H. (2018). The HAM10000 dataset, a large collection of multi-source dermatoscopic images of common pigmented skin lesions. *Scientific Data* 5, 180161. 10.1038/sdata.2018.161.

[14] Codella N. C. F., Gutman D., Celebi M. E., Helba B., Marchetti M. A., Dusza S. W., Kalloo A., Liopyris K., Mishra N., Kittler H., Halpern A. (2017). Skin lesion analysis toward melanoma detection: a challenge at the 2017 International Symposium on Biomedical Imaging (isbi), Hosted by the International Skin Imaging Collaboration (ISIC). arXiv:1710.05006.

[15] Combalia M., Codella N. C. F., Rotemberg V., Helba B., Vilaplana V., Reiter O., Halpern A. C., Puig S., Malvehy J. (2019). BCN20000: Dermoscopic lesions in the wild. arXiv:1908.02288.

[16] Gu J., Wang Z., Kuen J., Ma L., Shahroudy A., Shuai B., … Chen, T. (2018). Recent advances in convolutional neural networks. *Pattern Recognition* 77, 354–377.

[17] Kingma, D. P., Ba, J. (2014). Adam: a method for stochastic optimization. arXiv preprint arXiv:1412.6980.

[18] Deng J., Dong W., Socher R., Li L. J., Li, K., Fei-Fei L. (2009). Imagenet: a large-scale hierarchical image database. In: *IEEE Conference on Computer Vision and Pattern Recognition*, 248–255.

[19] Torrey L., Shavlik, J. (2010). Transfer learning. *Handbook of research on machine learning applications and trends: algorithms, methods, and techniques*, 242–264. IGI global.

[20] Chollet F. (2017). Xception: deep learning with depthwise separable convolutions. In: *IEEE Conference on Computer Vision and Pattern Recognition*, 1251–1258.

[21] Gessert N., Nielsen M., Shaikh M., Werner R., Schlaefer, A. (2020). Skin lesion classification using ensembles of multi-resolution Efficient Nets with meta data. *MethodsX 7*, 100864.

[22] Kassem M. A., Hosny K. M., Fouad, M. M. (2020). Skin lesions classification into eight classes for ISIC 2019 using deep convolutional neural network and transfer learning. *IEEE Access 8*, 114822–114832.

11 Application of Artificial Intelligence in Medical Imaging

Sampurna Panda
Assistant Professor, Department of EC&EE, Institute of Technology & Management, Gwalior, India

Rakesh Kumar Dhaka
Associate Professor, School of Nursing Sciences, ITM University, Gwalior, India

CONTENTS

11.1 Introduction......195
11.2 Machine Learning......196
11.2.1 Supervised Learning......197
11.2.2 Unsupervised Learning......197
11.2.3 Semi-supervised Learning......197
11.2.4 Active Learning......197
11.2.5 Reinforcement Learning......197
11.2.6 Evolutionary Learning......198
11.2.7 Deep Learning......198
11.3 Use of Machine Learning for Medical Imaging......199
11.4 Deep Learning in Medical Imaging......200
11.4.1 Image Categorisation......200
11.4.2 Object Classification......201
11.4.3 Organ or Region Detection......201
11.4.4 Data Mining......201
11.4.5 The Sign-up Process......201
11.5 Summary......201
References......202

11.1 INTRODUCTION

The computer system's machine learning algorithm is essential to improve its ability to make accurate predictions and make decisions. The area of study that teaches computers how to study without requiring them to be explicitly programmed is known as machine learning. [1] Deep learning is a machine learning category that allows systems to understand the world as regards a picture of ideas. [2]

DOI: 10.1201/9781003217497-11

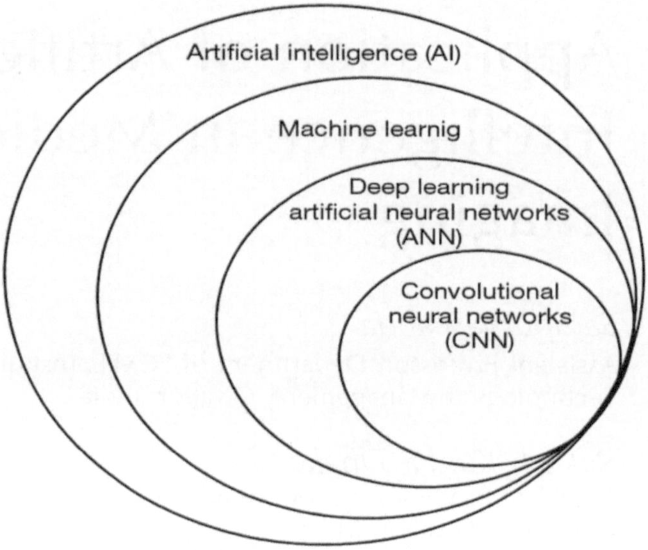

FIGURE 11.1 Relation if AI with ML, ANN, CNN [3].

The growing performance of neural networks propelled the growth of deep learning in computer vision.

11.2 MACHINE LEARNING

Machine learning describes methods that enable computers to learn on their own and solve problems. A mathematical model should be trained so that it can be fed useful input data and then produce valuable results. (Figure 11.1)

Machine learning models are provided with training data and optimised to yield accurate predictions. To put it simply, the models are developed to deliver predictions for new data with an unseen level of certainty. To estimate the generalisation ability of a model, you use a separate dataset called the validation set, and apply the model's predictions to that dataset as a form of feedback for tuning the model. The model is evaluated using test data against which it has been trained and fine-tuned, to see how it will perform with unseen data. It is possible to roughly categorise machine learning methods according to how the models' input data is utilised during training. An agent is built in reinforcement learning through trial and error, while one is optimising a particular objective function. The computer is assigned the task of learning on its own without guidance.

In a nutshell, grouping is the quintessential use case. Most of today's machine learning is done in real time algorithms such as supervised learning belongs to the class of supervised learning. Here, A set of already labelled or annotated images is given to the computer. Then challenged to assign correct labels to new, previously unseen data unseen datasets that are constructed according to the learned rules that were discovered dataset. This consists of a collection of input-output examples.

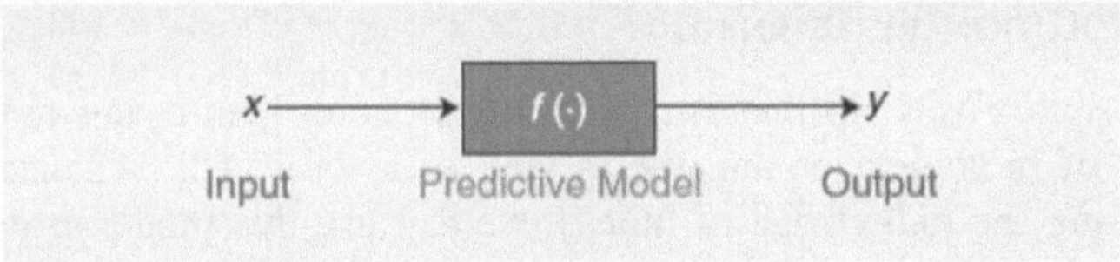

FIGURE 11.2 Supervised machine learning output is a function of input [4].

11.2.1 Supervised Learning

To perform specific data-processing tasks, the model is trained. Image annotation by applying labels such as "classify" to images estimating the amount of malignancy by measuring the severity of skin lesions [3] This describes a scenario in which a predicted output variable (y) is calculated on the basis of a vector of input variables (x). In Figure 11.2, it is assumed that the input and output conform to the functional relationship called the predictive model. Supervised learning, which is called discovery learning, is where a predictive model is discovered by data training with examples in which both y and x are known. I am made up of n (referred to as features), so x [Rn] For simplicity, only scalar outputs are concerned.

11.2.2 Unsupervised Learning

Decisions will be made autonomously, without requiring data to be processed. There are no labels that can be used for predictions made on the system. Feature learning enables us to obtain the hidden pattern using unsupervised learning. Unsupervised learning techniques are used to divide the input space into clusters. There is no way to identify these clusters earlier. Group formation is predicated on similarity.

11.2.3 Semi-supervised Learning

This learning assumes that the training data are incomplete. Typically this type of training is used with adequately trained data to improve performance in cases where a number of missing results are present. This kind of algorithm is used for training on unmarked information. The semi-controlled learning algorithm was developed on both etiquette and non-labelled data.

11.2.4 Active Learning

Training tags only appear a limited number of times in Active learning. It is utilised to help add tags to aid in the attainment of objectives. example: For example, a budget function in an organisation.

11.2.5 Reinforcement Learning

Reinforcement learning is applicable to real-world tasks that need guidance to successfully complete the goal, like driving a vehicle or playing a video game.

11.2.6 Evolutionary Learning

Biological research uses biospheres as learning tools for identifying and forecasting the lifespans of biological organisms, as well as to project the chances of having offspring. Using the knowledge of fitness, we can use this model to guess how to adjust the result.

11.2.7 Deep Learning

Neural networks are the most commonly used methods of machine learning in this phase, where they are used to learn and predict. A diversified group of algorithms is used. The aim is to establish a general system capable of addressing and predicting different kinds of problems. This graph has numerous processing layers, each of which contains several linear and non-linear conversions. (Figure 11.3)

Though they delivered on their promises, ML architecture increases the chance of failure in training dataset convergence and over-fitting. They are also time-consuming and require larger datasets for training. (Figure 11.4)

Today, illness diagnosis can be an extremely challenging mission in medical disciplines. Medical inspection and evaluation are important tasks to comprehend the accurate diagnosis of patients. A large amount of data concerning medical evaluation, a statement about the patient, treatment, supplements, prescriptions, and the like come from the healthcare sector. The main problem is that the reports appear to have a symbiotic relationship, caused by management errors in data management. [7] (Figure 11.5)

Today the diagnosis of disease in medical disciplines can be very challenging. Medical inspection and assessment are essential tasks for accurate diagnosis. The healthcare industry obtains data on medical assessment, as well as information on

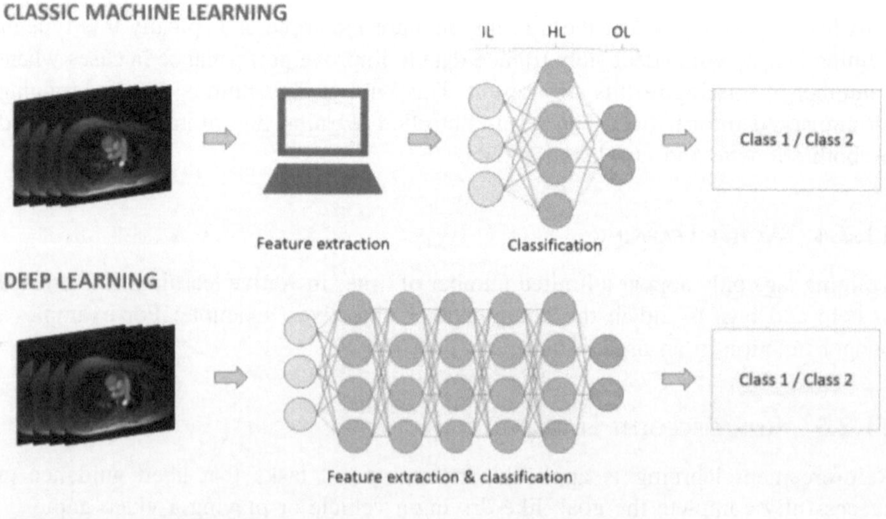

FIGURE 11.3 Traditional machine learning vs deep learning [5].

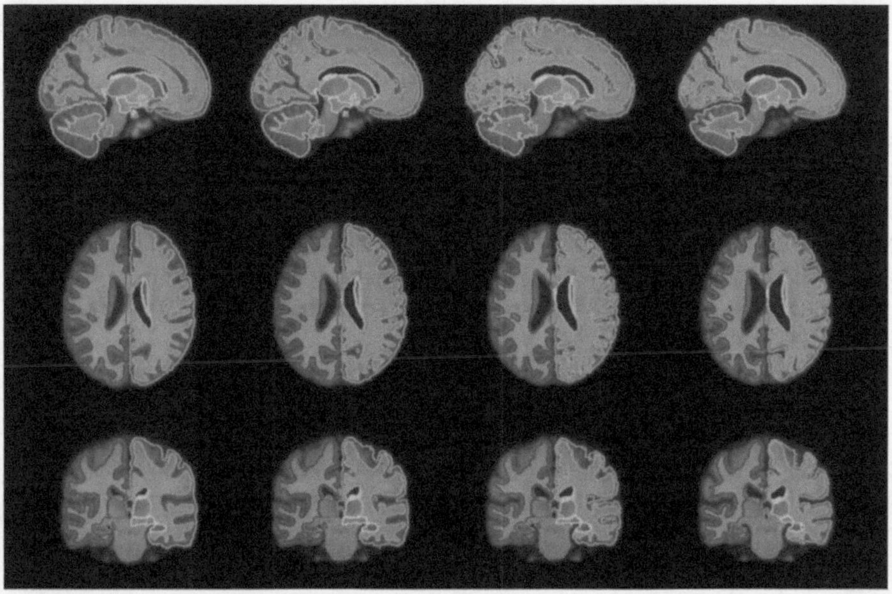

FIGURE 11.4 Traditional machine learning vs deep learning [6].

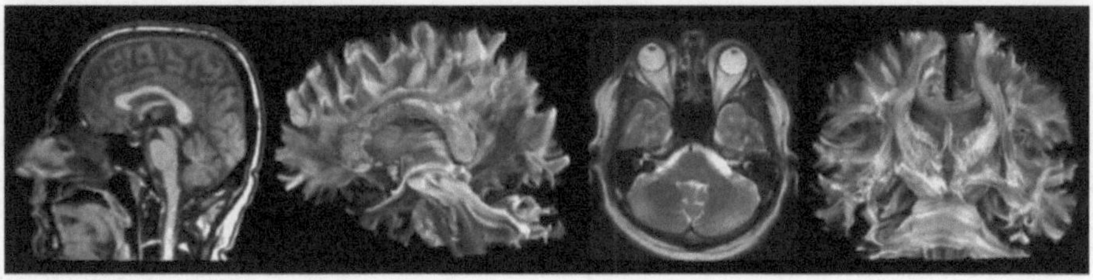

FIGURE 11.5 Traditional machine learning vs deep learning [8].

the patient, on therapy, on drugs and the like. The key problem is that the reports appear to be symbiotic due to data management errors. [4]

11.3 USE OF MACHINE LEARNING FOR MEDICAL IMAGING

Medical imaging is highly effective in using machine learning algorithms to study specific diseases. non-mathematical solutions are incapable of accurately representing certain entities in medical image processing such as lesions and organs. The pixel-based study was used for medical imagery diseases. Another example of machine-based extraction of learning features is the use of pixel analysis in machine learning. Instead of using a simple feature-based classifier for a given problem it can be more effective [5]. Due to its low contrast, it is difficult to test the image's properties. Functional calculation and segmentation do not require pixel based machine learning. [9] medical pixel analysis targeted low contrast pictures.

Histogram equalisation is the most effective technique for contrast improvement (HE), designed with the help of homomorphic image filtering to modify histogram based contrast enhancement techniques (MHFIL).

For global contrast improvement, histogram modification is employed in the first phase. Homomorphic filtering in the second phase is additionally used for image sharpening. This experiment investigates 10 chest X-ray images that have very low contrast. Using a minimum values approach across all ten images yields the MH-FIL. Radiologists bear the main responsibility for medical image clarification, with image analysis and quality assignments having equal importance. CAD has been developed for several years using computer-aided design.

Today's machine learning techniques need to focus on constructing and organising a relationship between unstructured, raw data and stories. By having such a large amount of data, the implementation of machine learning techniques in healthcare will yield major benefits. Although useful in helping physicians perform close to perfect diagnoses, identifying the best medications for patients, and reducing the number of patients who wind up on expensive medications, currently machine learning has limited capabilities. [6,10].

11.4 DEEP LEARNING IN MEDICAL IMAGING

The goal of this technique is to help computers find features that allow them to identify and characterise data that may apply to a given issue. This concept is fundamental to several machine learning algorithms. Increasingly detailed models, stacked on top of each other, transmute input images into outputs. Convolutional neural networks are the better model type for image analysis (CNNs). The CNNs utilise a number of filter layers to process the input. The medical field frequently employs deep learning methods to familiarise themselves with modern architecture by introducing them to various input formats, such as three-dimensional data. Previously, the CNNs avoided dealing with the large volume of Interest because of how big 3D convolutions are, along with the additional constraints that came along with them.

11.4.1 Image Categorisation

As one of the primary tasks in deep learning, the classification of medical images is focused on exploring clinical-related issues like earlier treatment for the patient. multi-image input; single diagnostic (disease yes or no). It is common to see that the number of different diagnostic tests used by a medical imaging method or software application is typically minor compared to the number of test models and sample sets utilised in computer vision. as seen in [11], it seems the fine modification, or feature extraction, did better, achieving 57.6% accuracy in evaluating knee osteoarthritis compared to 53.4% It seems that CNN feature extraction for cytopathology classification, as done by CNN feature extraction for cytology classification, yields accuracy levels between 69.1 percent and 70.5 percent [12].

11.4.2 Object Classification

The object classification is placed on small focused sections of the medical image, for those patients with a greater level of interest Projection into two or more classes is possible with these chunks. In order to obtain more accurate results, local facts, as well as global information, are critical. The results in [24] used three CNNs methods of deep learning to correct an image with respect to objects of differing sizes. After applying these three methods, the final image features matrix was calculated.

11.4.3 Organ or Region Detection

After classification, the next phase is object detection and localisation. Segmentation is a critical step where we can focus on only the important objects and discard the irrelevant ones. In response, we use deep learning algorithms to perform 3D data parsing in order to challenge this problem. Furthermore, three separate 2D and 3D image chunks were used in the image by the author. Its objective is to determine different regions linked to different diseases and focus on a particular one, such as the heart, the aortic arch and the descending aorta. [8,13]

11.4.4 Data Mining

Organ and substructure are extracted from medical images during the segmentation process. It is used to evaluate the clinical characteristics of the patient. An exam of the heart or brain, for example. It is also used for different functions in computer-aided design (CAD). The digital picture is defined by recognising the details that make up the topic of interest. This is the combination of upsamples and down-samples, where a certain data set is taken from and down each layer. It connected those two processes together by integrating convolution points and de-convolution samples of layers.[14]

11.4.5 The Sign-up Process

In the registration, multiple sets of data are each used to calculate a new coordinate. Providing comparison or integration of data from multiple viewpoints, times, depths, sensors, etc. is an important part of medical imaging.

11.5 SUMMARY

Machine learning capabilities have been cultivated over the past few years. In current practice, machine learning methods are robust to real-world applications, and the structures clearly enhance this advantage. Previously, this pertains to the preparation of medical imaging, and in the future, it will make a significant advancement at a swift pace. Machines that use machine learning can have important inferences for medication administration. It is an essential part of this research that patients will benefit from it. Verifying that the machines are used to their fullest potential is a huge part of the machine learning solution. The deep learning algorithms used in medical image analysis aid in classifying, categorising, and enumerating disease patterns. It also opens the door to exploring the boundary of analytical goals, which then helps to generate prediction models for treatment. Scientists in the imaging field are weighing these problems, deep learning in healthcare. It is rapidly improving, as deep learning is increasingly found in numerous other fields, especially those dealing with healthcare.

REFERENCES

[1] Valiant, Leslie G. "A theory of the learnable." *Communications of the ACM* 27, no. 11(1984): 1134–1142.

[2] Goodfellow, Ian, Yoshua Bengio, and Aaron Courville. *Deep Learning*. MIT Press, 2016.

[3] Esteva, Andre, Brett Kuprel, Roberto A. Novoa, Justin Ko, Susan M. Swetter, and Helen M. Blau. "Dermatologist-level classification of skin cancer with deep neural networks." *Nature* 542, no. 7639 (2017): 115–118.

[4] Warwick, William, Sophie Johnson, Judith Bond, Geraldine Fletcher, and Pavlo Kanellakis. "A framework to assess healthcare data quality." *The European Journal of Social & Behavioural Sciences* (2015).

[5] Suzuki, Kenji. "Pixel-based machine learning in medical imaging." *International Journal of Biomedical Imaging* 2012 (2012).

[6] Page D. Challenges in Machine Learning from Electronic Health Records. *MLHC* 2015.

[7] Schmidhuber, Jürgen. "Deep learning in neural networks: An overview." *Neural Networks* 61 (2015): 85–117.

[8] Wang, C.-W., et al., Evaluation and comparison of anatomical landmark detection methods for cephalometric x-ray images: a grand challenge. *IEEE Transactions on Medical Imaging* 34, no. 9 (2015): 1890–1900.

[9] Agarwal, Tarun Kumar, Mayank Tiwari, and Subir Singh Lamba. "Modified histogram based contrast enhancement using homomorphic filtering for medical images." In *2014 IEEE International Advance Computing Conference (IACC)*, pp. 964–968. IEEE, 2014.

[10] Maddux D. The Human Condition in Structured and Unstructured Data. *Acumen Physician Solutions*, 2014.

[11] Antony, J., et al. Quantifying radiographic knee osteoarthritis severity using deep convolutional neural networks. In Pattern Recognition (ICPR), 2016 23rd International Conference on. 2016. IEEE.

[12] Kim, E., M. Corte-Real, and Z. Baloch. A deep semantic mobile application for thyroid cytopathology. In Medical Imaging 2016: PACS and Imaging Informatics: Next Generation and Innovations. 2016. International Society for Optics and Photonics.

[13] De Vos, B.D., et al. 2D image classification for 3D anatomy localization: employing deep convolutional neural networks. In Medical Imaging 2016: Image Processing. 2016. International Society for Optics and Photonics.

[14] Çiçek, Ö. et al. 3D U-Net: learning dense volumetric segmentation from sparse annotation. In International Conference on Medical Image Computing and Computer-Assisted Intervention. 2016. Springer.

12 Machine Learning Algorithms Used in Medical Field with a Case Study

M. Jayasanthi
Associate Professor Department of ECE, PSG Institute of technology and applied research Coimbatore, Tamil Nadu, India

R. Kalaivani
Professor and Head Department of ECE, Erode Sengunthar Engineering College, Erode, Tamil Nadu, India

CONTENTS

12.1 Introduction........204
12.2 Machine Learning Algorithms........204
12.2.1 Supervised Learning........204
12.2.2 Unsupervised Learning........205
12.2.3 Reinforcement Learning........205
12.2.4 Semi-Supervised Learning........205
12.2.5 Regression Algorithms........205
12.2.6 Instance-based Algorithms........206
12.2.7 Regularization Algorithms........206
12.2.8 Decision Tree Algorithms........206
12.2.9 Bayesian Algorithms........207
12.2.10 Clustering Algorithms........207
12.2.11 Association Rule Learning Algorithms........207
12.2.12 Artificial Neural Network Algorithms........207
12.2.13 Deep Learning Algorithms........208
12.2.14 Dimensionality Reduction Algorithms........208
12.2.15 Ensemble Algorithms........209
12.3 ML Algorithms in Medical Diagnosis........209
12.4 ML Classifiers in Breast Cancer Diagnosis........211
12.4.1 Logistic Regression........212
12.4.2 K-Nearest Neighbor (k-NN) Algorithm........213
12.4.3 Support Vector Machine........213

DOI: 10.1201/9781003217497-12

12.4.4 Random Forest Classifier 214
12.4.5 Naive Bayes Classifier 215
12.4.6 Decision Tree Classifiers 216
12.4.7 Dimensionality Reduction Algorithms 216
12.5 Materials and Methods 216
12.6 Conclusion 218
References 220

12.1 INTRODUCTION

Artificial Intelligence (AI) is the intelligence demonstrated by machines, in comparison to the usual intelligence demonstrated by human beings and animals. The word AI is sometimes used for the machines that imitate cognitive functions like learning, decision-making, and problem-solving skills associated with human beings. AI techniques are prevalently applied in this world. Some major fields taking advantage of AI are healthcare, web search engines, recommendation systems, natural language processing, smart assistants, self-driving cars, social media monitoring, etc.

Machine learning (ML), which is a primary concept of AI research from its inception, is a branch that involves algorithms that improve themselves automatically through learning and experience. The algorithms can be categorized into different ways to model a problem. One way uses learning style and the other method uses similarity in the form or function. In the classification based on the learning style, three categories of problems are prevalent. It is built on its relationship with the environment or knowledge or whatsoever called the input data. This classification method of putting machine learning algorithms in order is very much constructive as it facilitates thinking about the accountability of the input data and the foundation practices involved in it. It also helps to select a model that is the most suitable for the given situation so as to get the best result. There are three types of ML algorithms based on broad classification. They are Supervised Learning, Unsupervised Learning and Reinforcement Learning.

12.2 MACHINE LEARNING ALGORITHMS

12.2.1 Supervised Learning

In the supervised learning model, predictors, referred to as training data, possess recognized outputs called labels for each instance. A machine learning model is developed as a result of a training process, during which it is expected to predict an output. When the predictions are wrong, training is performed again and again. The training practice keeps on moving till the model attains a preferred value of exactness on the training set of data. Supervised learning requires labeling and the method includes numerical regression and classification. Some of the examples of algorithms include Support Vector Machine, Linear Regression, Logistic Regression Algorithm, and Artificial Neural Network Algorithm.

The Regression methods shot to construct a function that depicts the association of inputs with the outputs and forecasts how the outputs should vary with respect to change in inputs. Classification is a method of determining the class or category that something belongs to. This classification will excel after a program undergoes a number of examples of stuff from several groups. Once training by a program or model for different groups is completed, the program is called the trained model.

12.2.2 Unsupervised Learning

Unsupervised learning involves finding the patterns in a stream of input, without requiring any labels or outputs. Input data do not have a known result or any label. By realizing the structures present in the inputs, general rules are extracted and unsupervised model is developed. This might be done by a mathematical process to organize data on a similarity basis or to steadily diminish the redundancy. The problems may be of association rule learning type or dimensionality reduction or clustering types. The algorithms may include K-Nearest Neighbor, K-Means algorithm, and Apriori algorithm.

12.2.3 Reinforcement Learning

While data are chomped to develop models for commercial decisions, supervised learning or unsupervised learning algorithms are, in general, used. When huge dataset exists with only some degree of labeled examples, semi-supervised learning algorithms are used.

12.2.4 Semi-Supervised Learning

In **Semi-Supervised Learning model,** Input data may or may not have targets. The model must learn the organization and structure of the data to make predictions and it is similar to a prediction problem.

Algorithms are frequently clustered by knowing how they carry out to do a successful work or how similar the algorithms are in terms of functionality. Example methods include tree-based methods, support vector-based methods, and neural networks inspired methods. Though it is a convenient grouping scheme, it is not flawless. There are algorithms that might merely apt into several classes similar to Learning Vector Quantization. There is a scheme inspired by neural network in addition to instance-based method. Regression and clustering are the algorithmic types that have indistinguishable names, which can be handled by arranging the algorithms twofold or by selecting the set that fits most perfectly.

12.2.5 Regression Algorithms

Regression is the process of estimating the association among variables that are iteratively developed with reference to error calculations prevalent in the model. Regression methods are pillars of information and are chosen for statistical machine learning. The most frequently used regression algorithms are:

- Logistic Regression algorithm
- Linear Regression algorithm

- Stepwise Regression algorithm
- Ordinary Least Squares Regression (OLSR) algorithm
- Locally Estimated Scatter plot Smoothing (LOESS) algorithm
- Multivariate Adaptive Regression Splines (MARS) algorithm

12.2.6 Instance-based Algorithms

In instance-based learning method, the predictors that are considered to be significant or mandatory to the model for decision making are taken into account. These methods naturally form a record of sample data and balance fresh data using a similarity extent so as to catch the greatest match and make an estimate. Intended for this purpose, instance-based approaches are termed winner-take-all methods. They are also called memory-based learning. Concentration is put on the expression of the stored occurrences and similarity processes used between occasions. The most commonly used instance-based algorithms are:

- k-Nearest Neighbor (kNN)
- Self-Organizing Map (SOM)
- Learning Vector Quantization (LVQ)
- Support Vector Machines (SVM)
- Locally Weighted Learning (LWL)

12.2.7 Regularization Algorithms

Regularization is an addition carried out in regression methods. The models are dealt with according to the complexity. Some simpler models that are better in generalization are also favored in this method. The most commonly used regularization algorithms are:

- Elastic Net algorithms
- Ridge Regression algorithms
- Least-Angle Regression (LARS) algorithms
- Least Absolute Shrinkage and Selection Operator (LASSO)

12.2.8 Decision Tree Algorithms

A model for making a decision is made with definite assessment of features in the dataset. The judgments or decisions divide the tree structures in anticipation of making a predictive decision for a given dataset. The decision trees are made trained on the data for the kind of regression and classification problems. The decision tree methods work fast and provide perfect solution and are largely preferred in machine learning.

The most commonly used decision tree algorithms include:

- Iterative Dichotomiser 3 (ID3)
- Classification and Regression Tree (CART)

- Chi-squared Automatic Interaction Detection (CHAID)
- C4.5 and C5.0 (different versions of a powerful approach)
- M5
- Decision Stump
- Conditional Decision Trees

12.2.9 Bayesian Algorithms

Bayes' Theorem is applied in Bayesian methods for solving the classification and regression type problems. Mainly used Bayesian algorithms are:

- Gaussian Naive Bayes
- Naive Bayes
- Averaged One-Dependence Estimators (AODE)
- Bayesian Belief Network (BBN)
- Bayesian Network (BN)
- Multinomial Naive Bayes

12.2.10 Clustering Algorithms

Clustering methods are naturally structured by hierarchal modeling and centroid-based approaches. All of the clustering methods take the inherent features of the records to organize them into the collection of greatest harmony in the best manner.

The most popular clustering algorithms are:

- k-Means
- Expectation Maximization (EM)
- k-Medians
- Hierarchical Clustering

12.2.11 Association Rule Learning Algorithms

The set of rules that best explain observed relationships among the variables in data record are extracted in Association rule learning methods. Important and commercially useful associations are discovered by the rules even in huge multi-dimensional datasets in this algorithm.

The commonly used algorithms based on association learning rule are:

- Eclat algorithm
- Apriori algorithm

12.2.12 Artificial Neural Network Algorithms

Artificial Neural Networks mimic the functions of biological neural networks and provide results for pattern matching. These algorithms are used for classification and regression in general. There are various subfields in the artificial neural networks and they include hundreds of algorithms and variants for all categories of problems.

The commonly used artificial neural network algorithms are:

- Multilayer Perceptrons (MLP)
- Perceptron
- Hopfield Network
- Stochastic Gradient Descent
- Radial Basis Function Network (RBFN)
- Back-Propagation

12.2.13 Deep Learning Algorithms

Deep Learning has been gaining massive growth and popularity and it is an emerging area in almost all the fields not limited to healthcare. The algorithms are state-of-the-art methods and they make use of plenty of low-cost computations. A large number of datasets with labels as output are required for processing images, texts, audio signals, and video signals.

The most fashionable and commonly used deep learning algorithms are:

- Convolutional Neural Network (CNN)
- Deep Belief Networks (DBN)
- Long Short-Term Memory Networks (LSTMs)
- Recurrent Neural Networks (RNNs)
- Deep Boltzmann Machine (DBM)
- Stacked Auto-Encoder

12.2.14 Dimensionality Reduction Algorithms

Dimensionality reduction methods search for and make use of the inherent constitution of the data, like the clustering methods, particularly for medical information in an unsupervised manner that uses less information. Data are transferred from a high-dimensional space into a low-dimensional space in the technique such that low-dimensional representation clasp some considerable possessions of the original data, rather close to its intrinsic measurements. This might be constructive to anticipate low dimensional data or to make simpler data that may be utilized in supervised machine learning processes afterward. A lot of these techniques may be settled in for use in regression and classification.

- Principal Component Regression (PCR)
- Principal Component Analysis (PCA)
- Partial Least Squares Regression (PLSR)
- Sammon Mapping
- Multidimensional Scaling (MDS)
- Linear Discriminant Analysis (LDA)

- Projection Pursuit
- Quadratic Discriminant Analysis (QDA)
- Mixture Discriminant Analysis (MDA)
- Flexible Discriminant Analysis (FDA)

12.2.15 Ensemble Algorithms

In Ensemble methods, several delicate and self-sufficient models are trained. The predictions of these simpler models are collectively arranged to make the overall forecast in any one of the ways. A number of works are performed to find out the category of weak learners which may be grouped and to find the technique in which to group them. These are very popular and very powerful classes of methods. The following techniques are involved in these ensemble algorithms.

- Boosting
- AdaBoost
- Weighted Average
- Bootstrapped Aggregation
- Stacked Generalization
- Gradient Boosted Regression Trees
- Random Forest
- Gradient Boosting Machines

There are other machine learning algorithms, such as Feature Selection Algorithms, Performance Measures, and Optimization Algorithms. Various other sub-categories of machine learning algorithms are:

- Natural Language Processing (NLP)
- Computational intelligence
- Computer Vision
- Recommender Systems
- Graphical Models
- Reinforcement Learning

All these algorithms can be used in one or the other way in computer-aided diagnosis systems or detection systems.

12.3 ML ALGORITHMS IN MEDICAL DIAGNOSIS

Machine learning is a technique that develops a model or an inference from data samples and it is a subset of Artificial Intelligence (AI) [1–3]. Learning entails two different phases: (i) Dependencies are evaluated in the given dataset and (ii) Output of the system is predicted by the application of the estimated dependencies. With different algorithms and techniques, Machine Learning has demonstrated its significant role in biomedical research, wherein an appropriate generalization is achieved by probing all the parameters or features in an n-dimensional space for identified samples along with various algorithms and their techniques [4]. As discussed already, training data sets are labeled in supervised learning whereas unsupervised learning works on unlabeled data to find the patterns and structures. So in unsupervised learning, learning scheme/model determines the pattern from the specified input data without any labels or outputs. Clustering and Regression are the two frequently found unsupervised learning tasks. The supervised learning procedure is defined as a classification problem, which characterizes a learning procedure for the classification of the data into a fixed number of groupings.

A different type of commonly applied learning method which is a combination of both supervised and unsupervised learning is semi-supervised learning. It blends the labeled and unlabeled data to build a precise learning algorithm or model. Compared to labeled datasets, this semi-supervised learning is frequently used for the unlabeled datasets. Each dataset is described with many features and all the features are of different values and types. Knowledge about the detailed kind of data in advance facilitates the right choice of tools and techniques for exploration.

Occurrence of noise, outliers, missing or duplicate data and biased data are misleading in the classification. Numerous strategies and preprocessing methods could be applied in preprocessing of medical signals, to obtain better data quality and for appropriating the dataset to a particular learning model. The (i) feature extraction (ii) feature selection and (iii) dimensionality reduction are the most significant preprocessing methods.

The ML techniques intend to construct a solution for classification and estimation or prediction. The most commonly performed task in machine learning is classification. Here the learning function aims to categorize the data into one of the pre-defined groups. The training data may lead to misclassification errors and test data may lead to generalization errors during the improvement stage in the classification model. A high-quality classifier should analyze the training set finely and it must precisely categorize each occurrence of data in the dataset. The best significant as well as stimulating stage in constructing a solution model is the selection of algorithm.

Computer-aided diagnosis (CADx) or Computer-aided detection (CADe) systems assist physicians in the interpretation of medical signals and images. Medical images like MRI, X-ray, and ultrasound images provide a large amount of information about the patients' condition. The radiologist or other qualified persons or physicians analyze the image and diagnose the discrepancy in the images if any, in a short period of time. The computer-aided design for medical diagnosis is an interdisciplinary technique that combines the essentials of AI technique and computer vision with radiological image processing methods. Detection of blocks in heart chambers or valves is the representative application. CAD tools are used in the preventive medical check-ups, such as the cases in mammography, lung cancer, and detection of polyps in the colon. These systems mark conspicuous structures and sections and evaluate them. For instance, in mammograms, CAD systems are used, which highlight micro-calcification segments or clusters and hyper-dense portions of the structures in the soft tissues. This helps the physicians or radiologists to describe conclusions about the condition of the patients. In another application, quantification can be performed where the tumor's manners in contrast medium or dimension of a tumor or can be retrieved.

In computer-aided simple triage (CAST) type of computer-aided diagnosis, a completely automatic opening version and triage of studies can be categorized into some significant groups like negative or positive). In urgent situation, where an exact diagnosis of life-threatening critical situation is required to be identified, CAST is predominantly relevant.

Although computer-aided methods are used in clinical environment for several decades, they cannot replace doctors or other professionals. They rather play a supporting role and the professional is in general accountable for the final analysis of a medical image. On the other hand, some CAD systems are used to detect the most basic signs of defects in patients, which the human professionals are not able to predict like architectural distortion in mammograms, diabetic retinopathy, ground-glass nodules in thoracic CT, and non-polypoid lesions in CT colonography.

Healthcare domain has created a remarkable place for Machine learning (ML) and its subset deep learning (DL) [5–9]. Although lots of traditional computer-aided detection (CAD) systems are increasingly used in analysis of healthcare data, the efficacy of these, is a topic of controversy [10–12] in this artificial intelligence world. A machine or deep learning algorithm can be applied to identify breast cancer as good as radiologists and can be accepted and incorporated into clinical practice. The purpose of work is to assess the performance of ML models with Preprocessing technique called PCA and to deal with the outliers to improve the accuracy and to analyze the dataset with ML techniques to identify which suits better for the real-world scenario.

12.4 ML CLASSIFIERS IN BREAST CANCER DIAGNOSIS

A worldwide significant health issue among women in current scenario is breast cancer. It represents the majority of the cancer problems and cancer-related diseases and deaths. Early prognosis of these types of cancer could promote timely clinical treatment and improve the chance of survival significantly. Further, undergoing unnecessary treatments can be avoided by accurate classification of benign tumors in an early stage. Prompt diagnosis of breast cancer and classification of the tumor cells into malignant or benign groups is to a great extent needed and is now an important area of research. As machine learning techniques has exceptional compensation like serious features recognition particularly in medical field, they are extensively chosen for breast cancer classification and forecast modelling. The research work in this chapter aims to experiment the cancer dataset for prediction of malignant and benign cells using the classifiers such as Decision Tree Classifier, Random Forest Classifier, Naive Bayes Classifier, Support Vector Machines, Logistic Regression, and K Nearest Neighbor. Training time and dimensionality can be reduced by machine learning models with preprocessing techniques. The effect of outliers has also been analyzed and reduced. The accuracy and other performance metrics of machine learning algorithms are compared and an optimal algorithm is suggested.

Breast cancer is the most commonly diagnosed illness among women across the world and it is the second most important basis of death [13]. Digital mammography (DM) is the most important screening test that could identify the breast cancer two years ahead of the cell growth felt by women or physician.

In investigative workup environment [14], DM has been made known to diminish the breast malignancy. In standard medical practice, mammograms are evaluated by the radiologists and Classification is done based on the American College of Radiology Breast Imaging Reporting and Data System (BI-RADS) lexicon [15]. If any abnormality is detected in mammogram, a diagnostic workup that includes imaging modalities or additional mammographic views is typically required. Further evaluation using biopsy is recommended when lesion is suspicious. There are some risk factors which might raise the possibility of getting affected with breast cancer. Roughly about 80 percent of breast cancers are found in women neighboring the age of 50. Family history and Personal history may also raise the risk. Women who are with definite genetic mutations, as well as changes to the Breast Cancer (BRCA1 and BRCA2) genes, are at increased risk of having breast cancer during their life. Childbearing and menstrual history and other gene changes may also raise the risk. Due to the subtle difference between lesions and background fibro-glandular tissue, non-rigid nature of the breast and different lesion types, analysis of these images is difficult which leads to significant inter-observer and intra-observer variability [16].

In this work, six commonly used Machine Learning techniques are used for classification of cancer cells as malignant or benign. They are: 1. Decision Tree Classifier, 2. Random Forest Classifier, 3. Naive Bayes Classifier, 4. Support Vector Machines, 5. K Nearest Neighbor, and 6. Logistic Regression

The number of features used in this dataset is 32 and some of them include radius, smoothness, compactness, concavity, symmetry, and texture-perimeter. There are totally 600 datasets considered in this research work among which 20% are considered for testing and evaluation of algorithm.

12.4.1 Logistic Regression

The supervised machine learning technique, Logistic Regression, is generally used in estimation based on possibilities. The effect of regression models is a numerical value whereas the effect of logistic regression is an unconditional variable. Sigmoid function or logistic function, a more complex cost function, is used by Logistic Regression. The theory of logistic regression states that the hypothesis function will have the values varying from 0 to 1 as given in the equation (12.1).

$$0 \leq h_\theta(x) \leq 1 \tag{12.1}$$

Sigmoid function is used to map the predicted values to various probabilities $(Z) = \sigma(\beta_0 + \beta_1 X)$ *with* $Z = \beta_0 + \beta_1 X$. Accordingly the hypothesis is stated by equation (12.2),

$$h\theta(X) = \frac{1}{1 + e^{-(\beta 0 + \beta 1 X)}} \quad (12.2)$$

Optimization objective is represented by cost function $J(\theta)$. Cost function must be minimalized to build an exact model with smallest error. The function given in equation (12.3) represents the cost function

After calculation of the cost, the cost should be reduced.

$$J(\theta) = -\frac{1}{m} \sum [y^{(i)} \log(h\theta(x(i))) + (1 - y^{(i)}) \log(1 - h\theta(x(i)))] \quad (12.3)$$

Gradient Descent method is used for cost reduction. It is done by calculating the gradient descent function on each parameter as mentioned in equation (12.4).

$$\theta_J := \theta_J - \alpha \frac{\partial J(\theta)}{\partial \theta_J} \quad (12.4)$$

Gradient descent method is similar to imagining ourselves at mountain top with a plan to reach the bottom of the hill when left stranded or blindfolded. Taking a move is analogous to one iteration to revise the parameters.

12.4.2 K-Nearest Neighbor (k-NN) Algorithm

A supervised machine learning algorithm, K-Nearest Neighbor which presume related things are present in close proximity. Similar choice of this algorithm is to calculate the Euclidean distance between points. For a chosen number of neighbors, K is initialized as soon as training data is loaded. Then, the distance between the current sample and the query is calculated for each sample in the data. Then to an ordered collection, the index and the distance of the sample are added and sorted based on the distance values. The first K records in the sorted group are picked along with their labels. For classification/regression problems, mode/mean of K labels is returned. When the value of k is 1, the data point is categorized into a group that has one adjoining neighbor alone. Several values of k are tried for classification or regression, and the best one that fits is chosen as the right K. It's simple to realize but becomes slow significantly as the data grows in size

12.4.3 Support Vector Machine

Support vector machine is applied to both classification and regression tasks. This algorithm provides considerable accuracy with minimum computation power. The aim of the SVM is to use support vectors to separate data points into two classes and to locate an N dimensional hyperplane for N features. The prime motto is to locate the plane with maximum margin between the possible hyperplanes. Upcoming data point classification is made confidently by making the margin distance maximum amongst the support vectors. As the count of hyperplanes equals the count of features, envisioning the plane with feature count greater than 3 is not easy. The position of the hyperplane changes due to the deletion of the support vectors. When the output parameter exceeds 1, the corresponding data is categorized as one of the classes and when the output is –1, it is recognized as an alternative class. To exploit the margin linking the hyper plane and the data points, the hinge loss function is employed which is shown in equation (12.5).

$$c(x, y, f(x)) = (1 - y*f(x))_{+} \tag{12.5}$$

When the actual and the predicted value are of the identical sign, the cost is 0. Otherwise, the loss value is computed. To set equilibrium on the margin maximization and loss, regularization constraint is included with the cost function. Once the regularization parameter is included, the cost functions looks like the equation shown in (12.6).

$$min_w \ \boldsymbol{\lambda}\|\boldsymbol{w}\|^2 + \sum_{i=1}^{n} (1 - y_i < x_i, w >)_{+} \tag{12.6}$$

Computing partial derivatives with reference to the weights and making the weights updated,

$$w = w - \alpha(2.\ \boldsymbol{\lambda}.\ w) \tag{12.7}$$

$$w = w + \alpha(y_i.\ x_i - 2.\ \boldsymbol{\lambda}.\ w) \tag{12.8}$$

When the model correctly predicts the class, and there is no misclassification in the model, only the gradients have to be updated. Otherwise, if misclassification is there and the model composes a mistake during the prediction, the error needs to be added with the regularization constraint as shown in equations (12.7) and (12.8) during gradient update is performed.

12.4.4 Random Forest Classifier

Decision Trees are the basic blocks of the random forest algorithms or models. Random forest is a compilation of huge quantity of discrete decision trees which functions as a group. Every singular tree in the random forest contributes in estimation of class. The class with large number of participation is the model's calculation. The main concept in random forest classification is that a large number of moderately uncorrelated trees functioning in a group will surpass any of the individual component trees or models. The little association amongst the models has a large amount of importance and it is a helpful thing as they can make ensemble calculation. This provides more accurate result compared to individual predictions. The rationale behind this brilliant outcome is that the trees keep each other from their individual misconceptions. So the nuts and bolts to carry out random forest fit are:

1. A number of definite signals need to be there in features, which would help the models to be built with good results compared to that with random guessing.
2. The predictions and hence the miscalculations must have minimal correlations to all others.

12.4.5 Naive Bayes Classifier

Naive Bayes classifier is a machine learning probabilistic model used for classification of tasks. It has a core representation from Bayes theorem as shown in equation (12.9).

$$P(y|X) = \frac{P(X|y)P(y)}{P(X)} \tag{12.9}$$

Bayes theorem can be used to know the probability of what has happened to X, When Y has occurred. Here the variable Y is substantiation and the variable X is hypothetical. Since assumptions are made as predictors/features are independent, it is called naive. The parameters/features represented as Variable X are shown in equation (12.10).

$$X = (x1,\ x2,\ x3,\ \ldots\ \ldots\ xn) \tag{12.10}$$

By substituting X value and expanding Probability using the chain rule equation (12.11) is retrieved.

$$P(y|x_1,x_2 \ldots ..x_n) = \frac{P\ (x_1,|y) \ldots \ldots \ldots \ldots \ldots\ P(x_n|y)P(y)}{P(X_1)P(X_2) \ldots \ldots \ldots P(X_n)} \tag{12.11}$$

Since for all entries of the dataset, there is no change in the denominator of (11), it can be removed. Introducing proportionality, we get equation (12.12)

$$P(y|x_1,x_2 \ldots ..x_n) \alpha\ P(y) \prod_{i=1}^{n} P(x_i|y) \tag{12.12}$$

As the classification can be multivariate, the class y with maximum value of probability is given by equation (12.13)

$$\mathrm{y} = \mathrm{argmax}_y\, P(y) \prod_{i=1}^{n} P(x_i|y) \tag{12.13}$$

The above function can be used to obtain the class when given with the predictors. Though Naive Bias classifiers are working fast and they are straightforward to put into practice, there is a requirement that the predictors must be independent. But in many cases, the predictors are not independent and so hindrance occurs in the performance of the classifier.

12.4.6 Decision Tree Classifiers

Decision tree classifier is an accurate potential classification model appropriate for diverse applications. This classifier is used in energy-based applications also. All the nodes in the decision tree represent a check on features and each subdivision coming down after the node keeps up a correspondence with one of the possible values of particular feature. Each leaf characterize the class labels connected to each occurrence. By directing from the topmost of the tree to a leaf at the end, classification of instances is done. The classification is established from the outcomes alongside the conforming path.

Starting from the root node of the tree, the instance gap is divided by each node into two or more sub-spaces dependent on the feature test situation. Then a new node is created by moving down the tree branch matching to the attribute value. This procedure is frequent for all the subtrees, until all statistics in the training data are classified. Gini index impurity-based criterion can be used to divide the records and developing the tree uses [17].

12.4.7 Dimensionality Reduction Algorithms

Principal Component Analysis (PCA) and Linear Discriminant Analysis (LDA) are the two algorithms used for dimensionality reduction. Information of classes is analyzed in LDA, to extract the different features in order to exploit the ability of separation. The ability of separation is maximized by inspecting the variance of each and every feature in PCA. Data is summarized in PCA by a set of values with low dimension. PCA looks for the variances in every feature that presents great variance to make a reasonable splitting amid the classes. Statistically, it accomplishes a linear transformation of unique features to a new subordinate dimensional space composed of principal components. This will be then used in reducing overfitting and dimensionality reduction.

12.5 MATERIALS AND METHODS

The dataset used in this work was obtained from the University of Wisconsin, where the features are calculated from a digitized picture of a fine needle aspirate (FNA) of a breast mass. Biopsy procedure in FNA, place a thin needle into an area of unusual cells at the time of monitoring by ultrasound monitors or CT scan. These collected data sample are then transferred to examine if cells in the biopsy are normal or not. The data set attributes have the information about Diagnosis (M = malignant, B = benign) and ID number. or each sample of the cell nucleus, 10 real-valued features considered are texture, area, radius, perimeter, compactness, smoothness, concave points, concavity, fractal dimension and symmetry. The mean, standard error and worst of features are calculated, which results in distinct

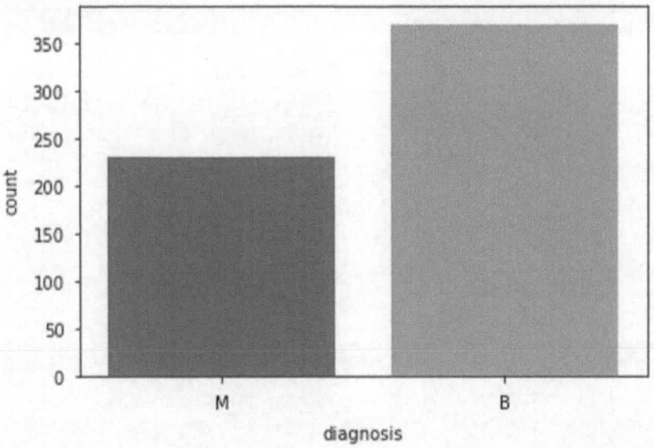

FIGURE 12.1 Number of malignant and benign cases.

30 features. Figure 12.1 shows the classification data for the entire dataset. The number of cases with Malignant and Benign is represented with M and B, respectively. Medical records, significant to breast cancer, are taken from database to model, train, and predict whether a tumor is benign or malignant.

In this retrospective study, datasets of 600 women are considered with 32 features. The correlation among the 32 features is represented as heat map and is shown in Figure 12.2 in which the features that are highly correlated and lightly correlated and uncorrelated are shown. Training is done with the most popular machine learning algorithms like Logistic regression, Support vector machine, KNN algorithm, Random forest decision tree, Decision tree classifier and Naïve bias classifier. Testing of the trained model has been performed with the 20% of the dataset.

Histograms in Figure 12.3 show the overall data distribution of the features radius, area, texture, and concavity.

The boxplot shown in Figure 12.4 displays the distribution of data and also it provides information about outliers. To deal with outliers, the data size has been increased with the additional features like standard error and worst values. The figures also describe that most benign cells have smaller area and radius and concavity than malignant cells. It is essential to assess the performance of the classifiers once the model is obtained using machine learning techniques. Sensitivity, specificity and accuracy are the parameters used in evaluating performance of the ML models.

Sensitivity measures how far the classifier classify the true positives correctly. Specificity is the classifier measures the ability of the classifier to identify true negatives correctly as negatives. Accuracy is a measure of correct predictions over the total number of predictions. To obtain trustworthy results from the model, training samples and testing samples should be suitably large and they must be independent.

The performance measures like True positive, False positive, True negative, and False negative are taken from the confusion matrix. Sensitivity, Specificity and

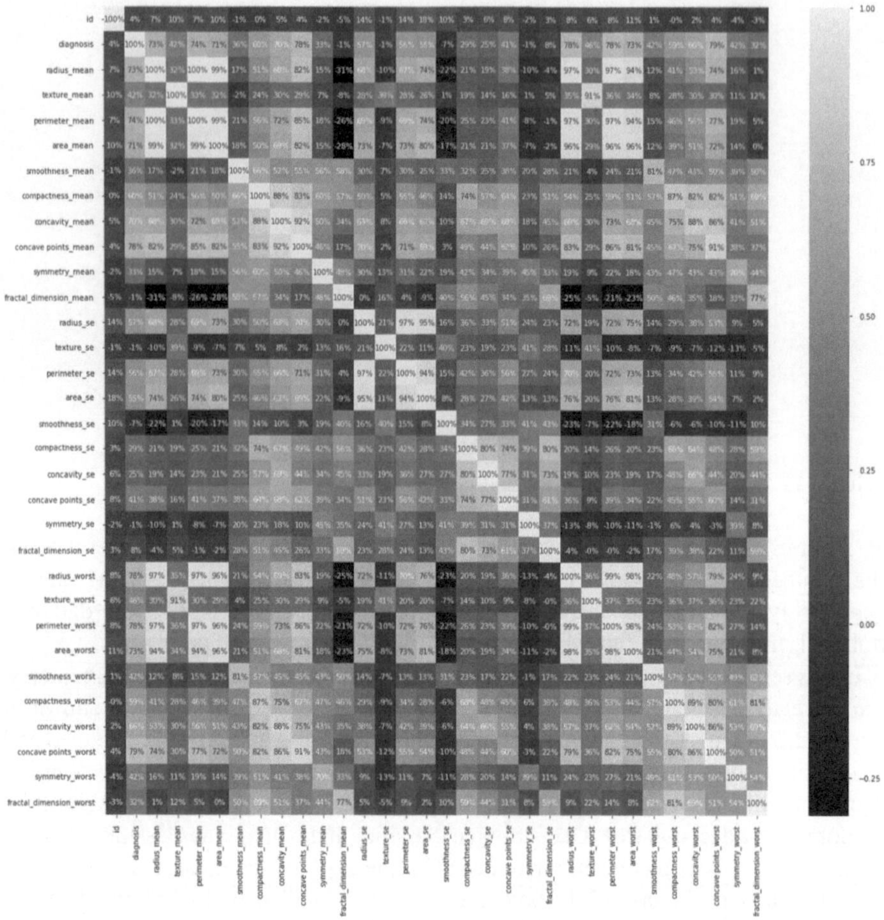

FIGURE 12.2 Heatmap showing correlation of features.

precision are also calculated. The results make it evident that the random forest classifier provides better performance in classification of malignant and benign. The accuracy of different algorithms are K Nearest Neighbor-81.8, Logistic Regression-63.8, Naive bias classifier-65.5, Support Vector Machines-64.7, Decision tree classifier-92.4 and Random forest classifier-95.68

12.6 CONCLUSION

This work for the most part is focused on the available predictive models and improvement in these models to accomplish good quality accuracy. The random forest model has attained an accurateness of 95%, which is the maximum one compared to the other mentioned algorithms. This improvement is attained by preprocessing the data before the processes of testing and training. By raising the dimension of the dataset, the outlier issues have been eliminated. Result analysis

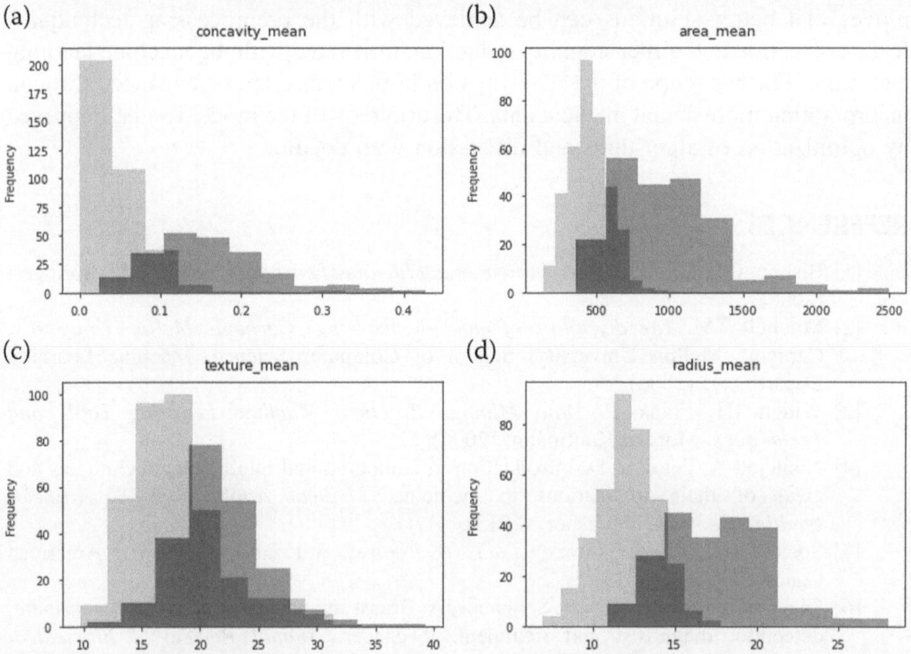

FIGURE 12.3 Overall data distribution for the features radius, area, texture, and concavity.

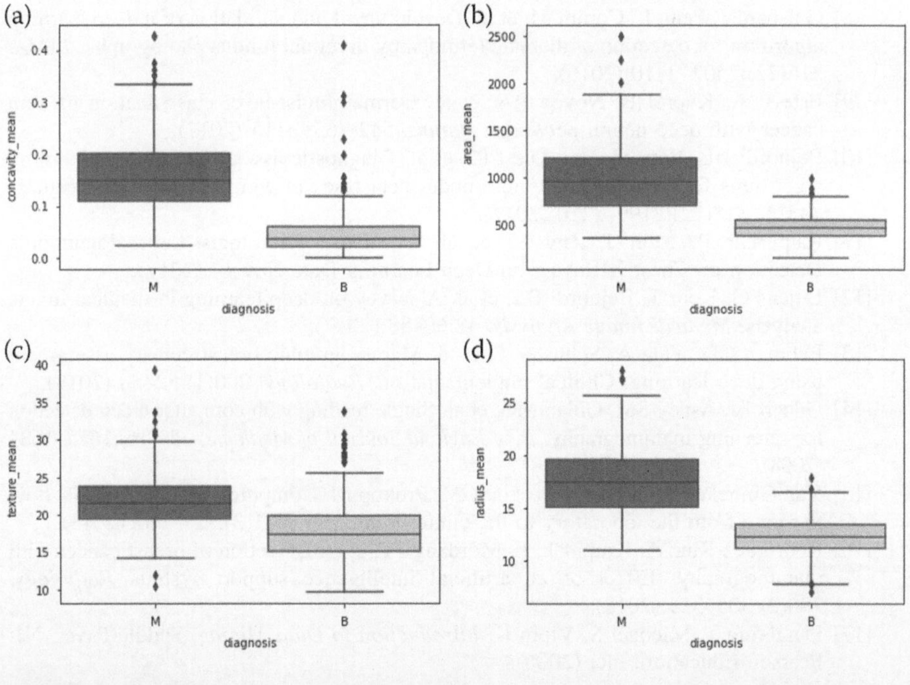

FIGURE 12.4 Distribution of data with outliers.

proves that better solutions can be achieved with the preprocessing techniques-feature selection and dimensionality reduction, integrated with the machine learning algorithm. Further scope of the investigation in this arena can be enhanced through incorporating more actual medical data. The accuracy of the model can be improved by optimization of algorithms and discussion with doctors.

REFERENCES

[1] Bishop CM. *Pattern Recognition and Machine Learning*. New York: Springer; (2006).

[2] Mitchell TM. *The discipline of machine learning: Carnegie Mellon University*. Carnegie Mellon University, School of Computer Science, Machine Learning Department; (2006).

[3] Witten IH, Frank E. *Data Mining: Practical Machine Learning Tools and Techniques*. Morgan Kaufmann; (2005).

[4] Niknejad A, Petrovic D. Introduction to computational intelligence techniques and areas of their applications in medicine. *Medical Applications of Artificial Intelligence*. CRC Publisher; (2013).

[5] Society AC. *Global Cancer Facts & Figures*. 3rd Edition. Atlanta: American Cancer Society; (2015).

[6] Giger ML, Karssemeijer N, Schnabel JA. Breast image analysis for risk assessment, detection, diagnosis, and treatment of cancer. *Annual Review of Biomedical Engineering*. 15:327–357 (2013).

[7] Sickles EA, D'Orsi CJ, Bassett LW. *American College of Radiology Breast Imaging Reporting and Data System Atlas Reston*, VA: American College of Radiology; (2013).

[8] Gulshan V, Peng L, Coram M, et al. Development and validation of a deep learning algorithm for detection of diabetic retinopathy in retinal fundus photographs. *JAMA*. 316(22):2402–2410 (2016).

[9] Esteva A, Kuprel B, Novoa RA, et al. Dermatologist-level classification of skin cancer with deep neural networks. *Nature*. 542(7639):115 (2017).

[10] Bejnordi BE, Veta M, Van Diest PJ, et al. Diagnostic assessment of deep learning algorithms for detection of lymph node metastases in women with breast cancer. *JAMA*. 318(22):2199–2210 (2017).

[11] Rajpurkar P, Irvin J, Zhu K, et al. CheXNet: Radiologist-Level Pneumonia Detection on Chest X-Rays with Deep Learning Date Nov 14 (2017).

[12] Litjens G, Kooi T, Bejnordi BE, et al. A survey on deep learning in medical image analysis. *Medical Image Analysis*. 42:60–88 (2017).

[13] Lehman CD, Yala A, Schuster T, et al. Mammographic breast density assessment using deep learning: Clinical implementation. *Radiology*. 290(1):52–58 (2018).

[14] Gilbert FJ, Astley SM, Gillan MG, et al. Single reading with computer-aided detection for screening mammography. *New England Journal of Medicine*. 359(16):1675–1684 (2008).

[15] Van Ginneken B, Schaefer-Prokop CM, Prokop M. Computer-aided diagnosis: how to move from the laboratory to the clinic. *Radiology*. 261(3):719–732 (2011).

[16] Rodríguez-Ruiz A, Krupinski E, Mordang J-J, et al. Detection of breast cancer with mammography: Effect of an artificial intelligence support system. *Radiology*. 290(2):305–314 (2018).

[17] PangNing T, Michael S, Vipin K. *Introduction to Data Mining*. Saddle River, NJ: Pearson Education, Inc; (2006).

13 Dual Customized U-Net-based Automated Diagnosis of Glaucoma

C. Thirumarai Selvi
Professor, Department of ECE, Sri Krishna College of Engineering and Technology, Coimbatore, Tamil Nadu, India

J. Amudha
Associate Professor, Department of EEE, Dr Mahalingam College of Engineering and Technology, Pollachi, Tamil Nadu, India

R. Sudhakar
Professor and Head, Department of ECE, Dr Mahalingam College of Engineering and Technology, Pollachi, Tamil Nadu, India

CONTENTS

13.1 Introduction......221
13.2 Literature Review......224
13.3 Proposed Work......226
13.4 Performance Measures......229
13.5 Simulation Results......230
13.5.1 Optic Disc Segmentation......230
13.6 Conclusion......240
References......240

13.1 INTRODUCTION

In our nation, diagnosis of disease severity is done generally by the expertise and experienced doctors, but still, there are situations of incorrect diagnosis and treatment are being reported. Patients have to undergo several tests that are very costly and occasionally all of them are not necessary but are forced needlessly into patients to increase the bill. Glaucoma is one of the optic nerve diseases reasoned due to a rise in intraocular pressure and affects the capacity of human vision. Due to a lack of detailed information, each fundus image takes an expert eight minutes to

DOI: 10.1201/9781003217497-13

annotate. Glaucoma is the second most common cause of vision loss after cataracts. Quigley et al [1] reported that around 60 million patients were diagnosed worldwide in 2010 and it is estimated that 80 million individuals would be affected by glaucoma by 2020. Glaucoma can cause irreversible damage to the optic nerve, leading to blindness if it is not correctly diagnosed. As a result, early detection of glaucoma is critical for the management of the disease's first-line remedial treatment. Figure 13.1 gives the details of eye image with normal and glaucoma. It also represents the optic cup and disc areas. The clarity of vision of a particular scenario is represented both without glaucoma and glaucoma is depicted in Figure 13.1. The Glaucoma detected eye focuses only on the center part and boundaries are darkened.

As a result, a boundary-marking system that is automated will be incredibly useful. Despite the existence of a number of segmentation algorithms, generating a reliable cup boundary from the CFI remains a difficult issue due to the lack of a distinct visual demarcation between the cup and the disc. At present, there are two existing approaches available named as classical and deep learning (DL). To parameterize disc and cup boundaries, the traditional method employs a combination of image processing techniques such as edge detection, wavelets, Hough transforms, and active contours. The DL-based technique, on the other hand, uses pipelines to segregate cup and disc and also necessitates additional pre-processing for considerable image resizing. Image-net pre-trained models with layers for disc and blood vessel segmentation, but not for cup segmentation, are used to obtain features.

The main focus of computer vision is to model and imitate human vision with the help of computer software and hardware. Computer vision worked together with graph theory has been popularized and successful in low-level tasks and high-level tasks. The low-level task includes object tracking, image segmentation, stereo matching, etc. On the contrary, high-level tasks are involved as object recognition, image classification, image parsing, etc. The goal of picture segmentation is to divide the input image into non-overlapping parts that are meaningful. In graph cut theory, the very first step is to map the image pixels on a graph. The graph is modeled by a set of nodes and edges. Automated type of segmentation algorithm finds applications in a variety of situations such as multimedia retrieval which requires faster, coarser, and region-based segmentation. Some applications entail accurate semantic objects, such kind of segmentation necessitates fully automated segmentation which is not possible. Interactive segmentation provides a solution for the above.

U-Net owns its name because of its symmetrical structure. Contracting (Down-sampling path), Bottleneck, and Expansive are the three sections (Up-sampling path). Here, the contracting path consists of four blocks and each block includes a convolutional layer and pooling layer. The bottle network is built up with two convolutional layers for normalization and dropout paths. Each of the four blocks in the expanding route consists of a de-convolutional unit, concatenation, and convolutional layer.

The following is a breakdown of the paper's structure: Section 13.2 explains the cutting-edge techniques of our proposed method. Section 13.3 enumerates the

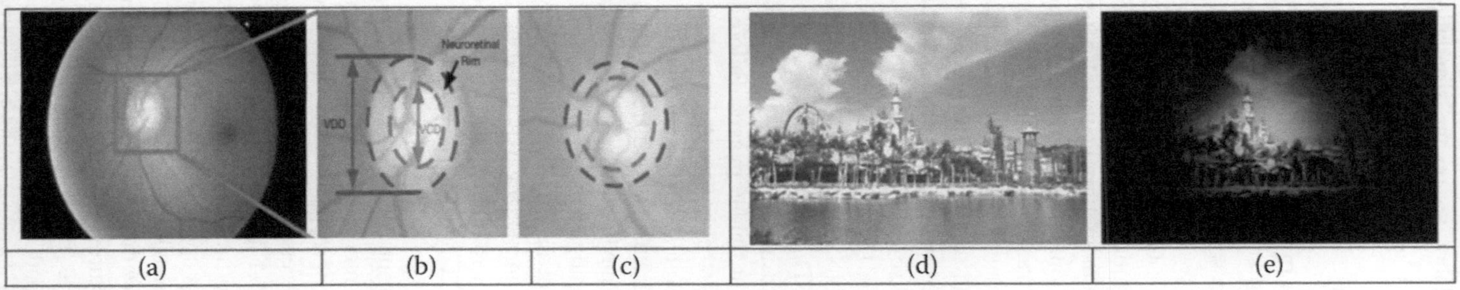

FIGURE 13.1 *Basics of Normal (absence of disease) and Glaucoma vision* (a) Fundus Image (b) Normal (c) Glaucoma (d) No Vision Loss (Normal) (e) Vision Loss (Glaucoma).

proposed work. Section 13.4 elaborates on the simulation results of the experimentation and finally, in Section 13.5, the conclusion and future work are discussed.

13.2 LITERATURE REVIEW

For retinal pictures, Sharath et al [2] studied retinal depth estimate as well as optic cup-disc segmentation. For depth segmentation, this method uses a fully convolutional network, and for multiple scale feature extraction, it uses dilated residual interception.

The inception module includes Google-net with slight modification in the convolution known as dilated convolution. Also, a residual function is employed in the network which overcomes the vanishing gradients introduced in the deep networks. For optic cup and disc segmentation, Huazhu Fu et al [3] used a multi-label network with polar transformation. This transformation has advantages like balancing cup proportion, augmentation equivalence, and spatial constraint. AUC of 0.6 arrives after the segmentation of cup and disc in ORIGA data sets.

Aquino et al [4] has segmented optical cup and disc using Convolutional Neural Network. CNN emphasizes the disc pallor without blood vessel obstruction. Coarse localization is performed using the Daubechies wavelet. It is used to skeletonize the vessel masks. Three classes of CNN are used for segmentation. CNN is trained with features exaggerated and original. This results in AUC value of 0.84and the sensitivity level is between 0.4-0.75. Gilbert Lim [5] has discussed automatic optic detection to verify the abnormality detection in fundus images. Before training this method performs whitening for normalizing the image. A cascaded classifier is involved in segmentation. The experiment is tested on different datasets that are publically available. Hannan et al [6] have discussed the different state-of-the-art techniques for optic cup and disc segmentation methods as a survey. Almazroa et al [7] have developed a pipelined fully convolutional neural network combined with a residual network for medical image segmentation. The model fully convolutional network operates for low capacity which normalizes its input data. Next, the prediction procedure is measured with a fully convolutional residual network Drozdol et al [8]. This novel method is tested for both CT and MRI data sets. The model is trained for 50 epochs in the Keras framework.

Vorontsov et al [9] have presented liver lesion segmentation by joint segmentation. It uses a simple one-stage model that can train end to end. The segmentation algorithm is tested with a dataset of metastatic lesions of 200 numbers in volume. In the 200 volume of data, only 130 sets are given for public verification. The network is trained using 115 examples, and the network is tested using 15 data sets. Three stages of segmentations are performed in this work. The very first segmentation is the rough one. Second, 2D FCN is applied for segmenting liver and lesions. Finally, 3D FCN segmentation is done by taking the input from the first stage of segmentation. Ronneberger et al [10] have discussed biomedical image segmentation based on U-Net. In general U-Net captures, the context through contraction and localization, using expansion structure. This net conventionally uses FCN with modification in the up-sampling path. The network uses the Caffe model for implementation. The model achieves an average IoU of 77.5%.

Harry Pratt et al. [11] have briefed about convolutional neural networks for diabetic retinopathy. This work decided to increase in convolutional layer to learn more features. The first CNN layer learns the features and the last layer of it is used mainly for classification. Training of 10,290 images is performed with 120 epochs. On the Kaggle dataset, it determined its accuracy value of about 95%. Diabetic retinopathy identification and classification of microaneurysms for early detection has been explored by Usman Akram et al [12]. Three-stage filter banks are used for identification. The model is supported by Gaussian and SVM classifier, which results in more accuracy.

Khaled [13] has reviewed the different states of methods for early identification of diabetic retinopathy's numerous eye ailments. This study helps to fill the gap between various diabetic-affected eye diseases with many local search techniques using deep learning. Habib et al. [14] suggested an ensemble classifier for detecting microaneurysms. This method detects the initial sets by a Gaussian mixture model. After that, a tree ensemble classifier with 70 features is used to classify the data. This works scores the ROC of 0.415. Also, this classifier exhibits consistent results across various data sets.

Wong et al [15] have discussed a work to compute the optic disc to cup ratio using the level set method. This method is tested for 104 image data sets and presented the CDR value by 0.2 units for the given ground truth. The main limitations of the techniques, which are analyzed for handcrafted measures (CDR, ACDR, ISNT rule, and vessel kinks) is not matching with the human expert's estimation. Bock et al [16] have presented a data-driven-based algorithm whose results are very closer to estimation be human experts. A system discussed by Joshi et al [17] is based on finding vessels bend at the boundary of optic disc and cup. The size of the vessel and the circular Hough transform were used to find the optic disc. The computed CDR error ranges from 0.12+/0.10. Also, Lin et al [18] employed the circular Hough transform to segment the optic cup and disc. With an average dice coefficient of 0.92, they tested their methods on 325 image data sets. Diaz et al [19] have worked on an automatic segmentation algorithm for measuring the handcrafted features, such as rim thickness by inferior superior nasal temporal rule, CDR and area CDR ratio. The computed sensitivity and specificity values for 53 pictures data set were 0.81 and 0.87, respectively, according to the experimented results. Cheng et al [20] used 650 images to test superpixel classification-based optic cup and disc segmentation. For two separate databases, they tested and attained an area under the curve of 0.8, 0.822. They have combined the area under the curve from fundus images with glaucoma screening methods and achieved AUC of 0.866. They evaluated their performance by utilizing the patient's personal data and patient's genome data.

Artem Sevastopolsky [21] has developed alterations to the U-Net convolutional neural method for detecting glaucoma using the optic cup and disc segmentation. This deep learning methodology has experimented on DRISHTI-GS, DRIONS-DN, RIM ONE v.3 publically available data sets. This technique outperforms the other state of art techniques by prediction time. Maninis et al [22] have demonstrated deep-learning-based optic disc segmentation of retinal images. This technology applies a transfer learning procedure and VGG16 based fully convolutional neural network. They achieved human expert quality of dice score and boundary error. Zilly et al [23] have recorded the fundus image optic-cup and disc segmentation by employing improvement in the convolutional filter with entropy sampling. Adaboost classifier has used in the hierarchical network for mosaic slab classification was found by Dogan and Akay [24]. Maninis [22] method has the drawback of longer execution time for training, large model size, and requires more General Processing Unit (GPU) memory. Zilly [23] techniques are more complicated, difficult to program and to produce results. In the entropy sampling method, images have to be cropped for the optic disc area before the training. Artem's [21] work has focused on lesser prediction time, but the edges are more delicate to bring more accurate classification. It further requires some enhancement in optic cup segmentation.

The architecture presented in the work resembles the original U network, which includes, on the left, there is a contracting path, and on the right, there is an expanded path. Information from the left side layers is merged in the expansive path with different scales like appropriate resolution and low resolution. Then rectified linear unit function is applied. Finally, a max-pooling operation is used to reduce image height and width. Then, the image is processed multiple times through the above-mentioned steps until low resolution is obtained.

13.3 PROPOSED WORK

This model depicts in Figure 13.2 accepts an image as input of glaucoma or normal patient. In the pre-processing, step image is enhanced after the homomorphic filtering process with contrast stretching using histogram equalization. Then the augmented data are collected after the application of a dual customized U deep learning network for a single image. By averaging these high-resolution feature maps, we can perform the image classification as glaucoma or normal patient. Using this stratagem, we have assessed our model and modified U-Net with various performance indicators.

The proposed model's block diagram is shown in Figure 13.3. RIM ONE V3 fundus image data sets in the pre-processing stage are read by the OpenCV and converted into NumPy array. For the optic cup, segmentation is properly done to crop the area of the optic disc. The proposed model can work either through cropping or without cropping. Cropping can be only done for optic cup segmentation. Images are cropped for the optic cup by 256 × 256 and for optic disc by 512 × 512. Then region of interest is done through the bilinear interpolation. The images were prepared for training after the pre-processed steps. The dataset contains 159 images, of which 127 are utilized for training and the remaining are applied for testing. The performance of the neural network degrades with respect to an increase in data. Hence data

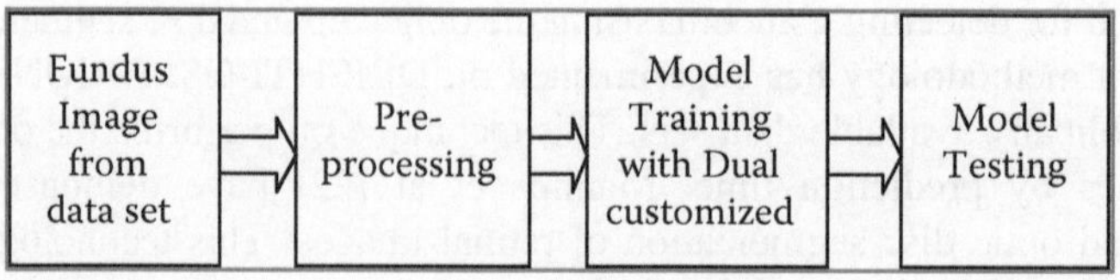

FIGURE 13.2 Workflow of the proposed model.

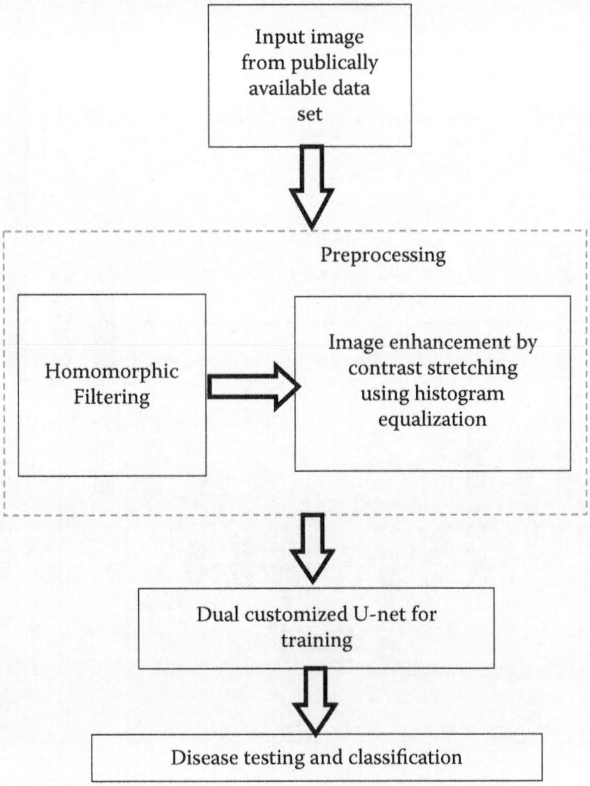

FIGURE 13.3 Block diagram of the proposed model.

augmentation based deep learning technique is used for training and classification. The convolutional neural network is more popular in data segmentation and classification.

VGG-16 net gains are used to create a fully conventional neural network. The original U-Net has an overall total of 5888 filters. The modified U-Net that was used in the existing methods has an overall total of 1024 filters. The proposed U-Net that was modified from the original U-Net has an overall total of 1216 filters.

The updated U-Net is superior to the original U-Net. U-Net that was proposed by Artem [21] as discussed earlier in the existing method has a a smaller number of filters in all convolutional layers and does not possess an increasing number of filters for decreasing resolution.

Compared to the modified U-Net that was used in the existing method, the presented modification has much greater number of filters in all convolutional layers and does not possess an increasing number of filters for decreasing resolution.

In comparison to the existing method, our proposed method has more filters. As a result, it is clear that the performance of our proposed approach may be superior to that of the present method. But the real question is about the training time and the

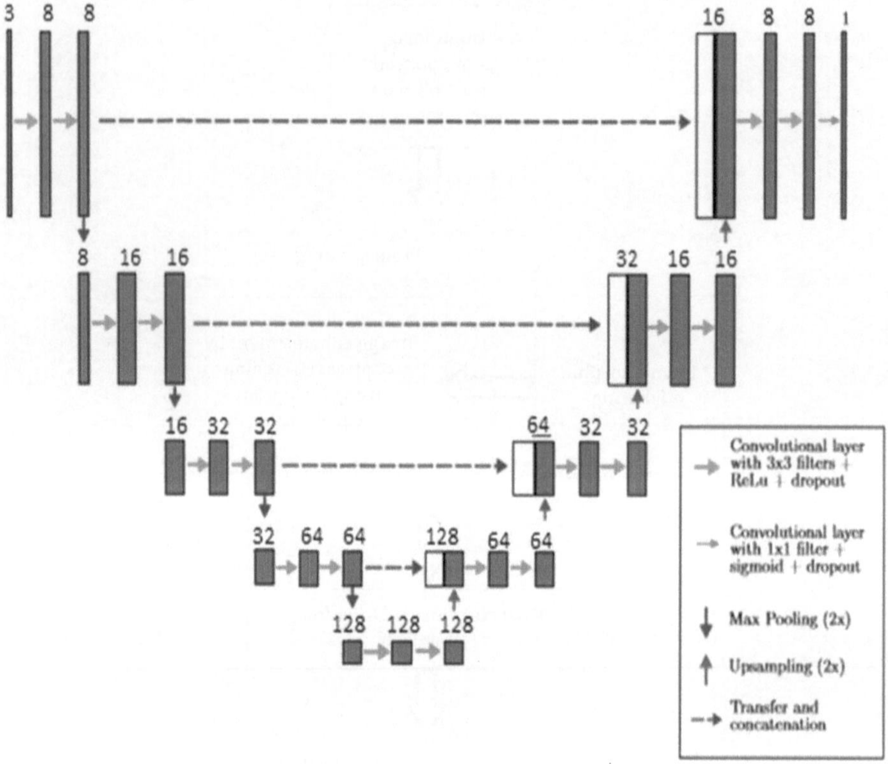

FIGURE 13.4 Architecture of neural network employed in proposed method.

prediction time of our method. Because our suggested method in Figure 13.4 has a much smaller number of filters than the original U-Net model, it is evident that our proposed model's prediction and training times beat the original U-Net model's training and prediction times.

The eye fundus images of the human eye along with the ground truth form the dataset for our project. There are many databases of eye fundus images that are available in public such as DRIONS-DB, RIM-ONE v.1, RIM-ONE v.2, RIM-ONE v.3, DRISHTI-GS, etc. We used RIM-ONE v.3 database for all the tests that are performed in this project. Keras and Open CV software are used to test this work. Numpy also supports several operations to be performed on its data.

Pandas is an open-source, BSD-licensed library for the Python programming language that provides high-performance, easy-to-use data structures, and data analysis tools. Pandas are used to view the results of our experiments. It is also used to export the results to the disc. Matplotlib is a Python 2D plotting package that generates high-quality figures in a range of hardcopy and interactive formats across platforms. With just a few lines of code, it can generate plots, histograms, power spectra, bar charts, error charts, scatter plots, and more. The plotting graphs are used for performance comparison and also to display the resulted in segmentation masks.

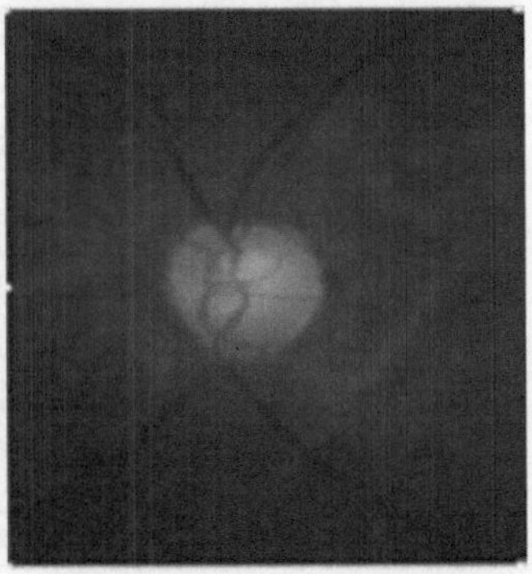

FIGURE 13.5 RIM-ONE V3 fundus image.

13.4 PERFORMANCE MEASURES

There are two metrics that we used in these experiments. They are the Dice score and Intersection over Union (IoU) score. The Jaccard index, commonly known as the Intersection over Union (IoU) measure, is a way for quantifying the percent overlap between the target mask and our forecast output. This metric is similar to the Dice coefficient, which is frequently used as a training loss function. Figures 13.5–13.7 depicts the RIM ONE data set used for testing the proposed method.

$$J(A, B) = x = \frac{|A \cap B|}{|A \cup B|} = \frac{|A \cap B|}{|A| + |B| - |A \cap B|} \tag{13.1}$$

Where A is the predicted output map with foreground information and B is the correct binary map.

Dice Score for the given two sets X and Y is given as DSC

$$\mathrm{DSC} = \frac{2|X \cap Y|}{|X| + |Y|} \tag{13.2}$$

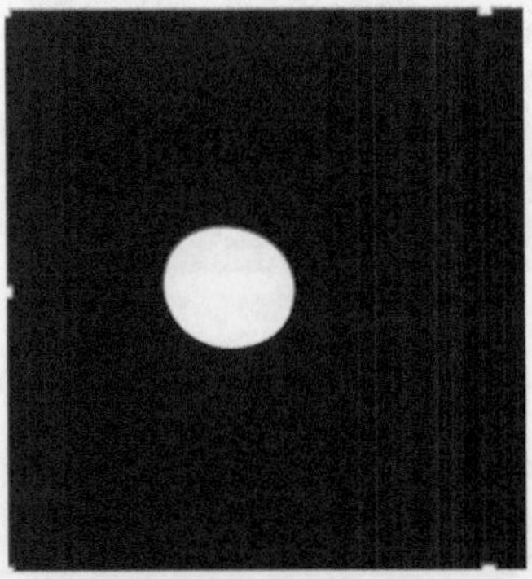

FIGURE 13.6 RIM-ONE V3 disc mask.

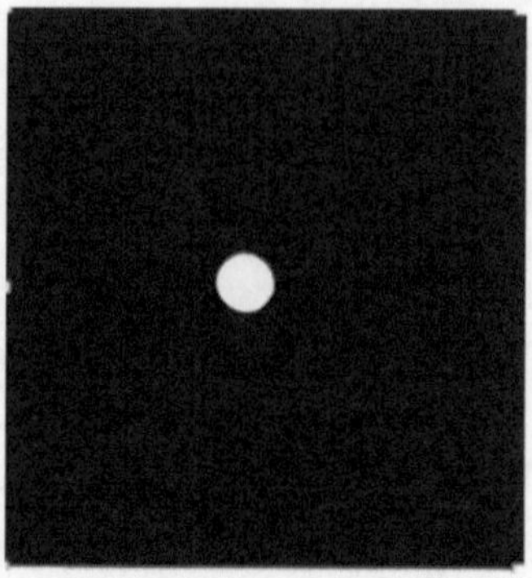

FIGURE 13.7 RIM-ONE V3 cup mask.

13.5 SIMULATION RESULTS

This section compares our proposed approach to existing methods for both of the tasks under consideration, namely segmentation of the optic disc and segmentation of the optic cup. Results are reported for publicly available dataset RIM-ONE v.3 that contains ground truth segmentation for optic disc and optic cup as well.

13.5.1 Optic Disc Segmentation

The proposed U-Net model for optic disc segmentation was trained using 127 training set images and then tested using the remaining 32 test images. Figure 13.8 shows the disc segmentation result of one of the test set images. The proposed model predicts a segmentation mask as shown in Figure 13.8.

The prediction time of the proposed model is also noted which is 560 milliseconds in this case. The predicted mask and ground truth mask that come with the RIM-ONE V3 dataset were used to determine the IoU and Dice scores. The ground truth mask is also shown in Figure 13.8. For the image in Figure 13.8, the IoU score and the dice score were calculated to be 0.82 and 0.91, respectively as shown.

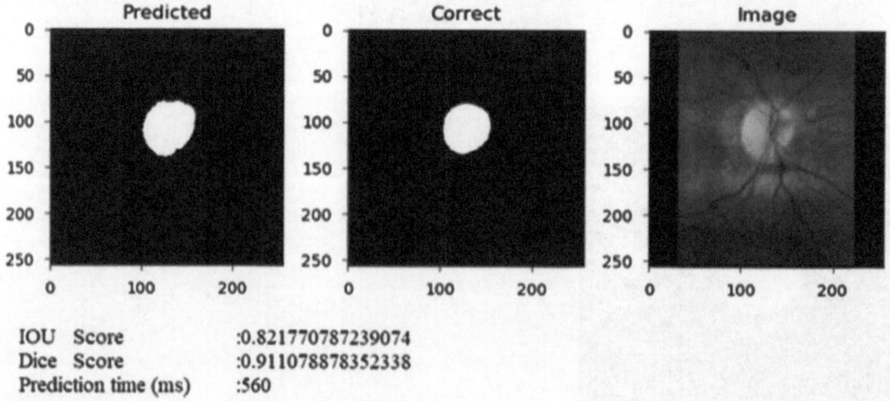

FIGURE 13.8 Disc segmentation result.

TABLE 13.1
Tabulation of Disc Segmentation Results

Image	IoU	Dice score	Prediction time(ms)
Image #01	0.85545224	0.929178253	762
Image #02	0.821770787	0.911078878	560
Image #03	0.769230783	0.876563985	556
Image #04	0.721121311	0.846701692	541
Image #05	0.829770088	0.912882638	563
Image #05	0.869002283	0.935515595	547

In the same way, segmentation mask is predicted by the proposed model for all the 32 test images and their corresponding IoU scores, Dice scores, and prediction time is tabulated. The tabulation for a few of those images is shown in Table 13.1.

Then the mean of IoU scores, Dice scores, and the prediction time is obtained using the tabulated data. The mean results are as follows: Mean IoU Score: 0.8317708, Mean Dice Score: 0.9131283286215005, and Mean Prediction Time (ms): 676.8125. Our proposed model predicts a segmentation mask as shown in Figure 13.9.

The prediction time of the proposed model is also noted which is 153 milliseconds in this case. The anticipated mask and the ground truth mask that come with the RIM-ONE V3 dataset were used to determine the IoU and Dice scores. The ground truth mask is also shown in Figure 13.9. For the image in Figure 13.9, the IoU score and the dice score were calculated to be 0.74 and 0.87.

In the same way, segmentation mask is predicted by our model for all the 32 test images and their corresponding IoU scores, Dice scores, and prediction time is tabulated. The tabulation for a few of those images is shown in Table 13.2.

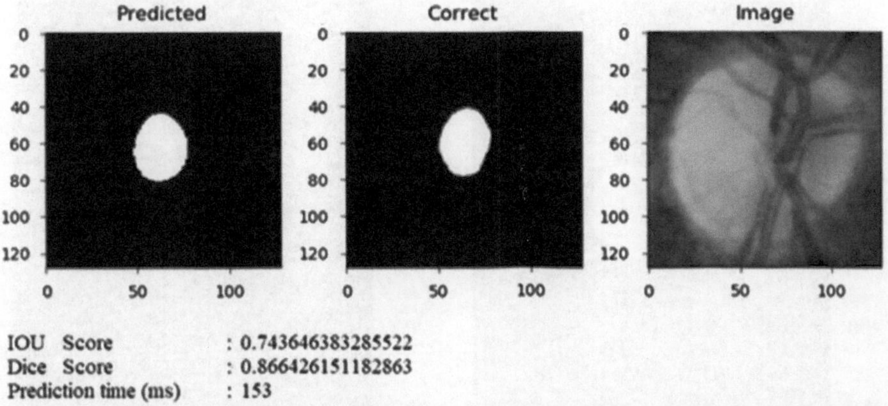

FIGURE 13.9 Cup segmentation result.

TABLE 13.2
Tabulation of Cup Segmentation Results

Image	IoU	Dice score	Prediction time(ms)
Image #01	0.758278	0.872556	342
Image #02	0.743646	0.866246	153
Image #03	0.708034	0.841902	135
Image #04	0.906774	0.960889	168
Image #05	0.813544	0.906206	152
Image #05	0.761986	0.875184	134

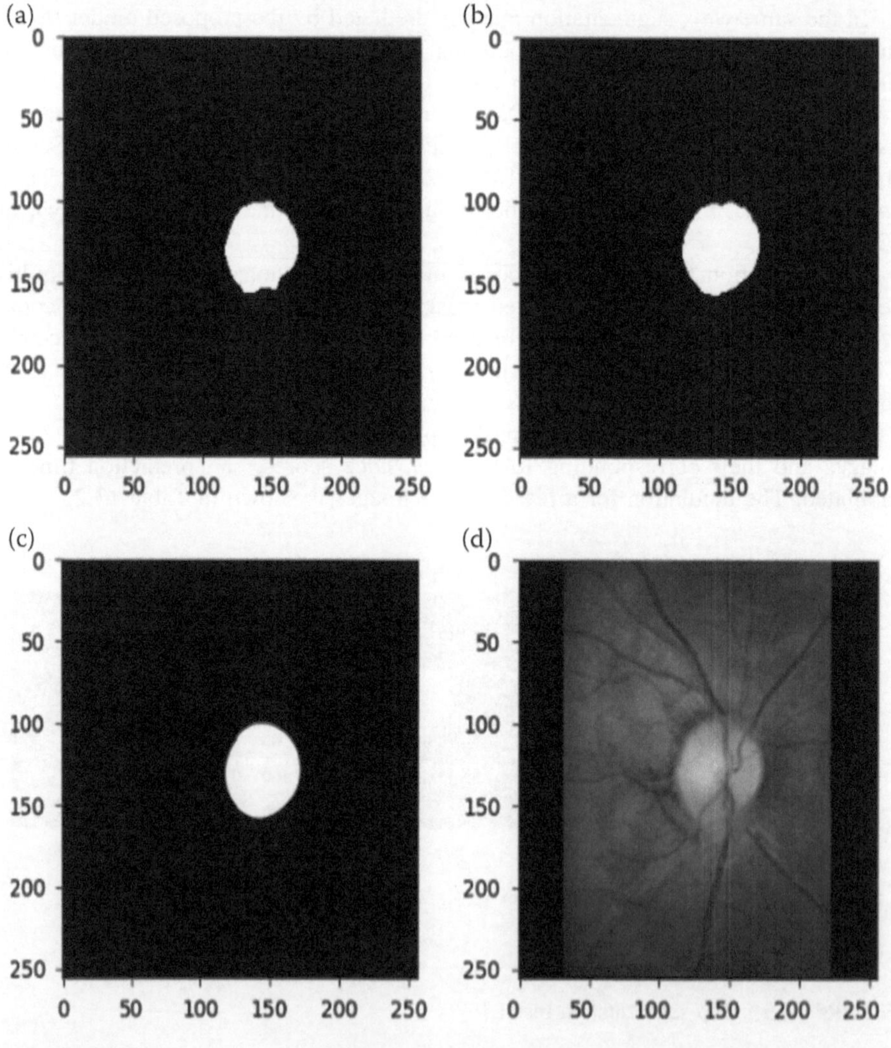

FIGURE 13.10 Comparison results of disc segmentation (a) Predicted-Existing Model (b) Predicted-Proposed Model (c) Correct (d) image.

The mean results are as follows: Mean IoU Score:0.7456728, Mean Dice Score:0.8598172241072453, and Mean Prediction Time (ms):144.78125.

Model-1 was the U-Net with the existing method's design, while model-2 was the U-Net with the proposed method's architecture. For optic disc segmentation, both the model-1 (existing model) and model-2 (previous model) was tested using the remaining 32 test images. The disc segmentation result of one of the test set photos is shown in Figure 13.9.

The prediction time of the existing model and the proposed model is also noted. The IoU and Dice scores were calculated using the predicted mask and the ground truth mask which comes along with the RIM-ONE V3 dataset. The ground truth mask is also shown in Figure 13.10. Dice scores and prediction time is calculated and tabulated. Table 13.3 shows the tabulation for a couple of the images.

Table 13.3 clearly shows that our method outperforms the prior methods in terms of forecast time. The plot representing the IoU and Dice scores of all 32 images using both the models is shown in Figure 13.11.

From Figure 13.11, we can see that the plot of the existing model and our proposed model almost overlap each other, this means that our proposed method is as efficient as the existing method in terms of IoU and Dice scores. Our proposed method outperforms the existing method in terms of prediction time. The mean of the IoU scores, Dice scores, and the prediction time for disc segmentation is given in Table 13.4.

As can be seen from the average results, the existing technique marginally beats the proposed method in terms of IoU and Dice scores, but the suggested method outperforms the existing method in terms of training and prediction time, as shown in Figure 13.12. Table 13.5 compares the diameters of the segmentation masks for a few of the test set images.

The suggested approach outperforms the present model in terms of IoU and dice scores, as shown in Table 13.6. The segmented boundaries are represented in

TABLE 13.3
Evaluation of Model Performance for Disc Segmentation

Image	Model	IoU	Dice Score	Prediction Time (ms)
Image #6	Existing	0.831354	0.915275	1840
Image #6	Proposed	0.895899	0.951075	539
Image #7	Existing	0.852156	0.928918	2087
Image #7	Proposed	0.912052	0.962761	575
Image #8	Existing	0.936205	0.971991	1821
Image #8	Proposed	0.877329	0.942663	540
Image #9	Existing	0.866203	0.937538	1829
Image #9	Proposed	0.786546	0.888701	555
Image #10	Existing	0.715842	0.841081	1831
Image #10	Proposed	0.817525	0.906095	538

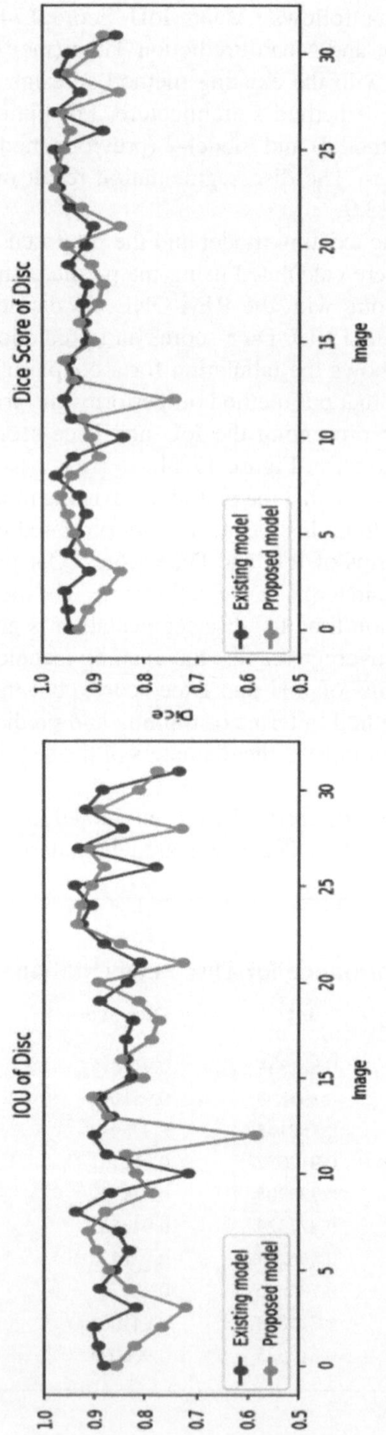

FIGURE 13.11 Plot of the IoU and dice score of proposed method and existing method for disc segmentation (Image #01).

TABLE 13.4
Performance Assessment of the Proposed with the Present Method for Image #01

Performance metrics	Existing	Proposed
Mean IoU	0.8617342	0.8317708
Mean Dice Score	0.9318939	0.9131283
Prediction time(ms)	2384.1875	676.8125

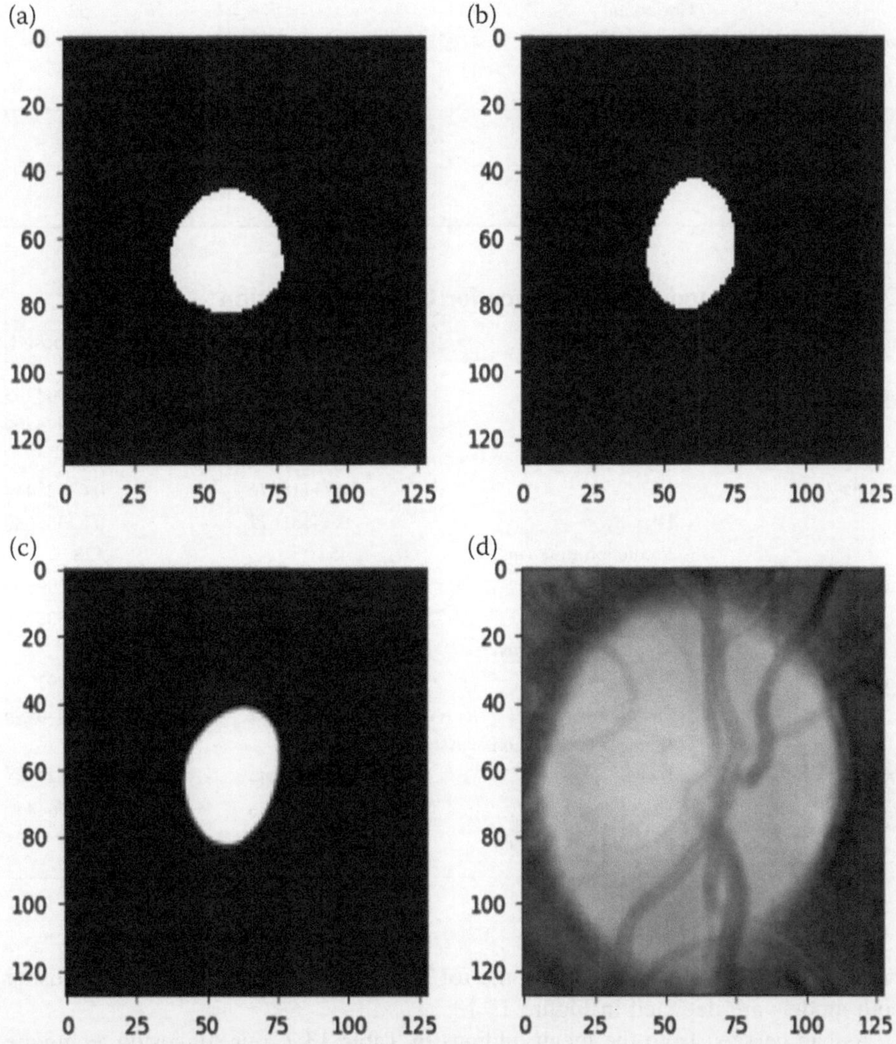

FIGURE 13.12 Comparison of the cup segmentation masks: (a) Predicted-Existing Model (b) Predicted-Proposed Model (c) Correct (d) image.

TABLE 13.5
Comparison of Disc Diameters

Image	Diameter	Original	Existing	Proposed
Image#6	Vertical	56	55	56
	Horizontal	51	53	55
Image#7	Vertical	48	53	49
	Horizontal	43	46	47
Image#8	Vertical	49	52	54
	Horizontal	43	46	46
Image#9	Vertical	52	52	47
	Horizontal	50	51	52
Image#10	Vertical	47	57	54
	Horizontal	44	46	50

TABLE 13.6
Comparison of Model Performance for Cup Segmentation

Image	Parameters	Existing	Proposed
Image#6	IoU	0.74224341	0.87904763
	Dice Score	0.8646322	0.94895499
	Prediction time (ms)	453	130
Image#7	IoU	0.71118176	0.68625444
	Dice Score	0.84156672	0.82367686
	Prediction time (ms)	453	128
Image#8	IoU	0.90402073	0.68199396
	Dice Score	0.96137379	0.97338739
	Prediction time (ms)	468	133
Image#9	IoU	0.68199396	0.71797234
	Dice Score	0.82013477	0.84440996
	Prediction time (ms)	438	133
Image#10	IoU	0.75651044	0.71337581
	Dice Score	0.88021366	0.8476444
	Prediction time (ms)	460	133

Figure 13.12. The plot representing the IoU and dice scores of all 32 images using both models are depicted in Figure 13.13.

As can be seen from the mean findings in Table 13.7, our suggested technique beats the existing method in terms of IoU scores, dice scores, training time, and

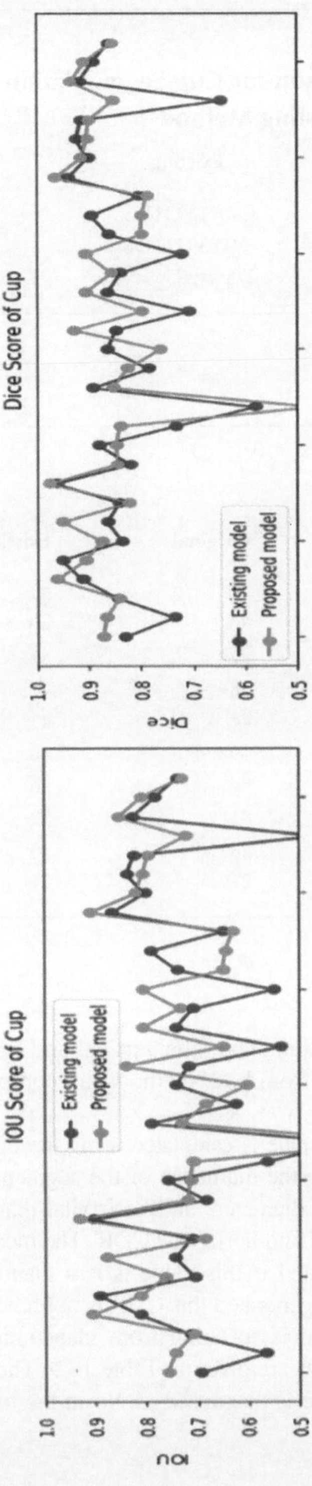

FIGURE 13.13 Plot of the IoU and dice score of proposed method and existing method for cup segmentation.

TABLE 13.7
Performance Comparison for Cup Segmentation of the Proposed with the Existing Method

Performance metrics	Existing	Proposed
Mean IoU	0.7148247	0.7456728
Mean Dice Score	0.839324496	0.85981722
Prediction time(ms)	475.84375	144.78125

TABLE 13.8
Comparison of Cup Diameters

Image	Diameter	Original	Existing	Proposed
Image#6	Vertical	37	37	39
	Horizontal	30	40	31
Image#7	Vertical	47	45	45
	Horizontal	38	47	49
Image#8	Vertical	44	42	44
	Horizontal	39	42	40
Image#9	Vertical	44	56	54
	Horizontal	41	52	49
Image#10	Vertical	28	26	32
	Horizontal	27	31	36

prediction time for cup segmentation. Then the vertical and horizontal diameters of the segmentation masks obtained from both methods are computed and tabulated in Table 13.8.

The CDR (Cup to Disc Ratio) value is calculated using the optic disc and optic cup diameters discovered by computing the diameters of the segmentation masks provided by our suggested method. Vertical diameters and horizontal diameters of the cup and disc are used to generate the vertical and horizontal CDR. The mean value of the vertical and horizontal CDR is computed and if this value is less than 0.5, it means that the person whose retinal fundus image generated this CDR is not having glaucoma. If CDR is greater than 0.5, then the person is suffering from glaucoma. The final glaucoma results of a few of the test set images are given in Table 13.9. The severity of glaucoma is diagnosed as Yes and its absence is diagnosed as No in the tabulated results.

TABLE 13.9
Glaucoma Results

Image	Disc Vertical Diameter	Disc Horizontal Diameter	Cup Vertical Diameter	Cup Horizontal Diameter	Vertical CDR	Horizontal CDR	CDR	Glaucoma Present
Image#128	58	50	24.921875	23.4375	0.4296875	0.46875	0.55	Yes
Image#129	51	50	17.9296875	21.875	0.3515625	0.4375	0.49	No
Image#130	46	44	11.5	10.65625	0.25	0.2421875	0.35	No
Image#131	31	32	9.203125	9	0.296875	0.28125	0.39	No
Image#132	50	51	13.28125	15.140625	0.265625	0.296875	0.38	No
Image#133	57	52	20.9296875	18.6875	0.3671875	0.359375	0.46	No
Image#134	63	54	23.625	19.40625	0.375	0.359375	0.47	No
Image#135	46	45	17.25	15.8203125	0.375	0.3515625	0.46	No
Image#136	48	42	21.375	18.375	0.4453125	0.4375	0.54	Yes
Image#137	49	40	22.203125	18.4375	0.453125	0.4609375	0.56	Yes

13.6 CONCLUSION

The proposed work is designed using dual customized U-Net based deep learning method for glaucoma disease identification. The most important advantage of our proposed method is training time and prediction time. It has proven that the training time and prediction time of the proposed model are approximately four times better than the previously used models.

Both tasks were examined using the same method, and it was discovered that high-quality segmentation was obtained, demonstrating its applicability to a variety of picture identification challenges. The proposed solution also has the advantages of simplicity, easy programming with modern frameworks, and the shortest possible prediction time.

REFERENCES

[1] Quigley, H. A. and Broman, A. T., 2006. The number of people with glaucoma worldwide in 2010 and 2020. *British Journal of Ophthalmology*, 90(3), pp. 262–267.

[2] Shankaranarayana, S. M., Ram, K., Mitra, K., and Sivaprakasam, M., 2019. Fully convolutional networks for monocular retinal depth estimation and optic disc-cup segmentation. *IEEE Journal of Biomedical and Health Informatics*, 23(4), pp. 1417–1426.

[3] Fu, H., Cheng, J., Xu, Y., Wing Knee Wong, D., Jiang, L., and Cao, X., 2018. Joint optic disc and cup segmentation based on multi- label deep network and polar transformation. *IEEE Transactions on Medical Imaging*. https://arxiv.org/pdf/1801.00926.pdf.

[4] Aquino, A., Gegundez-Arias, M. E., and Marin, D., 2010. Detecting the optic disc boundary in digital fundus images using morphological, edge detection, and feature extraction Techniques. *IEEE Transactions on Medical Imaging*, 29(11), pp. 1860–1869.

[5] Lim, G., Cheng, Y., Hsu, W., and Lee, M. L.Integrated Optic Disc and Cup Segmentation with Deep Learning," IEEE 27th International Conference on Tools with Artificial Intelligence (ICTAI), Vietrisul Mare, 2015, pp. 162–169. doi: 10.1109/ICTAI.2015.36.

[6] Hanan S. Alghamdi, Hongying Lilian Tang, Saad A. Waheeb, and Tunde Peto "Automatic optic disc abnormality detection in fundus images: A deep learning approach," in Proceedings of the Opthalmic Medical Image Analysis International Workshop, pp. 17–24, 2016.

[7] Almazroa, A., Burman, R., Raahemifar, K., and Lakshminarayanan, V. 2015. Optic disc and optic cup segmentation methodologies for glaucoma image detection: A Survey. *Journal of Ophthalmology*. 10.1155/2015/180972.

[8] Drozdzal, M., Chartrand, G., Vorontsov, E., Shakeri, M., Di Jorio, L., Tang, A., Romero, A., Bengio, Y., Pal, C. and Kadoury, S., 2018. Learning normalized inputs for iterative estimation in medical image segmentation. *Medical Image Analysis*, 44, pp. 1–13.

[9] Vorontsov, E., Tang, A., Pal, C., and Kadoury, S., "Liver lesion segmentation informed by joint liver segmentation," in IEEE 15th International Symposium on Biomedical Imaging (ISBI 2018), pp. 1332–1335, IEEE, 2018.

[10] Ronneberger, O., Fischer, P., and Brox, T., "U-net: Convolutional networks for biomedical image segmentation," in International Conference on Medical Image Computing and Computer-Assisted Intervention, pp. 234–241. Springer, Cham, 2015.

[11] Pratt, H., Coenen, F., Broadbent, D. M. et al., 2016. Convolutional neural network for diabetic retinopathy. *Procedia Computer Science*, 90, pp. 200–205.
[12] Usman Akram, M., Kalid, S., and Khan, S. A., 2012. Identification and classification of micro aneursysms for early detection of diabetic retinopathy. *Pattern Recognition*, 10.1016/j.patcog.2012.07.002.
[13] Almejalli, K. A., 2018. Microaneurysms, Haemorrhages and exudates based diabetic retinopathy: Automatic early detection systems and the state of art. *International Journal of Computer Science and Network Security*, 18(6), pp. 43–48.
[14] Harefbib, M. M., Velikala, R. A., Hoppe, A., Owen, C. G., Rudnicka, A. R., and Barman, S. A., 2017. Detection of microaneursyms in retinal images using an ensemble classifier, *Informatics in Medicine Unlocked*, 9, pp. 44–57.
[15] Wong, D. W. K., Liu, J., Lim, J. H., Jia, X., Yin, F., Li, H., and Wong, T. Y. "Level-set based automatic cup-to-disc ratio determination using retinal fundus images in ARGALI," in 30th Annual International IEEE EMBS Conference, pp. 2266–2269, 2008. 10.1109/IEMBS.2008.4649648.
[16] Bock, R., Meier, J., Nyúl, L. G., Hornegger, J., and Michelson, G., 2010. Glaucoma risk index: Automated glaucoma detection from color fundus images. *Medical Image Analysis*, 14, pp. 471–481. 10.1016/j.media.2009.12.006.
[17] Joshi G. D., Sivaswamy J., and Krishnadas S. R., 2011. Optic disk and cup segmentation from monocular color retinal images for glaucoma assessment. *IEEE Transactions on Medical Imaging*, 30, pp.1192–1205. 10.1109/TMI.2011.2106509.
[18] Yin, F., Liu, J., Wong, D. W. K., Tan, N. M., Cheung, C., Baskaran, M., Aung, T., and Wong T. Y. "Automated segmentation of optic disc and optic cup in fundus images for glaucoma diagnosis," in 25th IEEE International Symposium on Computer Based Medical Systems (CBMS), pp. 1–6, 2012. 10.1109/CBMS.2012.6266344.
[19] Diaz-Pinto, A., Morales, S., Naranjo, V., Alcocer, P., and Lanzagorta, A. "Glaucoma diagnosis by means of optic cup feature analysis in color fundus images," in 24th European signal processing conference (EUSIPCO), vol. 24, pp. 2055–2059, 2016. 10.1109/EUSIPCO.2016.7760610.
[20] Cheng, J., Liu, J., Xu, Y., Yin, F., Wong, D. W. K., Tan, N.-M., Tao, D., Cheng, C.-Y., Aung, T., and Wong T. Y., 2013. Superpixel classification based optic disc and optic cup segmentation for glaucoma screening. *IEEE Transactions on Medical Imaging*, 32, pp. 1019–1032. 10.1109/TMI.2013.2247770.
[21] Sevastopolsky, A., 2017. Optic disc and cup segmentation methods for glaucoma detection with modification of U-Net convolutional neural network. *Pattern Recognition and Image Analysis*, 27, p. 618. 10.1134/S1054661817030269.
[22] Maninis K.-K., Pont-Tuset, J., Arbelaez, P., and Van Gool L. "Deep retinal image understanding," in International Conference on Medical Image Computing and Computer Assisted Intervention, pp. 140–148, Springer, 2016.
[23] Zilly, J. G., Buhmann J. M., and Mahapatra D., "Boosting convolutional filters with entropy sampling for optic cup and disc image segmentation from fundus images," in *International Workshop on Machine Learning in Medical Imaging*, pp. 136–143, Springer, 2015.
[24] Dogan H. and Akay, O., 2010. Using adaboost classifiers in a hierarchical framework for classifying surface images of marble slabs. *Expert Systems with Applications*, 37(12), pp. 8814–8821.

14 MuSCF-Net: Multi-scale, Multi-Channel Feature Network Using Resnet-based Attention Mechanism for Breast Histopathological Image Classification

Meenakshi M. Pawer, Suvarna D. Pujari, and Swati P. Pawar
Department of Electronics and Telecommunication Engineering, SVERIs College of Engineering, Pandharpur, University of PAH, Solapur, India

Sanjay N. Talbar
Department of Electronics and Telecommunication Engineering, SGGS, Nanded, Maharashtra, India

CONTENTS

14.1 Introduction 244
14.2 Related Studies 245
14.3 Contribution 246
14.4 Material and Methods 246
14.4.1 BREAKHIS Database 247
14.4.2 Methodology 247
14.4.3 Preprocessing 249
14.4.3.1 Patch Creation 249
14.4.3.2 Augmentation 249
14.4.3.3 MuSCF-Net Mechanism 249
14.4.4 Training Details 255
14.4.4.1 Adam Optimizer [37] 255

DOI: 10.1201/9781003217497-14

14.4.4.2 Activation Function 256
14.4.4.3 ReLU 256
14.4.4.4 Softmax Activation Function 256
14.4.4.5 Loss 256
14.5 Results and Discussion 256
14.6 Conclusion 259
References 260

14.1 INTRODUCTION

Breast cancer (BC) is one of the most frequently diagnosed cancers, especially in women worldwide. According to GLOBOCAN 2020, breast cancer in women left behind lung cancer with 2,261,419 new cases and 684,996 deaths were recorded worldwide [1]. To reduce the mortality rate, identification of cancer in its early stages is needed. There are different tests available for breast cancer detection that includes physical examination, mammography, tomosynthesis, magnetic resonance imaging (MRI), ultrasound, and biopsy [2–4]. Biopsy is considered the gold standard for cancer detection and treatment. The accuracy of tumor detection from histopathological images depends on radiologists' experience; high rate of making diagnostic error is due to less experience of oncologist in their field than experts [5–7], and difference of opinion between the oncologists' explanations and the expert agreement [8], [9]. For early stage cancer detection, computer-aided diagnosis can support physicians for fast and accurate diagnosis. For classification of cancerous tissues, existing CAD system makes use of hand-crafted features, such as wavelet coefficients, co-occurrence matrix features, and histogram of Shearlet coefficients, etc. Many researchers are developing computer-aided tools to categorize breast whole slide images as non-cancerous (benign) or cancerous (malignant) [10]. The feature extraction techniques, such as Haralick, wavelet-based, intensity-based, and morphological features, are used to extract meaningful features from segmented nuclei and their surroundings to classify histopathological image [11], [12]. Due to histopathological images' complex structure, the handcrafted feature extraction technique is fruitless [13].

Breast cancer usually comprises manifold subtypes in diverse molecular pathogenesis and clinical features, as it is not a single disease [14], [15]. Therefore, recognition of cancer subtype is very difficult to facilitate precise cancer diagnosis and treatment. Recently, the development of deep neural networks was easy due to availability of high computational facilities and large training databases [16]. Using nonlinear transformations the high-level abstractions were extracted directly from images in deep learning (DL) [17]. Supervised machine learning algorithms, such as Support Vector Machine (SVM), K-NN, Naïve Bayesian [18], [19] were used in breast cancer detection. When there is an intra-class and inter-class variation, the classical machine learning approaches degrade the system's performance regarding efficiency and accuracy [20]. The convolution neural network (CNN)-based classifier networks like BCNN [21], DCNN [22], ResNet152 [20], and the ensemble-based multi-scale CNNs (EMS-Net) [3], Xception [23], were used to classify histopathological microscopy breast images. The automated process for the analysis of breast cancer in this process feature extraction is a challenging task due to diversity in the structure of the breast images. Feature extraction from patches created from the images enables to design low-complexity CNN for feature extraction [24]. Our main contribution is to improve the accuracy of classification of histopathological patches created [25] from whole slide images (WSI), different filter sizes give multiple feature maps, and these features through CBMA integrated with ResBlock give Robust and Refined features.

14.2 RELATED STUDIES

In another study by Zanariah et al. [26], three Deep Layer Convolution neural network (DCNN) architectures were used to detect breast cancer. In this method, they initially created patches from whole slide image, where Mitosis and non-Mitosis were selected of size 64 × 64 × 3. These patches were given to 6-layer CNN, 13-layer CNN 17-layer CNN, and 19-layer CNN; these three different CNN architectures were performed for CNN-based algorithms for 5-fold. They achieved an accuracy of 84.49% by using 19-CNN layer, which was the highest among the three CNNs.

Wang et al. [21] proposed a deep learning-based bilinear CNN method to classify histopathological images. The convolution and pooling layers applied on hematoxylin and eosin (H & E) stained breast tissue images decompose into H & E parts and then on both of these images combined and learn more effective feature representation. These two features were fused by bilinear pooling. This proposed method got success of an average accuracy of 92.6 ± 1.2% across all folds to classify the H & E stained breast cancer images.

Gandomkar et al.'s [20] major objectives from this research work: (i) To classify histopathological breast images as cancerous (malignant) or non-cancerous (benign), (ii) To perform sub-classification of cancerous (malignant) images as DC, LC, MC, PC; and (iii) To perform sub-classification of non-cancerous (benign) images as A, F, PT, or TA. In this study, multi-category classification of breast histopathological image using Deep Residual Networks (MuDeRN) was a two-stage network approach used to classify patients with the use of H & E stained slides. In the first stage, histopathological breast image is detected either benign or malignant, and then at the second stage malignant and benign cancer were categorizing for each class into four subtypes. MuDeRN was a very Deep CNN comprising 152 layers (ResNet152). The proposed framework was trained for different MF× 40, ×100, ×200 and ×400. First stage of MuDeRN achieved classification rates (CCR) of 98.52%, 97.90%, 98.33% and 97.66% in ×40, ×100, ×200 and ×400 MF, respectively. For the eight-class categorization of images based on the output of MuDeRN in second stage, Correct Classification Rates were 95.40%, 94.90%, 95.70% and 94.60% in ×40, ×100, ×200 and ×400, respectively.

The research study conducted by SanaUllah et al. [27] developed deep learning approach using a CNN called the BreastNet. BreastNet module comprises convolutional block attention module (CBAM), ResBlock, dense block, and hypercolumn technique. This model was a multi-classification of breast histopathological image. They also trained the proposed model for distinct magnification factors (×40, ×100, ×200 and ×400).

Kalpana George et al. [28] for automated breast cancer detection proposed a method that extracts feature from a nucleus using a DCNN, i.e., "NucDeep". They designed simple CNN with less complexity for feature extraction from non-overlapping nuclei patches spotted over the images. A feature fusion (FF) approach with SVM classification framework was applied to categorize breast histopathological images from the extracted CNN features from nuclei. The FF method converts the local features from nuclei into a compact feature at image-level that improves the classifier performance. The success rate for cancer detection was recognition rate of 96.66 ± 0.77 %, specificity of 100%, and sensitivity 96.21%.

14.3 CONTRIBUTION

In various medical image applications, CNN models have achieved promising results [20,22]. CNN gives more robust and refined features. The aforementioned studies indeed motivated us to explore the performance of different deep CNNs and also to validate the accuracy and network parameters for assessment of breast cancer using histopathological images.

The major contributions of this study are given below:

1. The proposed a multi-scale filter bank with an attention mechanism for feature extraction.
2. The proposed network consists of CBMA block, to examine the feature maps: channel and spatial and to get refined features.
3. The CBMA is integrated with ResBlock in Resnet.
4. The proposed network consists of multi-streams for fine-level as well as course-level feature extraction.
5. The proposed network follows a knowledge-sharing strategy by sharing learned features at each stream across the network.
6. Our developed model is a lightweight model.
7. The proposed network is trained and validated for histopathological hematoxylin-eosin stained breast digital slides on BreakHis dataset.

The remaining chapter is organized as follows. Section 14.4 gives details of the proposed approach and the materials used. Section 14.5 offers the experimental results and discussions of proposed network architecture. Finally, Section 14.6 refers concluding remark.

14.4 MATERIAL AND METHODS

This section discusses the proposed approach for classification of breast histopathological images; further it provides a brief explanation of the dataset used for our work. As with the traditional pattern recognition pipeline, we extract robust and refined features followed by pattern classification. As we know, effective feature extraction is key to get higher accuracy. As discussed in previous sections, the existing handcrafted feature extractor fails to extract robust features when there is a complex image structure. In the past decade, the convolution neural network's feature learning ability attracted many researchers for incorporating CNN for

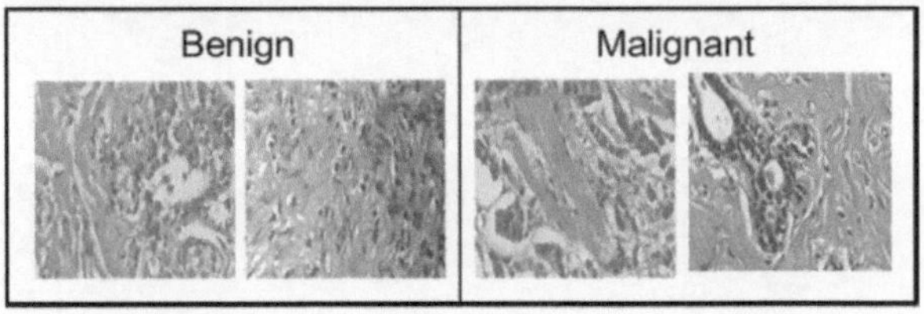

FIGURE 14.1 Sample images from BreakHis Dataset.

feature extraction. Thus, the CNN's robustness in feature extraction inspired us to propose a CNN network for breast image classification.

14.4.1 BREAKHIS DATABASE

BREAKHIS DATABASE contains 7,909 microscopic breast cancer histopathological RGB images of size 700 × 460 pixels from 82 patients with four visual MLs—×40, ×100, ×200 and ×400 as shown in Figure 14.1. Here, benign class consists of 2,480 images and malignant class of 5,426 images. The BREAKHIS database built-in P&D Laboratory Pathological Anatomy and Cytopathology, Parana, Brazil [29,30].

As shown in Table 14.1, benign is represented using four different subtypes: Adenosis (A), Fibroadenoma (F), Tubular Adenoma (TA), Phyllodes Tumor (PT). Whereas malignant subclasses are Ductal Carcinoma (DC), Lobular Carcinoma (LC), Mucinous Carcinoma (MC), Papillary Carcinoma (PC). The details about BreakHis database is given in Table 14.1.

From Table 14.1, it can be noted that at magnification level ×40, the database contains total 1,995 histopathological images. Next, at × 100 it has 2,081 images, at × 200 it consists of 2,013 images, and finally at ×400 it represents 1,820 images.

14.4.2 METHODOLOGY

In this work, we proposed a Multi-scale, Multi-Channel feature network using Resnet-Based Attention mechanism for breast histopathological image classification for training and prediction of breast cancer as shown in Figure 14.2. The proposed

TABLE 14.1
The Detailed Statics of BreakHis Database

Class	Benign				Malignant			
Sub-Classes	A	F	TA	PT	DC	LC	MC	PC
×40	114	256	109	149	864	156	205	145
×100	113	260	121	140	903	170	222	142
×200	111	264	108	150	896	163	196	135
×400	106	237	115	130	788	137	169	138
Total	444	1014	453	569	3451	626	792	560

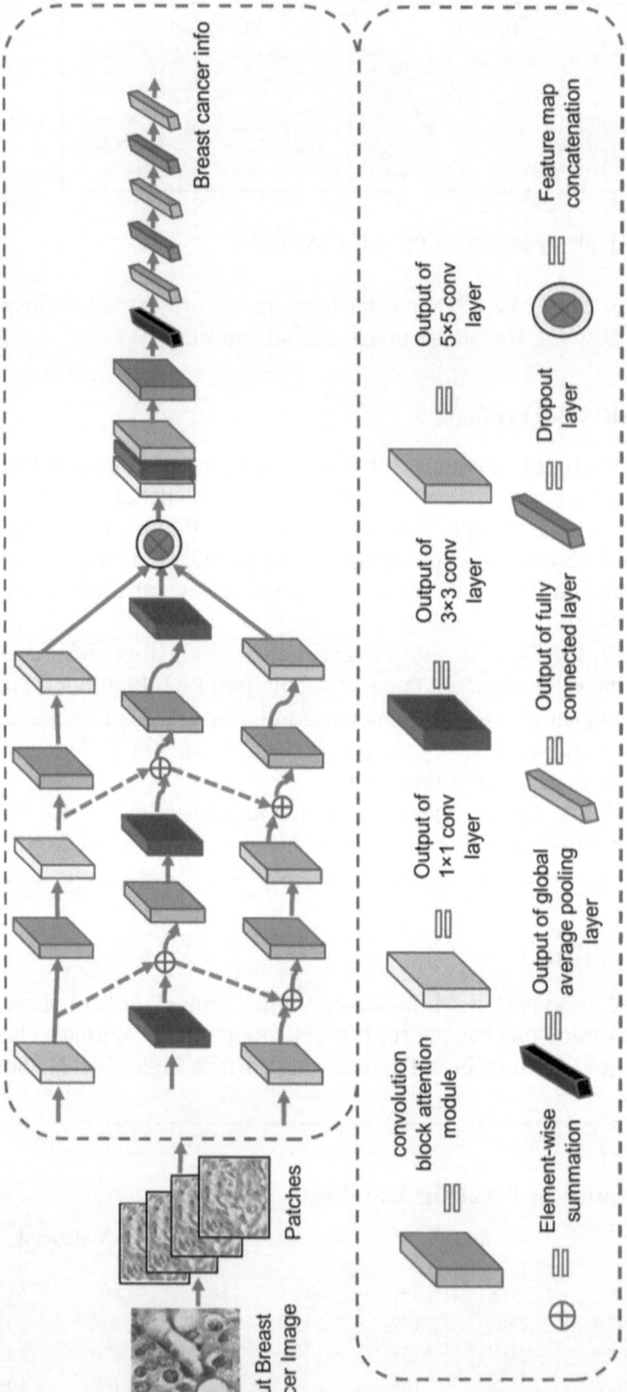

FIGURE 14.2 Block diagram of the proposed MuSCF-Net with Resnet-Based Attention mechanism.

network made up of three streams belong to a trail of convolution layer having filter size of 1×1, 3×3, and 5×5, respectively on CBMA [31] layer. Each convolution layer processes the patch from input breast histopathological image and extracts features at a particular scale; before the convolutional block, we used the CBMA block, which gives the focused region. For better feature learning, share the learned feature maps within the network stream. This was inspired by the work [32].

Element-wise addition and concatenation are two ways to share/integrate the learned feature maps. The feature map concatenation increases the number of network trainable parameters. Thus, keeping in mind the real-time use case of the proposed network, we use the element-wise addition operation to share the learned feature maps within the network streams. Figure 14.2 shows the feature map concatenation spikes the number of network trainable parameters. Thus, keeping in mind, we make use of element-wise addition operation to share the learned.

14.4.3 Preprocessing

14.4.3.1 Patch Creation

The whole slide image (WSI) of giga-pixel resolution is computationally hard for GPUs and cannot fit in GPU memory. There are three patch selection approaches i) Random selection, it is the simplest approach of patches from WSIs images are randomly [25]. ii) To Identify cancerous lesion in the image, machine learning algorithm for detection of cancer can be trained by randomly selected patches that can be patch-annotated lesion for cancerous part in WSIs by radiologist [33] or non-annotated patch as non-cancerous WSIs. iii) Cluster-based image patches approach, clustering of image patch is used to obtain variegated appearance of breast tissues. The cluster operation is carried out over 8 subtype image patches to represent WSI [34]. To identify subtype from image patch across whole training dataset centroid of image patch is calculated. Further, centroid of the 8 subtype clusters from database is compared and closest centroid of the cluster will be assign to the image patch. Along the side this process is repeated iteratively for every epoch of the training [35]. In this work due to simplicity we created patches using random selection approach.

14.4.3.2 Augmentation

Generally, augmentation was done on training data for better performance of network and keeps the network away from overfitting. Each image is rotated with different angles like 1,800, 2,700, or 900 and flipped with respect to horizontal or vertical axes along with random shift about ±10 pixels. While training of network for every epoch patches from images were augmented randomly and provided to the network.

14.4.3.3 MuSCF-Net Mechanism

It is the feature extractor model that consists of 1) convolution of filter bank for feature extraction and 2) CBMA integrated with ResBlock in Resnet.

14.4.3.3.1 Convolution of filter bank for feature extraction

We used CNN's basic building block, such as convolution, Relu, and batch normalization for feature extraction with different filter size. Figure 14.2 shows the block diagram of the proposed multi-scale multi-stream with attention mechanism deep neural network. Table 14.2 gives the detailed network architecture and parameter details of the proposed network. It is very difficult to choose a filter size for a particular convolution layer, and there is no universal rule for filter size selection. Thus, we choose filter size (1 × 1, 3 × 3, 5 × 5), multi-scale filter bank for feature extraction. This multi-scale filter bank helps tackle network design difficulties by letting the network decide the best route for itself.

14.4.3.3.2 Convolution Block Attention Module (CBMA) Integrated with ResBlock in ResNet

14.4.3.3.2.1 CBMA Integrated with ResBlockin Resnet As illustrated in Figure 14.3, the CBMA divided into sub models-channel sub-module uses both max-pooling outputs and average-pooling outputs with a shared network; this shared network is made up of multilayer perceptron (MLP) with one hidden layer. The ResBlock gives the class-wise input to the output.

14.4.3.3.2.2 Channel Attention (CA) Module The CA module produces feature map for each channel. It stresses on important parts of an input image. In CA module, average and maximum pooled features are extracted and processed together [31], [27]. In this module, average and max-pooling operations are used to combine spatial information of a feature map, which produces two spatial context descriptors: F^c_{max} and F^c_{avg} , as max-pooled features and average -pooled features, respectively. Then these spatial context descriptors are provided to the given shared network. This will generate the CA map as $M_c \in \mathbb{R}^{C\times1\times1}$. In this shared network, it consists of one hidden layer of MLP. The parameter overhead is reduced by setting hidden activation size as $\mathbb{R}^{C/r\times1\times1}$, here r denotes reduction ratio. The element-wise summation operation is performed on output feature vectors with the application of shared network over each spatial context descriptors.

Accordingly the CA can be calculated as follows:

$$M_c(F) = \sigma\,(\mathrm{MLP}(\mathrm{AvgPool}(F)) + \mathrm{MLP}(\mathrm{MaxPool}\,(F))) \tag{14.1}$$

$$= \sigma\left(W_1\left(W_0\left(F^c_{avg}\right)\right) + W_1(W_0(F^c_{max}))\right) \tag{14.2}$$

Where σ the sigmoid function, $W_0 \in \mathbb{R}^{C/r\times C}$, and $W_1 \in \mathbb{R}^{C\times C/r}$. Note that the multilayer perceptron weights, W_0 and W_1, are shared for both inputs. The activation function (ReLU) is followed by W_0.

14.4.3.3.2.3 Spatial Attention (SA) Module Along the channel axis in spatial sub-module two similar outputs pooled, concatenating them to generate an efficient feature descriptor and forwarding them to a convolution layer. The CBMA module not only gives the refine feature map but robust to the noise input. It decomposes the

TABLE 14.2
Network Architecture Details of the Proposed Network MuSCF-Net

Input	Input Image Size	Output Layer/Stride	Filter Size	Output Image Size	Parameters
Input Image	128 × 128 × 3	Conv1_1/2	1 × 1 × 3 × 64	64 × 64 × 64	256
Input Image	128 × 128 × 3	Conv1_3/2	3 × 3 × 3 × 64	64 × 64 × 64	1792
Input Image	128 × 128 × 3	Conv1_5/2	5 × 5 × 3 × 64	64 × 64 × 64	4864
Conv1_1, Conv1_3	64 × 64 × 64	Addition1_13	–	64 × 64 × 64	–
Conv1_1, Conv1_3, Conv1_5	64 × 64 × 64	Addition1_135	–	64 × 64 × 64	–
Conv1_1	64 × 64 × 64	CBMA1_1	–	64 × 64 × 64	8446
Addition1_13	64 × 64 × 64	CBMA1_13	–	64 × 64 × 64	8446
Addition1_135	64 × 64 × 64	CBMA1_135	–	64 × 64 × 64	8446
CBMA1_1	64 × 64 × 64	Conv2_1/1	1 × 1 × 64 × 64	64 × 64 × 64	4160
CBMA1_13	64 × 64 × 64	Conv2_3/1	3 × 3 × 64 × 64	64 × 64 × 64	36928
CBMA1_135	64 × 64 × 64	Conv2_5/1	5 × 5 × 64 × 64	64 × 64 × 64	102464
Conv2_1, Conv2_3	64 × 64 × 64	Addition2_13	–	64 × 64 × 64	–
Conv2_1, Conv2_3, Conv2_5	64 × 64 × 64	Addition2_135	–	64 × 64 × 64	–
Conv2_1	64 × 64 × 64	CBMA2_1	–	64 × 64 × 64	8446
Addition2_13	64 × 64 × 64	CBMA2_13	–	64 × 64 × 64	8446
Addition2_135	64 × 64 × 64	CBMA2_135	–	64 × 64 × 64	8446

(Continued)

TABLE 14.2 (Continued)

Network Architecture Details of the Proposed Network MuSCF-Net

Input	Input Image Size	Output Layer/Stride	Filter Size	Output Image Size	Parameters
CBMA2_1	64 × 64 × 64	Conv3_1/1	1 × 1 × 64 × 64	64 × 64 × 64	4160
CBMA2_13	64 × 64 × 64	Conv3_3/1	3 × 3 × 64 × 64	64 × 64 × 64	36928
CBMA2_135	64 × 64 × 64	Conv3_5/1	5 × 5 × 64 × 64	64 × 64 × 64	102464
Conv3_1, Conv3_3, Conv3_5	64 × 64 × 64	Concatenation	–	64 × 64 × 192	–
Concatenation	64 × 64 × 192	Conv4_1	3 × 3 × 192 × 128	64 × 64 × 128	221312
Conv4_1	64 × 64 × 128	Dropout_1	–	64 × 64 × 128	–
Dropout	64 × 64 × 128	Global Average Pooling(GAP)	–	128	–
GAP	128	FC_1	1 × 1 ×128 × 60	1 × 1 × 60	7740
FC_1	1 × 1 × 60	Dropout_2	–	1 × 1 × 60	–
Dropout_2	1 × 1 × 60	FC-2	1 × 1 ×1 × 4/2	60 × 8/2	244/122

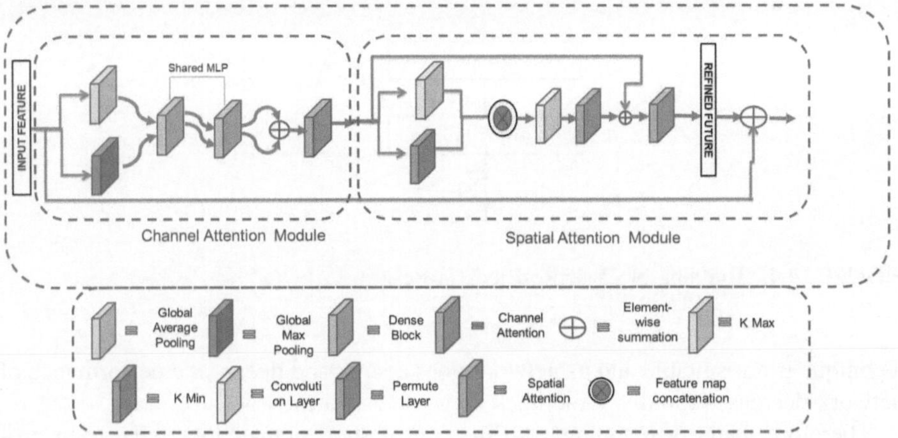

FIGURE 14.3 Convolution Block Attention Model (CBMA) integrated with ResBlock in Resnet.

process into a channel and spatial attention separately due to separation reduction in computation parameters [31], [27].

The highlighting informative regions are generated across channel axis with the use of pool operation over concatenated feature frames. The spatial attention map $M_s(F) \in R^{H\times W}$ is generated by applying a convolution layer, which encodes where to stress or suppress. Details of the operations have been shown below eqs. (14.3) and (14.4). By using two pooling operation we aggregated channel information of a feature map and generated two 2D maps: $F^c_{avg} \in \mathbb{R}^{1\times H\times W}$, and $F^c_{max} \in \mathbb{R}^{1\times H\times W}$ across the channel features as 1. Average pooled feature map and 2. Max pooled feature map. By a standard convolution layer these are then concatenated and convolved to produce 2 dimensional (2D) SA map. Accordingly, the SA can be calculated as follows:

$$M_s(F) = \sigma(f^{7\times7}([AvgPool(F);\ \ MaxPool(F)]) \tag{14.3}$$

$$= \sigma(f^{7\times7}\left(\left[F^c_{avg};\ \ F^c_{max}\right]\right) \tag{14.4}$$

Where σ represents the sigmoid function, $f^{7\times7}$ represents a convolution operation with the filter size of 7 × 7. These features are then transferred to CNN. Two attention modules, CA and SA, compute complementary attention, focusing on "what" and "where", respectively. These two modules placed sequentially.

14.4.3.3.2.4 ResBlock in Resnet [24] The training of DNN becomes difficult due to vanishing gradient problem. To tackle this problem, researchers have increased depth of the network by staking layers together. It is observed that this

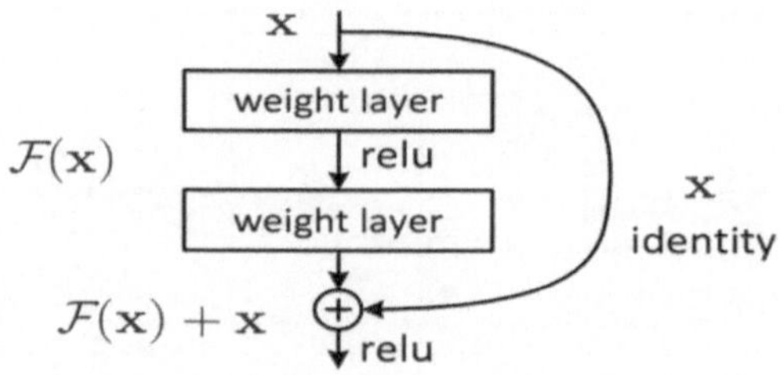

FIGURE 14.4 Building block of ResBlock in ResNet.

technique is not suitable and as network goes deeper and deeper the performance of network decreases rapidly sometimes network saturates.

Therefore, identity mapping with the use of short connections have been proposed [24], in this work the author has introduced skip connections that skip layers and join directly, where the connection is provided this network is known as Resnet, which is illustrated in Figure 14.4. As represented in Figure 14.4 the idea of skip connection while training, where it skips some layers and joins directly to output layer. The major benefit of using skip connection is performance degrading layer in the architecture can be skipped by regularization.

The vanishing gradient problem is overcome by introducing skip connection, i.e., deep residual learning framework in DNN. Let H(x) be a non-linear function that represents the mapping from input to output, F(x):= H(x) – x instead of F(x) + x.

14.4.3.3.2.5 Global Average Pooling Layer The global average pooling layer is used instead of the traditional, fully connected layer in CNN [32]. The last multi-perceptron convolution (mlpconv) layer generates one feature map for each corresponding class of the classification task; this feature map is a confidence map of classes due to mlpconv. The resulting vector is the average of each feature map and forwarded to the softmax layer shown in Figure 14.2. Due to no parameter to optimize overfitting is avoided in the global average pooling; thus, in this layer.

Let x; F represent the convolution layer's input and output in the proposed network, respectively.

$$\text{Thus,} \quad F_{ijN} = \textstyle\sum_{uvC} W_{uv}CN \times X_{i+u,\ j+v,\ C} \tag{14.5}$$

Where $W_{uv}CN$ denotes the filterbank having filters of spatial size M × N and locations

$$u \in \left[-\frac{(M-1)}{2}, \frac{(M-1)}{2}\right], \; v \in \left[-\frac{(K-1)}{2}, \frac{(K-1)}{2}\right]$$

C, N the number of channels and filters, respectively (i; j) denotes the image location. After instance normalization go through the ReLu as follows

$$F_{1ijk} = \frac{F_{ij} - \mu_k}{\sqrt{\sigma^2 + \varepsilon}} \tag{14.6}$$

$$\mu_k = \frac{1}{HW} \sum_{i=1}^{W} \sum_{j=1}^{H} F_{ijk}, \quad \sigma_k^2 = \frac{1}{HW} \sum_{i=1}^{W} \sum_{j=1}^{H} (F_{ijk} - \mu_k)^2 \tag{14.7}$$

Where, μ_k and σ_k represent the mean and variance of the kth feature map, W and H denotes the width and height of the feature map.

$$F_{2ijN} = \max\{0, \ F_{1ijN}\} \tag{14.8}$$

14.4.3.3.2.6 Dropout Layer The dropout layer is used for regularization in CNN and avoids the overfitting issue. It temporarily removes some units from the network and all its incoming and outgoing connections[36], used in the MuSCF-Net model of 0.2 dropout.

14.4.3.3.2.7 Dense Block Dense layer is widely used in the neural network and is used to change the vector dimension. In this layer, every neuron receives input from all neurons of its previous layer. So it is called a deeply connected layer. In the MuSCF-Net model three Dense Block, i.e., fully connected blocks are used.

14.4.4 Training Details

MuSCF-Net model trained on BreakHis dataset [29] details of the dataset given in Table 14.1. We created 64 × 64 size patches of an image from a given dataset and considered 80% patches as training and 20% as a validation set of each class; each magnification level. We trained our proposed model for ×40, ×100, ×200, and ×400 magnification factor. An Adam optimizer as optimizer and loss function as categorical cross-entropy are used to train a proposed breast histopathological image classification network. The network is trained on NVIDIA GeForce RTX 2060 super GPU for 10-fold cross-validation in each fold 10 epochs with a learning rate – Min 0.0001 to Max 0.001. We used Keras library on Tensorflow to design and train the proposed network.

14.4.4.1 Adam Optimizer [37]

It is a method that computes adaptive Learning (LR) for each parameter. In addition to storing an exponentially decaying average of Past Square of gradient. The mathematical representation of Adam optimizer shown in eq. (14.9)

$$m_t = \beta_1 m_{t-1} + (1 - \beta_1) * \left[\frac{\delta L}{\delta w_t}\right] v_t = \beta_2 v_{t-1} + (1 - \beta_2) * \left[\frac{\delta L}{\delta w_t}\right]^2 \tag{14.9}$$

Parameters Used:

$$m_t = Average \ \ of \ \ gradient;$$

$$v_t = variance\ \ with\ \ respect\ \ to\ \ momentum$$

$$\left[\frac{\delta L}{\delta w_t}\right] = \text{gradient}$$

β_1 & β_2 = decay rates of average of gradients in the above two methods ($\beta1 = 0.9$ & $\beta2 = 0.999$).

It is a momentum-based algorithm, with better control over regularization and average to variances and LR.

14.4.4.2 Activation Function

"A neural network without an activation function is essentially just a linear regression model". Thus activation function is most important feature of any neural network, to add non-linearity in the neuron, i.e., bias. In our module two activation function one is ReLu and another one is Softmax.

14.4.4.3 ReLU

ReLU (Rectified linear unit) is generaly used activation function right now, which ranges from **zero to** ∞, all less than zero values are converted into zero. As shown below.

$$\begin{aligned} F(t) &= t \quad \text{when } t > 0; \\ &= 0 \quad \text{when } t < 0. \end{aligned} \tag{14.10}$$

14.4.4.4 Softmax Activation Function

For decision-making, softmax activation function is useful, so it is used mainly at the last layer, i.e., output layer. It basically gives value to the input variable according to their weight and the sum of these weights is eventually one.

14.4.4.5 Loss

Categorical cross-entropy is log loss function, used for classification problem shown in (Eq. 14.10) [38].

$$\begin{aligned} \text{Categorical cross} - \text{entropy} = -\sum [(f(x)\log\widehat{f(x)}) \\ + (1 - f(x))\log(1 - \widehat{f(x)})] \end{aligned} \tag{14.11}$$

14.5 RESULTS AND DISCUSSION

In this section, we discussed the experimental analysis of the MuSCF-Net for breast histopathological image classification. For a classification problem, accuracy is not efficient as a performance measure; an alternative for classification accuracy is to use precision and recall metric. The performances measure parameters of the network like accuracy, precision (Pr), sensitivity (Se), specificity (Sp), and f1-score is shown in equations (14.12), (14.13), (14.14), and (14.15), respectively, and derived from the confusion matrix (CM) [39]. The formulations of the matrices are described as follows:

$$\text{Accuracy} = \frac{TP + TN}{TP + TN + FN + FP} \tag{14.12}$$

$$\text{Precision} = \frac{TP}{TP + FP} \tag{14.13}$$

$$\text{Se/Recall} = \frac{TP}{TP + FN} \tag{14.14}$$

$$\text{F1 Measure} = \frac{(2 \times Precision \times Recall)}{(Precision + Recall)} \tag{14.15}$$

Here,

TP (true positive) gives the number of malignant and their subclass images accurately predicted as malignant,

TN (true negative) gives the number of benign and their subclass images accurately predicted as benign,

FP (false positive) gives the number of benign and their subclass images inaccurately predicted as malignant,

FN (false negative) gives the number of malignant and their subclass images inaccurately predicted as benign.

The first part, the experimental result of our proposed method was compared with existing models like VGG16 and Xception model shown in Table 14.3, and the MuSCF-Net model achieved a superior, i.e., 98.07% and also less computational parameter 0.58 million result than the existing CNN models (Figure 14.5).

We got results at different magnification levels (×40, ×100, ×200, and ×400) of images but the proposed network gave best result at ×200. Figure 14.4 shows the

TABLE 14.3
The Accuracy and Loss of Existing CNN Models and the Proposed MuSCF-Net

Model		Acc(%)	Loss (%)	Computational Parameter in Million
VGG16	Multi-class	81.37	20.48	138
	Binary	92.58	10.20	
Xception	Multi-class	96.57	8.6	22.9
	Binary	99.01	1.68	
Proposed Model	Multi-class	**97.57**	**3.01**	**0.58**
	Binary	**98.92**	**1.09**	

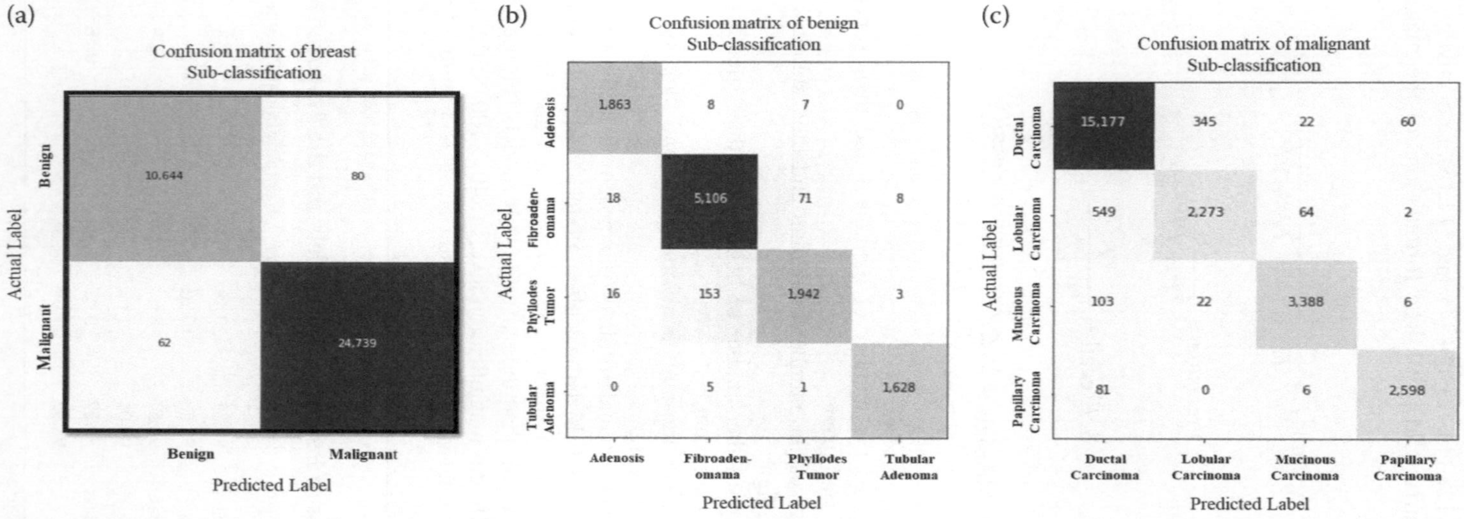

FIGURE 14.5 The confusion matrix of the MuSCF-Net model (a) CM of breast sub-classification (b) CM of benign sub-classification (c) CM of malignant sub-classification.

TABLE 14.4
Performances Measure Parameters of Proposed MuSCF-Net Module for Benign and Malignant Images at ×200 Magnification Level

Class	Sub-Classes	Acc (%)	Pr (%)	Recall (%)	F1 SC (%)	AvgAcc (%)
Benign	A	98.54	98.20	99.20	98.70	98.13
	F	97.07	97.10	98.14	97.62	
	PT	97.59	96.01	92.02	93.97	
	TA	99.01	99.33	99.63	99.47	
Malignant	DC	95.30	95.40	97.43	96.32	97.01
	LC	96.03	86.10	79.87	82.95	
	MC	99.15	97.01	96.55	97.32	
	PC	97.37	97.50	97.54	97.88	

confusion matrix of MuSCF-Net. The BreakHis contains benign and malignant and each into four subclasses. Table 14.4 examined the each subclasses performance measure; the average classification accuracy of subclasses of benign data is 98.13%. Similarly, the average classification accuracy of malignant data is 97.01%.

These superior results achieved by proposed MuSCF-Net model is due to robust feature of convolution of filter bank, which is then refined in CBMA. Multi-scale feature extraction as well as multi-stream network architecture and feature sharing strategy gives robust features, refines them channel attention, and spatial attention models.

14.6 CONCLUSION

In this work, we proposed the DCNN for H & E-stained breast histopathological image classification. The proposed Multi-scale, Multi-Channel feature network using Resnet-Based Attention mechanism for breast histopathological image classification consists multi-scale filter bank and composed of multiple streams for fine and cross level feature with attention mechanism to extract the robust features, and features are shared in between streams and ResBlock from Resnet. This study focused on improving classification accuracy and the classification has been carried out on BREAKHIS dataset. Patches of size 64 × 64 × 3 are created from histopathological images of BREAKHIS dataset. The classification accuracies and performance measure parameters of proposed model have superior 200x magnification level than previously available models. This model is lightweight with lower computational parameter of 0.58 million.

In BREAKHIS dataset only benign and invasive (malignant) cancer types were included; other cancer types such as HER_2, in situ cases, etc. were not included. We use different dataset to train the MuSCF-Net model. The proposed module can be generalized to the design of high-performance CAD systems for other bio-medical imaging processing tasks, in the future.

REFERENCES

[1] Sung, H., et al., Global cancer statistics 2020: GLOBOCAN estimates of incidence and mortality worldwide for 36 cancers in 185 countries. *CA: A Cancer Journal for Clinicians*, 2021.71(3): p. 209–249.

[2] Nover, A.B., et al., Modern breast cancer detection: a technological review. *International Journal of Biomedical Imaging*, 2009. 2009.

[3] Yang, Z., et al., *EMS-Net: Ensemble of multiscale convolutional neural networks for classification of breast cancer histology images. Neurocomputing*, 2019. **366**: p. 46–53.

[4] Screening, P. and P.E. Board, *Breast Cancer Screening (PDQ®), in PDQ Cancer Information Summaries [Internet]*. 2020, National Cancer Institute (US).

[5] Allison, K.H., et al., Trends in breast biopsy pathology diagnoses among women undergoing mammography in the United States: A report from the breast cancer surveillance consortium. *Cancer*, 2015. **121**(9): p. 1369–1378.

[6] Hamidinekoo, A., et al., Deep learning in mammography and breast histology, an overview and future trends. *Medical Image Analysis*, 2018. **47**: p. 45–67.

[7] Allison, K.H., et al., Understanding diagnostic variability in breast pathology: Lessons learned from an expert consensus review panel. *Histopathology*, 2014. **65**(2): p. 240–251.

[8] Elmore, J.G., et al., Variability in pathologists' interpretations of individual breast biopsy slides: a population perspective. *Annals of Internal Medicine*, 2016. **164**(10): p. 649–655.

[9] Coracin, F., et al., Diagnostic concordance among pathologists interpreting oral mucosal biopsies from individuals affected by GvHD. *Oral Surgery, Oral Medicine, Oral Pathology and Oral Radiology*, 2019. **128**(1): p. e36–e37.

[10] Gandomkar, Z., P.C. Brennan, and C. Mello-Thoms, Computer-based image analysis in breast pathology. *Journal of Pathology Informatics*, 2016. **7**.

[11] Niwas, S.I., P. Palanisamy, and K. Sujathan, *Wavelet based feature extraction method for breast cancer cytology images.* in *2010 IEEE Symposium on Industrial Electronics and Applications (ISIEA)*. 2010. IEEE.

[12] Weyn, B., et al., Automated breast tumor diagnosis and grading based on wavelet chromatin texture description. *Cytometry: The Journal of the International Society for Analytical Cytology*, 1998. **33**(1): p. 32–40.

[13] Liu, Z., X.-S. Zhang, and S. Zhang, Breast tumor subgroups reveal diverse clinical prognostic power. *Scientific Reports*, 2014. **4**(1): p.1–9.

[14] Guo, Y., et al., Improvement of cancer subtype prediction by incorporating transcriptome expression data and heterogeneous biological networks. *BMC Medical Genomics*, 2018. **11**(6): p. 87–98.

[15] Guray, M. and A.A. Sahin, Benign breast diseases: classification, diagnosis, and management. *The Oncologist*, 2006. **11**(5): p. 435–449.

[16] Bengio, Y., *Learning deep architectures for AI*. 2009: Now Publishers Inc.

[17] Ker, J., et al., Deep learning applications in medical image analysis. *IEEE Access*, 2017. **6**: p. 9375–9389.

[18] Gupta, P. and S. Garg, Breast cancer prediction using varying parameters of machine learning models. *Procedia Computer Science*, 2020. **171**: p. 593–601.

[19] Akay, M.F., Support vector machines combined with feature selection for breast cancer diagnosis. *Expert Systems with Applications*, 2009. **36**(2): p. 3240–3247.

[20] Gandomkar, Z., P.C. Brennan, and C. Mello-Thoms, MuDeRN: Multi-category classification of breast histopathological image using deep residual networks. *Artificial Intelligence in Medicine*, 2018. **88**: p. 14–24.

[21] Wang, C., et al., *Histopathological image classification with bilinear convolutional neural networks*. in *2017 39th Annual International Conference of the IEEE Engineering in Medicine and Biology Society (EMBC)*. 2017. IEEE.

[22] Hasan, S. Deep Layer CNN Architecture for Breast Cancer Histopathology Image Detection. *in The International Conference on Advanced Machine Learning Technologies and Applications (AMLTA2019)*. 2019. Springer.

[23] Pujari, S.D., M.M. Pawar, and M. Wadekar, Multi-Classification of Breast Histopathological Image Using Xception: Deep Learning with Depthwise Separable Convolutions Model, *in Techno-Societal 2020*. 2021, Springer. p. 539–546.

[24] He, K., et al., Deep residual learning for image recognition. in *Proceedings of the IEEE Conference on Computer Vision and Pattern Recognition*. 2016.

[25] Hou, L., et al., Patch-based convolutional neural network for whole slide tissue image classification. in *Proceedings of the IEEE Conference on Computer Vision and Pattern Recognition*. 2016.

[26] Zainudin, Z., S.M. Shamsuddin, and S. Hasan. *Deep layer CNN architecture for breast cancer histopathology image detection*. in *International Conference on Advanced Machine Learning Technologies and Applications*. 2019. Springer.

[27] Toğaçar, M., et al., *BreastNet: A novel convolutional neural network model through histopathological images for the diagnosis of breast cancer. Physica A: Statistical Mechanics and its Applications*, 2020. **545**: p. 123592.

[28] George, K. and P. Sankaran, *Computer assisted recognition of breast cancer in biopsy images via fusion of nucleus-guided deep convolutional features. Computer Methods and Programs in Biomedicine*, 2020. **194**: p. 105531.

[29] Benhammou, Y., et al., *BreakHis based breast cancer automatic diagnosis using deep learning: Taxonomy, survey and insights. Neurocomputing*, 2020. **375**: p. 9–24.

[30] Szegedy, C., et al., *Going deeper with convolutions*. in *Proceedings of the IEEE Conference on Computer Vision and Pattern Recognition*. 2015.

[31] Woo, S., et al., *CBAM: Convolutional block attention module*. in *Proceedings of the European Conference on Computer Vision (ECCV)*. 2018.

[32] Lin, M., Q. Chen, and S. Yan, *Network in network*. arXiv preprint arXiv:1312.4400, 2013.

[33] Feng, Z., J. Yang, and L. Yao. *Patch-based fully convolutional neural network with skip connections for retinal blood vessel segmentation*. in *2017 IEEE International Conference on Image Processing (ICIP)*. 2017. IEEE.

[34] Yao, J., et al., *Whole slide images based cancer survival prediction using attention guided deep multiple instance learning networks. Medical Image Analysis*, 2020. **65**: p. 101789.

[35] Xie, C., et al. *Beyond classification: Whole slide tissue histopathology analysis by end-to-end part learning. in Medical Imaging with Deep Learning*. 2020. PMLR.

[36] Srivastava, N., et al., *Dropout: a simple way to prevent neural networks from overfitting. The Journal of Machine Learning Research*, 2014. **15**(1): p. 1929–1958.

[37] Kingma, D.P. and J. Ba, *Adam: A method for stochastic optimization*. arXiv preprint arXiv:1412.6980, 2014.

[38] Ho, Y. and S. Wookey, *The real-world-weight cross-entropy loss function: Modeling the costs of mislabeling. IEEE Access*, 2019. **8**: p. 4806–4813.

[39] Powers, D.M., *Evaluation: From precision, recall and F-measure to ROC, informedness, markedness and correlation*. arXiv preprint arXiv:2010.16061, 20

15 Artificial Intelligence is Revolutionizing Cancer Research

B. Sudha, K. Suganya, K. Swathi, and S. Sumathi
Department of Biochemistry, Biotechnology and Bioinformatics, Avinashilingam Institute for Home Science and Higher Education for Women, Coimbatore, India

CONTENTS

15.1 Introduction 263
15.2 Development of Artificial Intelligence in Medical Research 264
15.3 AI in Different Cancer Treatment Modalities 265
15.3.1 Drug Development 265
15.3.2 Chemotherapy 266
15.3.3 Radiotherapy 266
15.3.4 Immunotherapy 267
15.3.5 Identifying Drug Targets 268
15.4 AI in Cancer Prediction at an Early Stage 268
15.5 Future Perspective in AI 270
15.6 Conclusion 271
References 271

15.1 INTRODUCTION

Artificial intelligence (AI) is one of the most common subjects of modern science. It is an evolving field that focuses on research and improvement in human intelligence modeling, extension, expansion hypotheses, processes, technology, and implementation systems. AI is a subdivision at its core, which is the science of computing (Bi et al. 2019; Abbasi, 2018). It is a broad phrase that includes machine learning and deep learning. Machine learning is an area of AI that focuses on deep artificial neural networks, while deep learning is a virtualization technology that concentrates on deep artificial neural networks. Due to its unique performance in computer vision tasks, such as face recognition and image categorization, among others, machine learning has acquired excellent output in recent years (LeCun, Bengio and Hinton, 2015).

Researchers seek to grasp the nature of intelligence and develop modern intelligent machines capable of responding to human intelligence. Advancements

DOI: 10.1201/9781003217497-15

in research and improvements in engineering extend toward medicine to encourage the progression of medical technologies (Sherbet et al. 2018). By edificing fast and precise intelligent medical systems, AI technology has been figured prominently in the medical industry. "Customisation, accuracy, low cost, and accessibility" are the four critical directions of future medical advancements. These paths have become highly evident with the guidance of computer technologies (Timp et al. 2010). Incorporating AI to analyze medical images minimizes the costs and increases the performance drastically. However, devices must be best positioned for the practical implementation of medical image processing to measure up the structural system of extracted images (Odle, 2020). Recently, the production of AI has hit a new eir characteristics like monitored, unera (Caobelli, 2020).

15.2 DEVELOPMENT OF ARTIFICIAL INTELLIGENCE IN MEDICAL RESEARCH

AI refers to the ability of a system to operate by itself. It guides to imitate some human reasoning patterns and intelligent actions to accomplish a specific objective in response to its surrounding background. It should have been acknowledged that several meanings presently subsist. Instead of applying directly programmable, Machine learning (ML), a subfield of AI technology, may change the subject's variables based on considerable amounts of exemplary performances (Deo, 2015). ML can be divided into hand-made and non-hand-made practical strategies based on their characteristics like monitored, unmonitored, and enhanced learning (Goldenberg et al. 2019). Manufactured functional ML techniques can derive various explicit characteristics such as what doctors usually search for during their diagnostics or decision-making procedures, as prescribed by the data collection. These ML techniques can measure the data in an intuitive approach from the samples using heuristic techniques that confide proven and known protocols, such as template matching in medical image analysis or signals (Deo, 2015). Non-handcrafted software ML approaches may handle the raw medical data and then they derive their characteristics by boosting the error rate or other categorization output metrics beyond different labeling from the data set. Learning algorithm relies upon such as aiding vector machines, Naive Bayes categorizations that specialists and protocols that have labeled. On the other hand, unmonitored practices, like critical component assessment, k-means grouping, and auto-encoders, individually separate the clinical samples into separate groups depending on the characteristics of the training results without relevant labels (Tshitoyan et al. 2019). A learning algorithm can be carried out to forecast the clinical examination feature which includes design-free and design-based deep learning, depending on past and present clinical features anticipated by optimizing the projected return at each point (Uehara et al. 2019).

AI has become a rapidly evolving weapon in biomedical applications. While many implementations are still far from feasible, they are quite likely to be realized in the next 10 to 15 years (Caobelli, 2020). A significant field of medical science is experimental medicine. Approximately 70 percent of the clinical judgment knowledge requirement arises from scientific experiments. Sample identification and interpretation are the key objectives of such research. Image recognition and decision-making mechanisms play a vital role in AI technology. At the pre-analysis level, AI implementation primarily concentrates on sample collection, storage, and detecting incompetent specimens. Blood drawing robots, sample distribution robots, automated sample distribution and automatic detection of unqualified samples (Naugler and Church, 2019). Image recognition is the most sophisticated technology in the diagnostic stage. In addition, an AI technology provides a route to the transition of diagnosis reports to test reports (Sun et al. 2017; Gruson et al. 2019).

AI is commonly used for rapid diagnosis (Orringer et al. 2017), prediction (Hornbrook et al. 2017), and treatment of tumors (Kuo et al. 2015). The accelerated growth of AI follows numerous opportunities and threats. One should hold the all-inclusive advantages of the possibilities to brace for the future to use AI technology to support the advancement of medicine and make rapid detection and treatment of diseases more effectively.

15.3 AI IN DIFFERENT CANCER TREATMENT MODALITIES

AI is a method for developing models that perform exceptionally well in preprocessing databases with the help of computer-based methodologies and high-throughput data (Kantarjian and Yu, 2015). Clinical oncology research highly focuses on decoding the molecular development of cancer through an understanding of its complicated biological architecture. It also aims at processing millions of relevant occurrences in Big Data and Biology to address the existing scenario for the growth in cancer mortality worldwide (Dlamini et al. 2020). In addition to it, the use of AI in clinical side increases the odds of NGS and high-resolution imagery techniques for early disease prediction and diagnosis. It would also lead to the evolution of new biomarkers for cancer diagnostics, the development of novel tailored medications, and the implementation of potential treatments utilizing specific bioinformatics tools (Iqbal et al. 2021).

15.3.1 Drug Development

AI is now being used to evaluate the efficacy of anticancer drugs or assist the production of anticancer drugs. Various cancer and the same medications have multiple action approaches, and data from comprehensive testing protocols also uncover the association between cancer cell genomic heterogeneity and drug activity. A random forest model was developed with the combination of artificial intelligence and screening data (Lind and Anderson, 2019). Based on the mutation status of the genomic DNA of cancer cells, the model may determine the behavior of anticancer agents. A machine learning methodology called elastic net regression which used to create a drug susceptibility prediction model (Wang et al. 2018). The drug susceptibility of patients including gastric cancer (Li et al. 2019; Taninaga et al. 2019; Liu et al. 2019), ovarian carcinoma (Paik et al. 2019; Hossain et al. 2019; McDonald, 2018), and endometrial cancer (Stanzione et al. 2021) are successfully predicted through machine learning models. It has been proven that all these patients have a terrible prognosis. This analysis indicates that there is tremendous potential for artificial intelligence to forecast the responsiveness of anticancer medicines.

AI is also used in the fight against cancer drug resistance (Beck et al. 2020). AI can easily explain how cancerous cells turn susceptible to improve healthcare by studying and evaluating information from large drug-resistance, which has the ability to strengthen drug discovery. AI can also reinstall the specialty by minimizing errors and enhancing parameters such as patient specificity monitoring due to its sophisticated computer technology (Thompson et al. 2018). Through amassing data and associated results, AI methods make it possible for devices to enhance a given mission's efficiency steadily and then produce decision support systems. It shows significant output in their precision to differentiate between different histopathological ratings, cancer subtypes, and biomarkers (Rajkomar et al. 2019).

15.3.2 Chemotherapy

In cancer treatment, AI mainly concentrates on the reaction between patients and medicines. The major role of AI includes estimation of drug resistance for chemotherapy, the control of drug use for chemotherapy, and the enhancement of chemotherapy (Chen et al. 2018; Levine et al. 2019; Smail-Tabbone et al. 2019; Zhu et al. 2012). AI could intensify and upgrade the objective functions of integrated treatments. The antagonists of poly ADP-ribose polymerase (PARP) could treat homologous recombination deficiency breast cancer cells. Gulhan et al. 2019, observed cancer cells with homologous recombination defects with 74 percent precision using a deep learning system. Researchers have developed an algorithm with machine learning that can determine the resistance of breast cancer to chemotherapy. The study, which looked at the relationship between patients, genes, and drugs was able to differentiate between effectiveness of multiple chemotherapy drugs, such as taxol and gemcitabine (Dorman et al. 2016). Tang et al. 2019 have reported that the deep learning system is substantially better than the Epstein-Barr DNA-based virus model in risk stratification and instruction for nasopharyngeal carcinoma induction chemotherapy. This implies that the leading function of deep learning can be used to forecast single induction chemotherapy as a possible predictor for advanced nasopharyngeal carcinoma (Peng et al. 2019). They are using an AI platform for breast core needle biopsies to forecast the exposure of high-risk tumors to neoadjuvant chemotherapy. The results provide the foundation for the continued creation of rapid and reproducible predictive methods that could be incorporated into the pathologist's procedure. Overall, they can revolutionize treatment and bring better outcomes for women with high risk and advanced breast cancer (Dodington et al. 2021).

15.3.3 Radiotherapy

The use of AI technologies is more precise throughout the process of cancer radiotherapy. It is designed to assist radiologists in automatically plotting target areas or scheduling radiation therapy for patients (Fiorino et al. 2020; Lou et al. 2019; Meyer et al. 2018). Radiomics is the term for AI-based radiology characterization, providing a more detailed picture than what can be seen with the naked eye (Su et al. 2020; Aerts, 2016). CT-derived radiomarkers were created and validated by creating a functional aerial description on the pretreatment contrast-enhancing CT imaging data for distinguishing immunotherapy responders from non-respondents in melanoma patients and non-small cell lung carcinomas (NSCLC). In this study, lesions with more diverse morphological features such as compact limits and uneven density patterns have been discovered which reacts better to immunotherapy (Forghani et al. 2019). Radiomics based on medical imaging could provide valid non-invasive biomarkers for therapeutic anti-PD1 prediction. It would suggest that AI-based models could be utilized for the assessment of cancer immunotherapy responses (Yan et al. 2019). Likewise, Sun et al. 2018 established the radiomic signatures in retrospective multi-cohort trials to predict clinical outcomes after anti-PD-L1 or anti-PD-1 immunotherapy for patients with highly advanced solid tumors. This methodology provides a potential method to evaluate tumor-infiltrating CD8 signatures and infer clinical results for cancer patients through the combination of RNA-seq genomic data from tumor biopsies and contrast-enhanced CT images. These investigations, therefore, suggested links between the responsiveness of immunotherapy and the properties of radiomics, showing uniform tendencies across cancer kinds as well as anatomical location. In order to obtain automatic differentiation of nasopharyngeal carcinoma with a precision of 79 %, which is equal to that of radiotherapy experts using the three-dimensional convolutional neural network (3D CNN) (Lin et al. 2019). Radiomics merged with deep learning technologies to create a theoretical framework that can determine the exposure to bladder cancer treatment (Cha et al. 2017). Deep learning technology-based automation software was developed to reduce the time to schedule radiation therapy to just a few hours. The AI program generates a treatment plan that is identical to patients typical, but it takes significantly less time (Babier et al. 2018).

15.3.4 Immunotherapy

Compared to conventional chemotherapy, radiotherapy, and surgery, immunotherapy plays a vital role in cancer care with the growing advancement of biotechnology and steady improvement in characteristics of tumor molecular mechanisms. Immunotherapy for cancer uses the patients' accessible immune system to treat cancer and has been known to be the first widely effective technique for multiple cancers (Looi et al. 2019; Fu et al. 2019). Immunotherapy is a significant milestone in developing medication for cancer; it is often confusing to determine whether a single patient can respond to treatment. AI focuses specifically on assessing the drug result and helping doctors change the treatment plan to implement cancer immunotherapy (Jabbari and Rezaei, 2019; Trebeschi et al. 2019; Abbasi, 2019; Tan et al. 2020). Immune checkpoints are repressive signaling pathways and groups of inhibitory receptors targeted by tumors to barricade the role of T lymphocytes and thereby contribute to resistant surveillance. In recent years, encouraging advancements have been made in the use of therapeutic immunotherapy, involving adoptive immunotherapy, immune checkpoint inhibitors, tumor vaccinations, and chimeric antigen receptor T cell therapies (Nishino et al. 2017). Clinical experience with immunotherapy can also be improved by enhancing its diagnosis efficacy and by selecting sick-person more prepared to respond to medications, in addition to tracking treatment outcomes. AI application services have appeared more regularly on the market, allowing natural language processing and vertical domain image algorithms and fulfilling the demands of the pharmaceutical sector and establishing a prime spot for the use of AI in medicine (Tang et al. 2019).

The implementation of AI increases the possibility of effective cancer immunotherapy by predicting the pharmacological activity based on the development of predictive immunotherapy ratings, including immunophenoscore and immunoscore (Angell and Galon, 2013). These two scoring systems have been designed to predict immune blocking point (ICB) reactions. Implementing an AI-based therapeutic framework with the descriptions of doctors can be strongly associated with improving diagnostic precision for indistinguishable subsets of cancer (Rajkomar et al. 2019). Consequently, the use of AI in cancer immunotherapy can bring oneself closer to good results in patients. A machine learning-based AI platform was created to accurately anticipate the therapeutic efficacy of programmed cell death protein 1 (PD-1) inhibitors (Sun et al. 2018). In patients with advanced solid tumors that are immune to PD-1 inhibitors, this platform can accurately measure the effects of immunotherapy. A machine learning method based on a human leukocyte antigen (HLA) mass spectrometry database was developed to enhance the detection of neoantigen cancer and the efficacy of cancer immunotherapy (Bulik-Sullivan et al. 2018).

15.3.5 Identifying Drug Targets

Machine learning technologies can provide a vital predictive and therapeutic prediction for patients with Epithelial Ovarian cancer before initial care. Predictive analytics can promote customized care choices by patient pre-treatment stratified (Kawakami et al. 2019). A comprehensive and entirely automatic system for the diagnosis and location of PTEN (Phosphatase and tensin homolog) loss in prostate cancer tissue samples has been demonstrated. AI-based algorithms can streamline sample evaluations in scientific and clinical laboratories (Harmon et al. 2021). ML-based collection of image retrieval approaches accompanied by survival analysis to predict particular miRNA biomarkers for breast cancer (Sarkar et al. 2021). A transformative interdisciplinary approach was proposed to identify early lung cancer diagnostic biomarkers with the association of integrating metabolomics and machine learning approaches. Metabolic biomarkers show significant diagnostic power for the early diagnosis of lung tumors (Xie et al. 2021).

15.4 AI IN CANCER PREDICTION AT AN EARLY STAGE

The timing of cancer identification, the accuracy of cancer diagnosis, and staging are all critical factors that influence clinical decision-making and outcomes. AI has made substantial contributions to this essential field of cancer in only a few years, with sometimes performance comparable to human specialists and with the added benefits of scalability and automation (Bhinder et al. 2021).

Digital photographs processing application was designed for women's cervix and reliably recognized the precancerous lesions that need to be handled to minimize patient over-diagnosis (Hu et al. 2019). A machine learning technique has been developed to reduce the unnecessary treatment of lesions suspected of becoming breast cancer. The method will predict the tumors are likely to become high-risk breast lesions, helping doctors choose the treatment choices and minimize needless surgeries (Bahl et al. 2018). Machine learning will predict average patients undergoing mortality results for hepatocellular carcinoma (Wang et al. 2021). Utilizing machine learning approaches, prediction models for early and late progression of first-line HR+/HER2-negative metastatic breast cancer have been developed. Based on professionally acquired data, the results of NLP-based machine learning models are somewhat better than predictive models (Ribelles et al. 2021).

Many studies have been published that deep learning-based models can diagnose cancer earlier and identify cancer subtypes directly from histopathologic and other medical images. Deep neural networks (DNNs) are potent algorithms applied to large images from biopsies or surgical resections with enough computing power. In addition, these model architectures have demonstrated their ability to classify images, such as determining whether or not a digitized stained slide contains cancer cells (Bejnordi et al. 2017; Khosravi et al. 2018; Liu et al. 2019; Al-Haija and Adebanjo 2020; Li et al. 2017; Korbar et al. 2017; Coudray et al. 2018; Iizuka et al. 2020; Campanella et al. 2019). The success of DNNs is not just limited to historic pathological photos. Still, it extends to other medical images acquired by non-invasive procedures like CT scans, MRIs, and mammograms and even suspected lesion photographs (Esteva et al. 2017).

The science of deep learning makes cancer care decisions more insightful. AI could find the most effective care strategy for physicians by knowing the medical data science of cancer patients (Meyer et al. 2018; Liu et al. 2018; Bogani et al. 2018; Walsh et al. 2019; Blackledge et al. 2019). A Clinical Decision Support System (CDSS) based on deep learning technologies was developed to collect and analyze a vast volume of clinical data from medical reports and create alternatives for cancer care. The study reveals the value of AI technologies in assisting oncologists in improvising patient cancer care strategies (Printz, 2017).

Thousands of cancer laboratories are now regularly sequencing cancer genes, genomes, and exomes due to the widespread availability of NGS. Still, they typically fail in specific situations, such as insufficient coverage and repeat-rich genome sections. Several computational approaches may be used to identify mutations and genetic variants in NGS data. The idea of recasting mutation detection as a machine learning problem has been investigated by several organizations (Poplin et al. 2018; Park et al. 2019). On high-throughput screening results, machine learning techniques can be equipped to create methods for predicting the reaction of patients and cancer cell lines to new drug substances and drug formulations (Simon et al. 2020; Meng et al. 2020; Goecks et al. 2020). Researchers are speeding up drug development using machine learning to produce and establish reverse synthesis pathways for molecules. A lot of data is created by the entire process of making a new medicine. Machine learning offers a fantastic opportunity to process chemical data and deliver outcomes that will assist us in producing drugs (Nascimento et al. 2019; Sharma and Rani, 2020; Watson et al. 2019). Machine learning will assist us in processing knowledge gathered over the years, if not decades, in a relatively short amount of time (Vamathevan et al. 2019). It would also assist us in making more rational choices that would otherwise have to be taken through prognostication and examination (Koromina et al. 2019; Klambauer et al. 2019; Ballester, 2019).

Deep learning (DL) has achieved top performance in drug investigation (Xia et al. 2020; Baskin, 2020; Stokes et al. 2020). These models have specific features that can make them more efficient for challenging operations in the modeling of drug interactions based upon chemical and biological information, but only in recent times have deep learning been investigated to predict drug reactions. DL has lately been utilized to create unprecedented gains in the way computers derive information from images. DL has been used to create attractive new medication reuse potential.

15.5 FUTURE PERSPECTIVE IN AI

While AI methods have a great promise in cancer immunotherapy, various challenges were faced during the initial launch of AI strategies into healthcare delivery. For example, missed assumptions in models and primary data could lead to the AI system generating harmful suggestions undiscerning local care systems (Crawford and Calo 2016; Cabitza et al. 2017). Most patients will quickly be impacted by problems with commonly used software. In addition, AI's involvement in therapy supervision may threaten some categories of medical employment, resulting in expertise and potential technological mistakes (Cabitza et al. 2017; Verghese et al. 2018). To manage these drawbacks efficiently, it is crucial to establish appropriate strategies as follows,

i. It is essential to understand and examine the types of socio-technical risks that AI strategies may pose in various healthcare aspects to create a coherent outline of the protected environment (Shameer et al. 2018).
ii. In order to rule and clarify the patient safety venture developed by AI systems, the development of socio-technical security models and related analytical methods is necessary (McCartney and Margaret McCartney 2018).
iii. In order to build institutional and social structures worthy of approval and support, people must first consider the viewpoints of patients, clinicians, and the general public concerning the acceptability, advantages, and risks of AI interventions in active therapeutics, as well as in developing institutional and social mechanisms deserving of recognition and support (Esteva et al. 2019).
iv. Developing on higher-level standards, checking the actual statutory responsibilities and basic organizational structure would allow the stability of evolving AI systems to be assured, while at the same time adapting to the unique challenges of technology governance, with the features of

continuous independent adaptation and development (Winfield and Jirotka 2018; Macrae 2019).

In addition, to enhance immunotherapy response prediction, new accurate computational models incorporating different biomarkers are required. Developers newly created a platform containing the entire biochemical indices of cancer patients, biomarkers, and radiography data to include some practical methods for improving AI-based frameworks (Zeng et al. 2019).

15.6 CONCLUSION

AI also makes extraordinary attention to the advancement and development of anticancer medications. Humans are constrained with their experience level, finding it impossible to devise the most appropriate therapy. From this perspective, patients will skip crucial care options if doctors seek ineffective treatment, which will also worsen the patient's condition. To conclude, AI is commonly used in the healthcare industry, and its production offers users improved healthcare services. It can have valuable ideas and insights which cannot be detected through personal authentication, and for each cancer patient, it can personalize treatment. The development of new technologies could be facilitated with AI, which might significantly step up the production of anticancer medicines. It is assumed that AI is expected to be a vital motivating factor in the study and treatment of human cancer. In the future, we think AI will make outstanding contributions to modern onco-medicine.

REFERENCES

[1] Abbasi J. "Electronic Nose" predicts immunotherapy response. *JAMA*. Nov. 2019; 322(18):1756.

[2] Abbasi J. Artificial intelligence tools for sepsis and cancer. *JAMA*. 2018 Dec. 11; 320(22):2303.

[3] Aerts HJ. The potential of radiomic-based phenotyping in precision medicine: A review. *JAMA Oncology*. Dec. 2016; 2(12):1636–1642.

[4] Al-Haija QA, Adebanjo A. Breast cancer diagnosis in histopathological images using ResNet-50 convolutional neural network. In 2020 IEEE International IOT, Electronics and Mechatronics Conference (IEMTRONICS) 2020 Sep 9 (pp. 1–7). IEEE.

[5] Angell H, Galon J. From the immune contexture to the Immunoscore: The role of prognostic and predictive immune markers in cancer. *Current Opinion in Immunology*. Apr. 2013; 25(2):261–267.

[6] Babier A, Boutilier JJ, McNiven AL, Chan TC. Knowledge-based automated planning for oropharyngeal cancer. *Medical Physics*. Jul. 2018; 45(7):2875–2883.

[7] Bahl M, Barzilay R, Yedidia AB, Locascio NJ, Yu L, Lehman CD. High-risk breast lesions: A machine learning model to predict pathologic upgrade and reduce unnecessary surgical excision. *Radiology*. Mar. 2018; 286(3):810–818.

[8] Ballester PJ. Machine learning for molecular modelling in drug design. *Biomolecules*. 2019; 9(6):E216.

[9] Baskin II. The power of deep learning to ligand-based novel drug discovery. *Expert Opinion on Drug Discovery*. Jul. 2020; 15(7):755–764.

[10] Beck JT, Rammage M, Jackson GP, Preininger AM, Dankwa-Mullan I, Roebuck MC, Torres A, Holtzen H, Coverdill SE, Williamson MP, Chau Q. Artificial intelligence tool for optimizing eligibility screening for clinical trials in a large community cancer center. *JCO Clinical Cancer Informatics*. Jan. 2020; 4:50–59.
[11] Bejnordi BE, Veta M, Van Diest PJ, Van Ginneken B, Karssemeijer N, Litjens G, Van Der Laak JA, Hermsen M, Manson QF, Balkenhol M, Geessink O. Diagnostic assessment of deep learning algorithms for detection of lymph node metastases in women with breast cancer. *JAMA*. Dec. 2017; 318(22):2199–2210.
[12] Bi WL, Hosny A, Schabath MB, Giger ML, Birkbak NJ, Mehrtash A, Allison T, Arnaout O, Abbosh C, Dunn IF, Mak RH. Artificial intelligence in cancer imaging: Clinical challenges and applications. *CA: A Cancer Journal for Clinicians*. Mar. 2019; 69(2):127–157.
[13] Binder A, Bockmayr M, Hagele M, Winenert S, Heim D, Hellweg K, Ishii M, Stenzinger A, Hocke A, Denkert C, Muller K R. Morphological and molecular breast cancer profiling through explainable machine learning. *Nature Machine Intelligence*. Apr. 2021; 3(4): 355–366.
[14] Blackledge MD, Winfield JM, Miah A, Strauss D, Thway K, Morgan VA, Collins DJ, Koh DM, Leach MO, Messiou C. Supervised machine-learning enables segmentation and evaluation of heterogeneous post-treatment changes in multi-parametric MRI of soft tissue sarcoma. *Frontiers in Oncology*. Oct. 2019; 9:941.
[15] Bogani G, Rossetti D, Ditto A, Martinelli F, Chiappa V, Mosca L, Leone Roberti Maggiore U, Ferla S, Lorusso D, Raspagliesi F, Artificial intelligence weights the importance of factors predicting complete cytoreduction at secondary cytoreductive surgery for recurrent ovarian cancer, *Journal of Gynecologic Oncology*. 2018; 29(5): e66.
[16] Bulik-Sullivan B, Busby J, Palmer CD, Davis MJ, Murphy T, Clark A, Busby M, Duke F, Yang A, Young L, Ojo NC. Deep learning using tumor HLA peptide mass spectrometry datasets improves neoantigen identification. *Nature Biotechnology*. Jan.. 2018; 37(1):55–63.
[17] Cabitza F, Rasoini R, Gensini GF. Unintended consequences of machine learning in medicine. *JAMA*. Aug. 2017; 318(6):517–518.
[18] Campanella G, Hanna MG, Geneslaw L, Miraflor A, Silva VW, Busam KJ, Brogi E, Reuter VE, Klimstra DS, Fuchs TJ. Clinical-grade computational pathology using weakly supervised deep learning on whole slide images. *Nature Medicine*. Aug. 2019; 25(8):1301–1309.
[19] Caobelli F. Artificial intelligence in medical imaging: Game over for radiologists?. *European Journal of Radiology*. May 2020; 126:108940.
[20] Cha KH, Hadjiiski L, Chan HP, Weizer AZ, Alva A, Cohan RH, Caoili EM, Paramagul C, Samala RK. Bladder cancer treatment response assessment in CT using radiomics with deep-learning. *Scientific Reports*. Aug. 2017; 7(1):1–2.
[21] Chen G, Tsoi A, Xu H, Zheng WJ. Predict effective drug combination by deep belief network and ontology fingerprints. *Journal of Biomedical Informatics*. Sep. 2018; 85:149–154.
[22] Coudray N, Ocampo PS, Sakellaropoulos T, Narula N, Snuderl M, Fenyö D, Moreira AL, Razavian N, Tsirigos A. Classification and mutation prediction from non–small cell lung cancer histopathology images using deep learning. *Nature Medicine*. Oct. 2018; 24(10):1559–1567.
[23] Crawford K, Calo R. There is a blind spot in AI research. *Nature News*. Oct. 2016; 538(7625):311.
[24] Deo RC. Machine learning in medicine. *Circulation*. Nov. 2015; 132(20):1920–1930.
[25] Dlamini Z, Francies FZ, Hull R, Marima R. Artificial intelligence (AI) and big data

in cancer and precision oncology. *Computational and Structural Biotechnology Journal*. 2020; 18: 2300–2311.
[26] Dodington DW, Lagree A, Tabbarah S, Mohebpour M, Sadeghi-Naini A, Tran WT, Lu FI. Analysis of tumor nuclear features using artificial intelligence to predict response to neoadjuvant chemotherapy in high-risk breast cancer patients. *Breast Cancer Research and Treatment*. Apr. 2021; 186(2):379–389.
[27] Dorman SN, Baranova K, Knoll JH, Urquhart BL, Mariani G, Carcangiu ML, Rogan PK. Genomic signatures for paclitaxel and gemcitabine resistance in breast cancer derived by machine learning. *Molecular Oncology*. Jan. 2016; 10(1):85–100.
[28] Esteva A, Kuprel B, Novoa RA, Ko J, Swetter SM, Blau HM, Thrun S. Dermatologist-level classification of skin cancer with deep neural networks. *Nature*. Feb. 2017; 542 (7639):115–118.
[29] Esteva A, Robicquet A, Ramsundar B, Kuleshov V, DePristo M, Chou K, et al. A guide to deep learning in healthcare. *Nature Medicine*. Jan. 2019; 25(1): 24–29.
[30] Fiorino C, Guckenberger M, Schwarz M, van der Heide UA, Heijmen B. Technology-driven research for radiotherapy innovation. *Molecular Oncology*. Jul. 2020; 14(7):1500–1513.
[31] Forghani R, Savadjiev P, Chatterjee A, Muthukrishnan N, Reinhold C, Forghani B. Radiomics and artificial intelligence for biomarker and prediction model development in oncology. *Computational and Structural Biotechnology Journal*. 2019; 17:995.
[32] Fu Y, Liu S, Zeng S, Shen H. From bench to bed: the tumor immune microenvironment and current immunotherapeutic strategies for hepatocellular carcinoma. *Journal of Experimental & Clinical Cancer Research*. Dec. 2019; 38(1):1–21.
[33] Goecks J, Jalili V, Heiser LM, Gray JW. How machine learning will transform biomedicine. *Cell*. Apr. 2020; 181(1):92–101.
[34] Goldenberg SL, Nir G, Salcudean SE. A new era: Artificial intelligence and machine learning in prostate cancer. *Nature Reviews Urology*. Jul. 2019; 16(7):391–403.
[35] Gruson D, Helleputte T, Rousseau P, Gruson D. Data science, artificial intelligence, and machine learning: opportunities for laboratory medicine and the value of positive regulation. *Clinical Biochemistry*. Jul. 2019; 69:1–7.
[36] Gulhan DC, Lee JJ, Melloni GE, Cortes-Ciriano I, Park PJ. Detecting the mutational signature of homologous recombination deficiency in clinical samples. *Nature Genetics*. May 2019; 51(5):912–919.
[37] Günakan E, Atan S, Haberal AN, Küçükyıldız İA, Gökçe E, Ayhan A. A novel prediction method for lymph node involvement in endometrial cancer: machine learning. *International Journal of Gynecologic Cancer*. Feb. 2019; 29(2): 320–324
[38] Harmon SA, Patel PG, Sanford TH, Caven I, Iseman R, Vidotto T, Picanco C, Squire JA, Masoudi S, Mehralivand S, Choyke PL. High throughput assessment of biomarkers in tissue microarrays using artificial intelligence: PTEN loss as a proof-of-principle in multi-center prostate cancer cohorts. *Modern Pathology*. Feb. 2021; 34(2):478–489.
[39] Hornbrook MC, Goshen R, Choman E, O'Keeffe-Rosetti M, Kinar Y, Liles EG, Rust KC. Early colorectal cancer detected by machine learning model using gender, age, and complete blood count data. *Digestive Diseases and Sciences*. Oct. 2017; 62(10):2719–2727.
[40] Hossain MA, Islam SM, Quinn JM, Huq F, Moni MA. Machine learning and bioinformatics models to identify gene expression patterns of ovarian cancer associated with disease progression and mortality. *Journal of Biomedical Informatics*. Dec. 2019; 100:103313.
[41] Hu L, Bell D, Antani S, Xue Z, Yu K, Horning MP, Gachuhi N, Wilson B, Jaiswal MS, Befano B, Long LR. An observational study of deep learning and automated

evaluation of cervical images for cancer screening. *JNCI: Journal of the National Cancer Institute*. Sep. 2019; 111(9):923–932.

[42] Iizuka O, Kanavati F, Kato K, Rambeau M, Arihiro K, Tsuneki M. Deep learning models for histopathological classification of gastric and colonic epithelial tumours. *Scientific Reports*. Jan. 2020; 10(1):1–1.

[43] Iqbal MJ, Javed Z, Sadia H, Qureshi IA, Irshad A, Ahmed R, Malik K, Raza S, Abbas A, Pezzani R, Sharifi-Rad J. Clinical applications of artificial intelligence and machine learning in cancer diagnosis: Looking into the future. *Cancer Cell International*. Dec. 2021; 21(1):1–1.

[44] Jabbari P, Rezaei N. Artificial intelligence and immunotherapy. *Expert Review of Clinical Immunology*. Jul. 2019; 15(7):689–691.

[45] Kantarjian H, Yu PP. Artificial intelligence, big data, and cancer. *JAMA Oncology*. Aug. 2015; 1(5):573–574.

[46] Kawakami E, Tabata J, Yanaihara N, Ishikawa T, Koseki K, Iida Y, Saito M, Komazaki H, Shapiro JS, Goto C, Akiyama Y. Application of artificial intelligence for preoperative diagnostic and prognostic prediction in epithelial ovarian cancer based on blood biomarkers. *Clinical Cancer Research*. May 2019; 25(10):3006–3015.

[47] Khosravi P, Kazemi E, Imielinski M, Elemento O, Hajirasouliha I. Deep convolutional neural networks enable discrimination of heterogeneous digital pathology images. *EBioMedicine*. Jan. 2018; 27:317–328.

[48] Klambauer G, Hochreiter S, Rarey M. *Machine Learning in Drug Discovery*. 2019; 59(3) 945–946.

[49] Korbar B, Olofson AM, Miraflor AP, Nicka CM, Suriawinata MA, Torresani L, Suriawinata AA, Hassanpour S. Deep learning for classification of colorectal polyps on whole-slide images. *Journal of Pathology Informatics*. 2017; 8:1–9.

[50] Koromina M, Pandi MT, Patrinos GP. Rethinking drug repositioning and development with artificial intelligence, machine learning, and omics. *Omics: A Journal of Integrative Biology*. Nov. 2019; 23(11):539–548.

[51] Kuo RJ, Huang MH, Cheng WC, Lin CC, Wu YH. Application of a two-stage fuzzy neural network to a prostate cancer prognosis system. *Artificial Intelligence in Medicine*. Feb. 2015; 63(2):119–133.

[52] LeCun Y, Bengio Y, Hinton G. Deep learning. *Nature*. May 2015; 521(7553): 436 10.1038/nature14539.

[53] Levine MN, Alexander G, Sathiyapalan A, Agrawal A, Pond G. Learning health system for breast cancer: pilot project experience. *JCO Clinical Cancer Informatics*. Aug. 2019; 3:1–1.

[54] Li Q, Qi L, Feng QX, Liu C, Sun SW, Zhang J, Yang G, Ge YQ, Zhang YD, Liu XS. Machine learning–based computational models derived from large-scale radiographic- radiomic images can help predict adverse histopathological status of gastric cancer. *Clinical and Translational Gastroenterology*. Oct. 2019; 10(10): 1–13.

[55] Li S, Jiang H, Pang W. Joint multiple fully connected convolutional neural network with extreme learning machine for hepatocellular carcinoma nuclei grading. *Computers in Biology and Medicine*. May 2017; 84:156–167.

[56] Lin L, Dou Q, Jin YM, Zhou GQ, Tang YQ, Chen WL, Su BA, Liu F, Tao CJ, Jiang N, Li JY. Deep learning for automated contouring of primary tumor volumes by MRI for nasopharyngeal carcinoma. *Radiology*. Jun. 2019; 291(3):677–686.

[57] Lind AP, Anderson PC. Predicting drug activity against cancer cells by random forest models based on minimal genomic information and chemical properties. *PLoS One*. Jul. 2019; 14(7):e0219774.

[58] Liu C, Liu X, Wu F, Xie M, Feng Y, Hu C. Using artificial intelligence (Watson for Oncology) for treatment recommendations amongst Chinese patients with lung cancer: feasibility study. *Journal of Medical Internet Research*. 2018; 20(9):e11087.
[59] Liu C, Qi L, Feng QX, Sun SW, Zhang YD, Liu XS. Performance of a machine learning based decision model to help clinicians decide the extent of lymphadenectomy (D1 vs. D2) in gastric cancer before surgical resection. *Abdominal Radiology*. Sep. 2019; 44(9):3019–3029.
[60] Liu Y, Kohlberger T, Norouzi M, Dahl GE, Smith JL, Mohtashamian A, Olson N, Peng LH, Hipp JD, Stumpe MC. Artificial intelligence–based breast cancer nodal metastasis detection: insights into the black box for pathologists. *Archives of Pathology & Laboratory Medicine*. Jul. 2019; 143(7):859–868.
[61] Looi CK, Chung FF, Leong CO, Wong SF, Rosli R, Mai CW. Therapeutic challenges and current immunomodulatory strategies in targeting the immunosuppressive pancreatic tumor microenvironment. *Journal of Experimental & Clinical Cancer Research*. Dec. 2019; 38(1):1–23.
[62] Lou B, Doken S, Zhuang T, Wingerter D, Gidwani M, Mistry N, Ladic L, Kamen A, Abazeed ME. An image-based deep learning framework for individualising radiotherapy dose: a retrospective analysis of outcome prediction. *The Lancet Digital Health*. Jul. 2019; 1(3):e136–e147.
[63] Macrae C. Governing the safety of artificial intelligence in healthcare. *BMJ Quality & Safety*. Jun. 2019; 28(6): 495–498.
[64] McCartney M. Margaret McCartney: AI in medicine must be rigorously tested. *BMJ*. Apr. 2018; 361.
[65] McDonald JF. Back to the future-The integration of big data with machine learning is reestablishing the importance of predictive correlations in ovarian cancer diagnostics and therapeutics. 2018; 230–231
[66] Meng C, Hu Y, Zhang Y, Guo F. PSBP-SVM: A machine learning-based computational identifier for predicting polystyrene binding peptides. *Frontiers in Bioengineering and Biotechnology*. Mar. 2020; 8:245.
[67] Meyer P, Noblet V, Mazzara C, Lallement A. Survey on deep learning for radiotherapy. *Computers in Biology and Medicine*. Jul. 2018; 98:126–146.
[68] Nascimento AC, Prudêncio RB, Costa IG. A drug-target network-based supervised machine learning repurposing method allowing the use of multiple heterogeneous information sources. In *Computational Methods for Drug Repurposing* 2019 (pp. 281–289). Humana Press, New York, NY.
[69] Naugler C, Church DL. Automation and artificial intelligence in the clinical laboratory. *Critical Reviews in Clinical Laboratory Sciences*. Feb. 2019; 56(2):98–110.
[70] Nishino M, Ramaiya NH, Hatabu H, Hodi FS. Monitoring immune-checkpoint blockade: response evaluation and biomarker development. *Nature Reviews Clinical Oncology*. Nov. 2017; 14(11):655–668.
[71] Odle T. The AI era: The role of medical imaging and radiation therapy professionals. *Radiologic Technology*. Mar. 2020; 91(4):391–400.
[72] Orringer DA, Pandian B, Niknafs YS, Hollon TC, Boyle J, Lewis S, Garrard M, Hervey- Jumper SL, Garton HJ, Maher CO, Heth JA. Rapid intraoperative histology of unprocessed surgical specimens via fibre-laser-based stimulated Raman scattering microscopy. *Nature Biomedical Engineering*. Feb. 2017; 1(2):1–3.
[73] Paik ES, Lee JW, Park JY, Kim JH, Kim M, Kim TJ, Choi CH, Kim BG, Bae DS, Seo SW. Prediction of survival outcomes in patients with epithelial ovarian cancer using machine learning methods. *Journal of Gynecologic Oncology*. Apr. 2019; 30(4): 1–13.
[74] Park H, Chun SM, Shim J, Oh JH, Cho EJ, Hwang HS, Lee JY, Kim D, Jang SJ, Nam SJ, Hwang C. Detection of chromosome structural variation by targeted next-

generation sequencing and a deep learning application. *Scientific Reports*. Mar. 2019; 9(1):1–9.
[75] Peng H, Dong D, Fang MJ, Li L, Tang LL, Chen L, Li WF, Mao YP, Fan W, Liu LZ, Tian L. Prognostic value of deep learning PET/CT-based radiomics: Potential role for future individual induction chemotherapy in advanced nasopharyngeal carcinoma. *Clinical Cancer Research*. Jul. 2019; 25(14):4271–4279.
[76] Poplin R, Chang PC, Alexander D, Schwartz S, Colthurst T, Ku A, Newburger D, Dijamco J, Nguyen N, Afshar PT, Gross SS. A universal SNP and small-indel variant caller using deep neural networks. *Nature Biotechnology*. Nov. 2018; 36(10):983–987.
[77] Printz C. Artificial intelligence platform for oncology could assist in treatment decisions. *Cancer*. Mar. 2017; 123(6):905.
[78] Rajkomar A, Dean J, Kohane I. Machine learning in medicine. *New England Journal of Medicine*. Apr. 2019; 380(14):1347–1358.
[79] Ribelles N, Jerez JM, Rodriguez-Brazzarola P, Jimenez B, Diaz-Redondo T, Mesa H, Marquez A, Sanchez-Muñoz A, Pajares B, Carabantes F, Bermejo MJ. Machine learning and natural language processing (NLP) approach to predict early progression to first-linetreatment in real-world hormone receptor-positive (HR +)/HER2-negative advanced breast cancer patients. *European Journal of Cancer*. Feb. 2021; 144:224–231.
[80] Sarkar JP, Saha I, Sarkar A, Maulik U. Machine learning integrated ensemble of feature selection methods followed by survival analysis for predicting breast cancer subtype specific miRNA biomarkers. *Computers in Biology and Medicine*. Apr. 2021; 131:104244.
[81] Shameer K, Johnson KW, Glicksberg BS, Dudley JT, Sengupta PP. The whole is greater than the sum of its parts: Combining classical statistical and machine intelligence methods in medicine. *Heart*, Jul. 2018; 4(14):1228.
[82] Sharma A, Rani R. Ensembled machine learning framework for drug sensitivity prediction. *IET Systems Biology*. Oct. 2019; 14(1):39–46.
[83] Sherbet GV, Woo WL, Dlay S. Application of artificial intelligence-based technology in cancer management: A commentary on the deployment of artificial neural networks. *Anticancer Research*. Dec. 2018; 38(12):6607–6613.
[84] Simon AB, Vitzthum LK, Mell LK. Challenge of directly comparing imaging-based diagnoses made by machine learning algorithms with those made by human clinicians. *Journal of Clinical Oncology*. Jun. 2020; 38(16):1868.
[85] Smail-Tabbone M et al., I.Y.S.O.B. Section Editors for the I. Translational, Contributions from the 2018 literature on bioinformatics and translational informatics, *Yearbook of Medical Informatics*. 2019; 28(1): 190–193.
[86] Stanzione A, Cuocolo R, Del Grosso R, Nardiello A, Romeo V, Travaglino A, Raffone A, Bifulco G, Zullo F, Insabato L, Maurea S. Deep myometrial infiltration of endometrial cancer on MRI: A radiomics-powered machine learning pilot study. *Academic Radiology*. May 2021; 28(5):737–744.
[87] Stokes JM, Yang K, Swanson K, Jin W, Cubillos-Ruiz A, Donghia NM, MacNair CR, French S, Carfrae LA, Bloom-Ackermann Z, Tran VM. A deep learning approach to antibiotic discovery. *Cell*. Feb. 2020; 180(4):688–702.
[88] Su X, Chen N, Sun H, Liu Y, Yang X, Wang W, Zhang S, Tan Q, Su J, Gong Q, Yue Q. Automated machine learning based on radiomics features predicts H3 K27M mutation in midline gliomas of the brain. *Neuro-oncology*. Mar. 2020; 22(3):393–401.
[89] Sun R, Limkin EJ, Vakalopoulou M, Dercle L, Champiat S, Han SR, Verlingue L, Brandao D, Lancia A, Ammari S, Hollebecque A. A radiomics approach to assess

tumourinfiltrating CD8 cells and response to anti-PD-1 or anti-PD-L1 immunotherapy: An imaging biomarker, retrospective multicohort study. *The Lancet Oncology*. Sep. 2018; 19(9):1180–1191.

[90] Sun Y, Liu Y, Wang G, Zhang H. Deep learning for plant identification in natural environment. *Computational Intelligence and Neuroscience*. May 2017; 2017.

[91] Tan S, Li D, Zhu X. Cancer immunotherapy: Pros, cons and beyond. *Biomedicine & Pharmacotherapy*. Apr. 2020; 124:109821.

[92] Tang X, Huang Y, Lei J, Luo H, Zhu X. The single-cell sequencing: New developments and medical applications. *Cell & Bioscience*. Dec. 2019; 9(1):1–9.

[93] Tang Z, Chuang KV, DeCarli C, Jin LW, Beckett L, Keiser MJ, Dugger BN. Interpretable classification of Alzheimer's disease pathologies with a convolutional neural network pipeline. *Nature Communications*. May 2019; 10(1):1–4.

[94] Taninaga J, Nishiyama Y, Fujibayashi K, Gunji T, Sasabe N, Iijima K, Naito T. Prediction of future gastric cancer risk using a machine learning algorithm and comprehensive medical check-up data: A case-control study. *Scientific Reports*. Aug. 2019; 9(1):1–9.

[95] Thompson RF, Valdes G, Fuller CD, Carpenter CM, Morin O, Aneja S, Lindsay WD, Aerts HJ, Agrimson B, Deville Jr C, Rosenthal SA. Artificial intelligence in radiation oncology: A specialty-wide disruptive transformation?. *Radiotherapy and Oncology*. Dec. 2018; 129(3):421–426.

[96] Timp S, Varela C, Karssemeijer N. Computer-aided diagnosis with temporal analysis to improve radiologists' interpretation of mammographic mass lesions. *IEEE Transactions on Information Technology in Biomedicine*. Apr 2010; 14(3):803–808.

[97] Trebeschi S, Drago SG, Birkbak NJ, Kurilova I, Calin A M, Delli Pizzi A, Lalezari F, Lambregts DMJ, Rohaan M W, Parmar C, Rozeman E A, Hartemink K J, Swanton C, Haanen J, Blank C U, Smit E F, Beets-Tan R G H, Aerts H, Predicting response to cancer immunotherapy using noninvasive radiomic biomarkers, *Annals of Oncology*. 2019; 30(6): 998–1004.

[98] Tshitoyan V, Dagdelen J, Weston L, Dunn A, Rong Z, Kononova O, Persson KA, Ceder G, Jain A. Unsupervised word embeddings capture latent knowledge from materials science literature. *Nature*. Jul. 2019; 571(7763):95–98.

[99] Uehara S, Mawase F, Therrien AS, Cherry-Allen KM, Celnik P. Interactions between motor exploration and reinforcement learning. *Journal of Neurophysiology*. Aug. 2019; 122(2):797–808.

[100] Vamathevan J, Clark D, Czodrowski P, Dunham I, Ferran E, Lee G, Li B, Madabhushi A, Shah P, Spitzer M, Zhao S. Applications of machine learning in drug discovery and development. *Nature Reviews Drug Discovery*. Jun. 2019; 18(6):463–477.

[101] Verghese A, Shah NH, Harrington RA. What this computer needs is a physician: Humanism and artificial intelligence. *JAMA*. Jan. 2018; 319(1):19–20.

[102] Walsh S, de Jong EE, van Timmeren JE, Ibrahim A, Compter I, Peerlings J, Sanduleanu S, Refaee T, Keek S, Larue RT, van Wijk Y. Decision support systems in oncology. *JCO Clinical Cancer Informatics*. Feb. 2019; 3:1–9.

[103] Wang Y, Ji C, Wang Y, Ji M, Yang JJ, Zhou CM. Predicting postoperative liver cancer death outcomes with machine learning. *Current Medical Research and Opinion*. Apr. 2021; 37(4):629–634.

[104] Wang Y, Wang Z, Xu J, Li J, Li S, Zhang M, Yang D. Systematic identification of noncoding pharmacogenomic landscape in cancer. *Nature Communications*. Aug. 2018; 9(1):1–5.

[105] Watson OP, Cortes-Ciriano I, Taylor AR, Watson JA. A decision-theoretic approach to the evaluation of machine learning algorithms in computational drug discovery. *Bioinformatics*. Nov. 2019; 35(22):4656–4663.
[106] Winfield AFT, Jirotka M. Ethical governance is essential to building trust in robotics and artificial intelligence systems. *Philosophical Transactions of the Royal Society A: Mathematical, Physical and Engineering Sciences*. Nov. 2018; 376(2133): 20180085.
[107] Xia X, Gong J, Hao W, Yang T, Lin Y, Wang S, Peng W. Comparison and fusion of deep learning and radiomics features of ground-glass nodules to predict the invasiveness risk of stage-I lung adenocarcinomas in CT scan. *Frontiers in Oncology*. Mar. 2020; 10:418.
[108] Xie Y, Meng WY, Li RZ, Wang YW, Qian X, Chan C, Yu ZF, Fan XX, Pan HD, Xie C, Wu QB. Early lung cancer diagnostic biomarker discovery by machine learning methods.*Translational Oncology*. Jan. 2021; 14(1):100907.
[109] Yan Y, Zeng S, Wang X, Gong Z, Xu Z. A machine learning algorithm for predicting therapeutic response to anti-PD1. *Technology in Cancer Research & Treatment*. Sep. 2019; 18:1533033819875766.
[110] Zeng S, Wang D, Yan Y, Zhu M, Liu W, Gong Z, Wang L, Sun S. Single-center analysis of the potential inappropriate use of intravenous medications in hospitalized patients in China. *Clinical Therapeutics*. Aug. 2019; 4(8):1631–1637.
[111] Zhu X, Lin MC, Fan W, Tian L, Wang J, Ng SS, Wang M, Kung H, Li D. An intronic polymorphism in GRP78 improves chemotherapeutic prediction in non-small cell lung cancer. *Chest*. Jun. 2012; 141(6):1466–1472.

16 Deep Learning to Diagnose Diseases and Security in 5G Healthcare Informatics

Partha Ghosh
Department of Computer Science and Engineering, Government College of Engineering and Ceramic Technology, Kolkata, West Bengal, India

CONTENTS

16.1 Introduction 281
16.2 Key Types of Learning Methods Used to Solve 5G Problems 282
16.2.1 Supervised Learning 283
16.2.2 Unsupervised Learning 283
16.2.3 Reinforcement Learning 283
16.3 Main Deep Learning Techniques Used in 5G Scenarios 283
16.3.1 Fully Connected Models 283
16.3.2 Recurrent Neural Networks 283
16.3.3 CNN 284
16.3.4 DBN 284
16.3.5 Autoencoder 284
16.3.6 Combining Models 285
16.4 Most Common Scenarios Used for 5G Assessment and Deep Learning Integration 285
16.5 Applications of Machine Learning and Deep Learning for 5G Security 285
16.6 Blockchain Technology in Healthcare 286
16.7 Evolution of Machine Learning in Disease Detection 287
16.7.1 Supervised Learning 287
16.7.1.1 K-Nearest Neighbour (KNN) 288
16.7.1.2 Support Vector Machine (SVM) 288
16.7.1.3 Decision Trees (DTs) 288
16.7.1.4 Classification and Regression Trees (CARTs) 288
16.7.1.5 Logistic Regression (LR) 288
16.7.1.6 Random Forest Algorithm (RFA) 288
16.7.1.7 Naive Bayes (NB) 288

DOI: 10.1201/9781003217497-16

16.7.1.8 Artificial Neural Network (ANN) 289
16.7.2 Unsupervised Learning 289
16.7.3 Semi-supervised Learning 289
16.7.4 Evolutionary Learning 289
16.7.5 Active Learning 290
16.7.6 Reinforcement Learning 290
16.7.7 Ensemble Learning 290
16.7.8 Deep Learning 290
16.7.9 Transfer Learning 291
16.7.9.1 Feature Extraction 291
16.7.9.2 Fine-tuning 291
16.8 Applications of Deep Learning in Disease Diagnosis 291
16.8.1 ML/DL in Healthcare: The Large Picture 292
16.8.2 A Look at the Healthcare Applications of ML and DL 293
16.9 Deep Learning in Disease Diagnosis: To Save Lives and Cuts Treatment Costs 296
16.9.1 Breast Cancer 297
16.9.2 Early Detection of Melanoma: Skin Cancer 297
16.9.3 Lung Cancer 298
16.9.4 Testing for Diabetic Retinopathy 298
16.9.5 Assessment of Cardiac Hazard from ECG Data 298
16.9.6 Using CT Scans of the Head to Detect Strokes Early 299
16.10 Benefits of Deep Learning 299
16.11 Scope of Deep Learning Techniques for Disease Diagnosis 300
16.12 A Deep Learning-Based Approach to Detect Neurodegenerative Diseases: Multiclass Classification (Case Study-1) 301
16.12.1 Material and Methods 302
16.12.1.1 ADPP Dataset Description 303
16.12.1.2 VGG 19 Architecture 303
16.12.2 Results and Discussion of the Above Discussed Framework 303
16.13 Pneumonia Detection using Deep Learning (Case Study-2) 307
16.13.1 Methodology 309
16.13.1.1 Structural Units 310
16.13.1.2 Architecture of CovXNet 312
16.13.1.3 Stacking of Multiple Networks 312
16.13.1.4 Transfer Learning Method of CovXNet for New Corona Virus Data 313
16.13.1.5 Network Training and Optimisation 314
16.13.2 Results and Discussions 314
16.13.2.1 Datasets 314
16.13.2.2 Evaluation of Performance 314
16.14 Early Detection of Deep Learning-based Diabetic Retinopathy (Case Study-3) 319
16.14.1 Datasets Used 319
16.14.2 Metric Assessment 320

16.14.2.1 Quadratic Weighted Kappa (QWK) 320
16.14.2.2 Intuition of Cohen's Kappa 320
16.14.2.3 Quadratic Weight Intuition in Ordinary Classes — Quadratic Weighted Kappa (QWK) 321
16.14.3 Method 322
16.14.3.1 Image Pre-processing and Augmentations 322
16.14.3.2 Network Architecture 322
16.14.3.3 Training Process 323
16.14.4 Results 324
16.14.4.1 Model Evaluation on Test Data 324
16.14.4.2 Other Transfer Learning Models 326
16.15 Conclusion 326
References 329

16.1 INTRODUCTION

Several diseases today are required to be diagnosed early in order to begin appropriate care. If not, they can become incurable and fatal. As a result, complicated medical data, medical reports, and medical pictures should be processed in less time, however with bigger precision. Humans may not be able to detect such anomalies in certain cases. However, because of its superior success in the field of data analysis beyond human experts, artificial intelligence (AI) has a lot of potential to advance medical diagnostic technology.

Despite its excellent success in the field of automated diagnosis using medical images, AI still faces significant challenges in terms of interpretability and text-based medical data analysis. On a global scale, researchers have increasingly combined DL technology with medical diagnosis to solve the problems described above. So, ML/DL strategies are being utilised in healthcare for computational selection making in conditions in which a crucial statistics evaluation on clinical statistics is wanted to show mystery relationships or anomalies that aren't obvious to humans.

As a subset of ML, DL is capable of learning multilevel representations from raw input data, removing the need for handcrafted features in traditional ML. It's a multilayer (deep) structure with nonlinear activation functions that has an extension of traditional linear models. The logic of moving "deeper" is connected to learning complex data structures, and it has been made possible by the development of more rigorous optimisation techniques for efficient training of these algorithms. ML/DL has been used in the healthcare sector for anything from extracting knowledge from medical records to predicting or diagnosing diseases. The application of deep learning algorithms to the sector of machine biology has considerably increased medical imaging. Medical image processing using ML/DL algorithms is now used to diagnose a wide variety of diseases.

In this context, the volume of data exchange on the Internet has increased significantly, mainly due to the development of high-speed broadband Internet, or rather the rapid introduction and massive use of smartphones and corresponding tariff plans.

According to Cisco, global Internet traffic will hit about 30 GB per capita by 2021, with wireless and handheld devices accounting for more than 63% of this traffic. The next generation of telecommunication (5G) is being considered for this reason, and both industry and researchers are enthusiastic about it. The 5G network has a wide range of specification criteria that are technologically demanding. High volumes of information per region, a large number of associated gadgets per area, high info speeds, length of battery life for low-power gadgets, and reduced dormance start are just a few of them.

In this particular situation, DL models can be seen as one of the essential technologies in the preparation of information for checking and informatics. Since these models can distinguish important provisions from the crude information (photos, messages and various types of unstructured information), 5G and DL reconciliation seems promising and requires further study.

In recent years, DL has outperformed traditional machine learning strategies in a number of areas, including computer vision, natural language processing, and genomics [1].

There are 2 distinct ways in which a clinical higher cognitive process answer interprets by examination previous data that's enclosed within the dataset. A fast, instinctive system based on the basic clinical example recognition and often used in health-related crises is essential. In any event, these people are more likely to be unbiased and have faulty insights.

The slow or reasoned solution is the alternative. It is deductive, deliberate, and necessitates more details in terms of intelligence, time, and expense. However, the decisions taken are more precise.

Since all of those choices are supported knowledge that's obtained, processed, and keep in complicated and heterogeneous formats, it's crucial to use algorithmic approaches so as to scale back the quantity of process power needed. ML/DL applications have already created a serious contribution to rising the potency of clinical higher cognitive process round the world, and that they can still do thus within the future.

This is not just identifying or predicting health care diseases; it also involves conducting health research, patient care, resource use, hospital capacity control, public health policy formulation, etc.

For example, given the current COVID-19 pandemic situation, health care should consider all of the above and these activities should be completed within a relatively short period. The safest way to do this is to leverage AI / ML / DL-based decision making in the healthcare space. This is why the field of "emergency machine learning" is in such high demand in today's world [2].

In addition, improved AI/ML/DL models also maintain data confidentiality, and improved end-to-end protection of communications and control would be advantageous. Some authentication issues for distributed ledger systems are supposed to be solved by blockchain-like processes, but further work is required to help machine-learning models predict incoming attacks [3,4].

Nonetheless, an AI-assisted diagnosis system can significantly streamline the process of patients needing treatment, alleviate the paradox of a lack of adequate resources, and enhance the overall survival of emergency patients. Following that, we'll go through the different forms of learning methods that can be used to solve 5G problems.

16.2 KEY TYPES OF LEARNING METHODS USED TO SOLVE 5G PROBLEMS

Three different learning techniques are used to solve 5G problems. Supervised Learning, Reinforcement Learning, and Unsupervised Learning are the most common learning types used in the deep learning models for 5G.

16.2.1 Supervised Learning

Despite the difficulty of finding labelled datasets in 5G environments, the supervised learning technique was used in the majority of the studies. This method is generally used to solve classification and regression problems [5].

16.2.2 Unsupervised Learning

Unsupervised learning occurs when a machine makes decisions instead of being trained by a dataset because it is not provided labelled data from which to make predictions. The model, which combines supervised learning and unattended training, can be used as a hybrid approach. The goal is to find an estimated solution for the best joint resource allocation technique and energy consumption [6]. For single associated connections, the model can be trained using a hybrid training procedure that combines supervised and unmonitored learning to identify errors and false alerts between connections [7]. A MU-SIMO framework was represented using an unsupervised deep learning model [8]. Its main aim is to cut the distance between signals received and transmitted.

16.2.3 Reinforcement Learning

Learning material is only provided in reinforcement of education as a response to the programme conduct in an arbitrary context for Associate Nursing. Continuous learning in the environment through a repetitive process of learning.

As in [9], for example, the author used reinforcing learning to improve URLLC (Ultra Reliable Low Latency Communication) energy efficiency and latency tolerance over distributed resources. In [10], authors learned to improve memory and hit the cache rate. Next, we will examine the deepest teaching methods used in 5G scenarios.

16.3 MAIN DEEP LEARNING TECHNIQUES USED IN 5G SCENARIOS

Classical neural networks with fully connected layers are a popular technique for deep learning to solve 5G problems. This is a technique of deep learning that is often applied at buildings. The following are short-term memory (LSTM) and CNN.

16.3.1 Fully Connected Models

In 5G systems, most studies using fully coupled levels focused on physical problems of the environment [11,12].

16.3.2 Recurrent Neural Networks

A recurrent neural network (RNN) is a form of neural network that can deal with sequential data including time series, voice, and language. It's because of its ability to store information from previous elements when given an element in a sequence. To deal with sequential data, one study used RNN [13] and several others used RNN variations (such as LSTM [14]).

16.3.3 CNN

CNN models are designed for data from multiple tables or multidimensional arrays to get related properties. This means that the convolutional layer is used to process data of different sizes, including simple and sequential signals, 2D images or 3D spectra for audio and video, or 3D images.

Input data for CNN models are represented in the form of images to take advantage of the natural features of convolutions used in CNN layers [15].

The use of DL techniques to achieve accurate outdoor positioning was made possible by the idea of beamformed fingerprints. [15] discusses the use of sequence-based DL architectures to capture the information contained in a device's movement. With temporal convolutional networks, the consequent predictions were not only more accurate, but also more stable, with less variance.

16.3.4 DBN

Deep belief networks (DBNs) are appealing for problems with a large range of unlabelled information and few labelled data. This is often thanks to the very fact that unlabelled data is employed to coach the model whereas labelled data is used to fine-tune the whole network throughout the coaching process. As a result, during the training phase, this deep learning methodology incorporates each supervised and unattended learning.

16.3.5 Autoencoder

The autoencoder network is trained to reproduce the input output. In these networks, the internal representation of the entrance is represented by a hidden layer. You can use this view to restore network input to output. As a result, [16] used an autoencoder architecture to encode and decode physical signal paths.

Sparse code multiple access (SCMA) is a technique that can help 5G wireless communication networks achieve higher spectral efficiency and huge connectivity. In [16], a deep learning-aided SCMA (D-SCMA) approach was discussed, in which an autoencoder-inspired framework was used to generate codewords and determine decoding strategy.

Using a deep learning technique, an effective codebook and decoding strategy for a sparse and multidimensional superimposed signal can be automatically deduced. In terms of bit error rate (BER) and computational complexity, this scheme outperforms traditional schemes.

16.3.6 Combining Models

The authors of [17], for illustration, suggested the use of an LSTM and a completely connected model together. A new theoretical model for holistic handover (HO) cost estimation has been proposed in [17], which incorporates signalling overhead, latency, call dropping, and radio resource wastage.

The mathematical model built here can be applied to a variety of cellular technologies, but the Control/Data Separation Architecture (CDSA) was the emphasis here. By novel implementation of a recurrent deep learning architecture, explicitly a stacked long-short-term memory (LSTM) system, a data-driven HO prediction is also developed and evaluated as part of the holistic cost.

In [18], an intelligent resource scheduling method (iRSS) for 5G radio access network (RAN) slicing that incorporated LSTM and reinforcement learning was presented.

In [19], reinforcement learning was combined with a fully connected model. In this paper, a DL architecture for user association was proposed, in which a digital twin of the network environment is created at the central server for off-line algorithm training. In [20], a hybrid model called generative adversarial network (GAN) was used, which merged LSTM and CNN layers. Following that, we'll go through some of the most common scenarios for evaluating 5G and DL integration.

16.4 MOST COMMON SCENARIOS USED FOR 5G ASSESSMENT AND DEEP LEARNING INTEGRATION

According to the study, the most common scenario is living in the city, which can be understood as dynamic, complex, and heterogeneous urban scenarios in which many obstacles (people, vehicles, etc.), objects, and structures must be overcome. represent extreme conditions that previous generations of cells could not cope with and where 5G requires unique solutions to fulfil its obligations, such as the use of millimetre waves, advanced beam forming, etc., NOMA, etc. problems.

Due to their low latency and high availability, 5G networks are an important part of autonomous vehicles and communications. Many researchers therefore consider profound learning a possible way of solving some of the more difficult challenges of 5G. Three of them are assessed. Several settings are mentioned in [20], namely medical video discussion and virtual procedures (unidirectional, real-time, downlink) and basic data. Different settings, such as medical (downlink) (uplink data exchange occurs in one direction only). Next, we see how 5G safety can be improved with machine learning and deep learning.

16.5 APPLICATIONS OF MACHINE LEARNING AND DEEP LEARNING FOR 5G SECURITY

By analysing network behaviour patterns and parameters, ML and DL models may be utilised to determine suspicious behaviours in real time. Cyber security solutions benefit from DL because it can automatically learn patterns from previous entries to prevent potential intrusion and recognize unusual patterns.

By monitoring network parameters namely throughput and network error logs, classification algorithms can be used to detect anomalies. Clustering algorithms may be used to categorize different forms of network security threats and vulnerabilities. Models like statistical inference attacks and generative adversarial networks (GAN) can build fake datasets to test and enforce new security protocols and algorithms, as well as establish and evaluate new security measures.

By integrating various protocols for faster computations, the protected computation field is making new progress. Gazelle, TAPAS, and Faster CryptoNets are three examples of stable computation with homomorphic encryption. SecureNN is an ML solution that uses comparison-based neural network operations to retrieve bits and share secrets.

Unsupervised algorithms like neural networks and clustering can be used to help humans in detecting suspicious behaviour. Denial-of-Service (DoS) and cyber-attacks would be more popular in 5G and beyond networks that rely on Service Based Architecture (SBA), independent decentralised network functions, and third-party servers. As a result, various ML and DL solutions for dealing with decentralised networks have been presented. To deal with such attacks, recent solutions have used a variety of reinforcement learning (RL) and deep reinforcement learning (DRL) techniques.

In the event of a hacker jamming radio frequency (RF) signals, DRL-based solutions have been established that select suitable frequency channels and escape attack using an optimal policy learned from previous observations.

DL has been used to detect anomalies on the physical network, malware, virus, and botnet detection in the mobile network, and user-level security (private information protection).

DL networks are used to classify malicious programmes, spam, unknown traffic, and botnets at the software level. In terms of user privacy, DL has demonstrated its usefulness in addressing issues such as data sharing, information leakage, and privacy protection. Following that, we'll talk about Blockchain Technology in Healthcare.

16.6 BLOCKCHAIN TECHNOLOGY IN HEALTHCARE

However, data sharing, data accessibility, data protection and accuracy, and convenience are all key criteria for human healthcare. These are the most relevant criteria for healthcare data to communicate with electronic medical records (EMR) systems. Blockchain technology allows for secure content-based storage. Through intelligent data processing, it ensures data protection and privacy. Healthcare could be revolutionised if AI and blockchain work together. A healthcare blockchain is thus another source of medical data. Since transactions are stored in a network of distributed servers, blockchains are becoming more popular in the medical field. This ensures a high level of availability.

This provides additional safeguards against network outages and hardware failure. Furthermore, the format of the transactions is stored in such a way that tampering with the data is practically impossible. Any healthcare solution must emphasize data integrity and accountability. Although the amount of data obtained by a medical blockchain does not compare to the amount of raw data collected by medical devices, the data received by a medical blockchain is detailed. If we expand the scope of a smart contract, the data obtained from smart contract transactions [3,21] can be extremely valuable.

Since existing EMR systems lack of consistent and reliable framework for data protection and reliability policies, they are ineffective in meeting these critical issues for an efficient method. As a result, a reliable and dependable infrastructure is needed to strengthen data protection and authoritative access to medical information in accordance with government privacy regulations to track clinic data use. By incorporating its unique and robust features related to data protection, data reliability, and accuracy, blockchain technology appears to improve the conventional healthcare industry [21]. Blockchain technology is a stable and decentralised ledger that stores and maintains immutable records of online financial transactions. It's also known as Distributed Ledger Technology (DLT) because it records signed transactions between two parties using decentralisation and cryptographic hashing mechanisms.

Since blockchain technology shares data with all parties concerned, it is likely to be used for spectrum and data exchange, improving the security of 5G networks and beyond. Next, the evolution of ML in disease detection is discussed.

16.7 EVOLUTION OF MACHINE LEARNING IN DISEASE DETECTION

ML may be represented as a discipline involved with however computers learn from knowledge and improve over time. It's primarily focussed on statistics and probability. When it comes to decision-making, however, it outperforms traditional statistical methodologies. The information gathered from a dataset and fed to the algorithm is referred to as features. A ML developer's job is to identify the subset of features that best suit the objective, improving the model's accuracy. There are 3- simple steps to follow when applying ML algorithms to applications: training, testing, and verification. The accuracy of the results depends on the training data set, so training is very important.

The algorithm's output will be evaluated using the test dataset. When using test data to assess performance, it's also critical to reduce bias and increase variance during the testing period. The bias-variance trade-off must be optimised by a successful ML algorithm. The validation dataset is used to evaluate the final machine learning algorithm's efficiency during the validation phase. It would be interesting to have a basic understanding of the different approaches machine learning approaches.

16.7.1 SUPERVISED LEARNING

Manually labelled records are used for supervised learning to build models to predict or classify future events, or to identify variables that are most important to the results. Supervised learning is divided into two categories: classification and regression.

When using classification methods for classification, the trained framework assigns inputs to classes. The origin of regression is continuous rather than discrete. Regression prediction uses square root error estimates, and classification prediction uses precision or precision estimates. A few supervised learning algorithms commonly used in health care and biomedicine are mentioned below.

16.7.1.1 K-Nearest Neighbour (KNN)

KNN may be an algorithm used in various fields, as well as for the recognition of patterns, the intrusion detection, etc.

16.7.1.2 Support Vector Machine (SVM)

SVM is a supervised algorithm used mainly for solving problems with classification but it can also be used for solving problems with regression. SVM has an easy feature that can map points to many other dimensions in front of other algorithms with nonlinear relationships. SVM can solve linear and non-linear issues, but non-linear SVM is better because it performs better than linear SVM.

16.7.1.3 Decision Trees (DTs)

DT is a supervised algorithm that uses a tree-like model that takes into account decisions, their potential consequences, and their outcomes. Every branch denotes a result, and every node corresponds to a query. The class labels are the leaf nodes. When dealing with imbalanced datasets, it has some drawbacks such as the over-fitting problem and biased outcomes.

16.7.1.4 Classification and Regression Trees (CARTs)

CART could be a prophetic model that predicts the output price supported the present values within the made tree. The CART model is delineated as a binary tree, with every root admire one input and a split purpose for that element. Predictions are made using the output from leaf nodes.

16.7.1.5 Logistic Regression (LR)

In the field of ML, LR is a common mathematical modelling technique for epidemiologic datasets. A hypothesis and a cost function are necessary for LR, which is a supervised ML algorithm. It's worth mentioning that optimisation the cost function is crucial.

16.7.1.6 Random Forest Algorithm (RFA)

The RF algorithm is a popular technique of ML that can regress and classify. This algorithm creates a set of decision trees and mainly for training the encapsulation method. RFA is noise insensitive to unbalanced datasets and can be used. Removal is not a problem in RFA, either.

16.7.1.7 Naive Bayes (NB)

The NB algorithm is a classification method used for two-class and multi-class problems. NB classifier is a group of classification algorithms based on Bayesian theory. However, they all obey the same rule: any pair of features being classified had to be distinct from one another.

16.7.1.8 Artificial Neural Network (ANN)

ANN is a well-known supervised ML method for image classification. Artificial neurons, which are analogous to biological neural networks, are considered the fundamental concept of ANN. An ANN has three layers, each of which is connected to all of the other layers' nodes. Deeper neural networks can be generated by growing the number of hidden layers.

16.7.2 Unsupervised Learning

Unsupervised learning clusters data points within a dataset that belong to similar classes by learning the similarities, patterns, and structures between them. Clustering issues are included in this group. In unsupervised learning, the scheme makes judgements without being trained by a dataset because the system is not given labelled data from which to make predictions. Precision medicine relies heavily on unsupervised learning.

For example, when individuals are grouped based on their genetics, atmosphere, and medical history, unsupervised ML algorithms can recognise previously undetectable relationships between them. K-means, mean shift, affinity propagation, DBSCAN, Gaussian mixture modelling, Markov random fields, ISODATA, and FCM systems are a few instances for unsupervised algorithms. For unsupervised learning, it should be noted that the use of unsupervised machine learning in healthcare when diagnosing specific diseases might also diagnose different diseases of the patient.

The explanation for this is that the algorithm has learned the information to be considered for different types of diseases, and based on this data, analyzes the data and classifies it as a disease. With regard to the above aspects, there is no question that the unsupervised machine learning approach greatly enhances healthcare decision-making.

Here are a few examples of machine learning applications in medical field: ML classifiers are being used in neuroscience to investigate the functional and structural complexities of the brain. In cancer detection and prognosis, ML methods are used. Prostate cancer is diagnosed using SVM classifiers. Alzheimer's disease has been studied using hierarchical clustering. Different subtypes of psychogenic non-epileptic seizures have been classified using ANN.

16.7.3 Semi-supervised Learning

For semi-instructive training, part of the training data set is used. This type of training is used if some training information is missing. Tagged and untagged information is used to form semi-controlled algorithms of learning. Machine learning functions monitored and unattended.

16.7.4 Evolutionary Learning

Evolutionary learning in biology is used mainly for the study and forecasting of biological organisms. The results can also be predicted for accuracy with this method. Evolutionary algorithms can be used to optimise the classification parameters for SVM and MLP to classify medical datasets for disease diagnosis.

16.7.5 Active Learning

In Active Learning (AL), the system only receives training tags for a limited set of occurrences. AL concept has been widely used in situations where manual annotation is time-consuming, as these strategies aim to optimise computer models while reducing the amount of required training data.

A labelled set of training data is used in supervised learning to estimate or map the desired output. This fact, however, can be resolved by AL, which learns incrementally by starting with a few examples and then asking the medical expert to label only the instance that the algorithm determines to be the most informative in each iteration.

In the medical sector, AL techniques have proven to be effective. Deep active learning algorithms can be used to identify white blood cells in microscopic images of leucorrhoea.

16.7.6 Reinforcement Learning

The learning data is only used for program operations in response to self-motivation and enhanced learning scenarios. It uses an iterative learning process to continually learn from the environment. It is a form of reward-based learning (commonly used in gaming and robotics) that is based on experiences with the environment, with positive and negative reinforcements both contributing to the predictive model's progress.

16.7.7 Ensemble Learning

Ensemble learning is a type of meta-algorithm that combines many ML algorithms and techniques into a single predictive model to reduce variance, bias, and improve accuracy. In ML, ensemble learning is commonly used to enhance model output and reduce decision risk. It can also be used to enhance the classification and prediction in healthcare.

As a result, it enhances efficiency by integrating and aggregating a number of different base learners using particular techniques. Ensemble learning methods can be loosely divided into two types: Bagging, which is a parallel process, and Boosting, which is a sequential method.

16.7.8 Deep Learning

Deep learning (DL) is a monitored technique that uses neural networks and automated algorithms to extract meaningful patterns from large datasets. By simulating the complexities of a human brain, you can explore complex hierarchical images of data with multiple abstraction levels. Neural networks learn from your experience, read data, create layers, and provide advanced input and output levels. You can reduce the average error in results and predictions by estimating the weights of the input and output data.

Doctors use their education, skills training, and cultural background to make the diagnosis. Deep learning can broaden and enhance medical knowledge, particularly for non-experiencing doctors. DL can access more complex nonlinear data patterns with more hidden layers than conventional neural networks.

Thus, the use of DL in medical research has recently been made popular with the increasing volume and complexity of data, especially in the field of image analysis. The most commonly used DL algorithms in medical applications are constitutional neural networks (CNNs), deep belief networks, repetitive neural networks and profound neural networks.

16.7.9 Transfer Learning

Transfer learning is a powerful technique for conducting computer vision applications on small datasets. A network is saved here that's been pre-trained on a very huge image dataset. "ImageNet (http://image-net.org/about-overview)" is one such database that offers tens of millions of hand-labelled images for computer vision applications.

The volume of available datasets in healthcare is a major concern. There are just a few hundred samples in several medical datasets. When large amounts of training data are unavailable, transfer learning algorithms are extremely successful. It has been widely used in medical imaging for disease diagnosis. Apart from the small size of available healthcare datasets, there is also "THE CURSE OF DIMENSIONALITY" to tackle in the context of ML. The "curse of dimensionality" simply means that the larger each sample is, the more data you'll need. To put it another way, the more pixels you have with an image, the more detail you can hold.

For example, if you compare a thumbnail of an image to the same full-resolution image, the thumbnail would have less detail. Although this appears to be an advantage, it is difficult for a ML model to learn how to interpret the additional detail. And more data is needed for the model to learn from this additional detail.

In healthcare, Transfer Learning can be used to apply DL to smaller datasets and solve the "curse of dimensionality." Feature extraction and fine-tuning are two popular methods for harnessing the power of transfer learning.

16.7.9.1 Feature Extraction

Feature extraction is the method of taking a pre-trained network's convolutional base and running it through a new classifier (dense layer) that has been trained from the scratch. Since the dense layer of a pre-trained model is specific to the task on which it was trained, it is not used.

16.7.9.2 Fine-tuning

Early layers in the convolution base tend to extract less-abstract concepts like edges and dots, whereas higher layers tend to extract task-specific features. Unfreezing a few of the top layers while keeping the rest of the foundation frozen allows you to fine-tune a pre-trained model. By modifying these abstract layers that are more important to the problem at hand, this could improve the model's efficiency. Now, we'll look at how deep learning can be used to diagnose diseases.

16.8 APPLICATIONS OF DEEP LEARNING IN DISEASE DIAGNOSIS

This section covers several key ML/DL applications in the healthcare sector.

16.8.1 ML/DL in Healthcare: The Large Picture

Healthcare services produce a huge volume of mixed data and information on a regular basis, making it impossible to analyse and process using "traditional methods." ML/DL approaches assist in the accurate analysis of this data for predictive analytics.

In addition, there are many data sources that can be used to enrich health data, including but not limited to genomics, health data, social media data, and environmental data. The following are examples of the main types of ML/DL that can be used in sanitary applications:

a. Unsupervised Learning
b. Supervised Learning
c. Semi-supervised Learning
d. Reinforcement Learning

a. **Unsupervised Learning:** Unsupervised learning techniques employ unlabelled data and are ML techniques. Unsupervised learning techniques include clustering data points based on a single similarity measure and dimensionality reduction to translate high-dimensional data to a lower-dimensional feature space (occasionally also referred to as feature selection).

Anomaly detection, brain tissue segmentation [22] and clustering [23] are examples of unsupervised learning applications. Unsupervised approaches to learning in healthcare include clustering to predict heart disease and Principal Component Analysis (PCA) to predict hepatitis disease.

b. **Supervised Learning:** Using labelled training data to create or show the relationship between input and output is called supervised learning. When the result is discrete, it is called a classification problem, and when the output is continuous, it is called regression.

Two notable samples of supervised learning approaches in care are the detection of varied varieties of respiratory organ diseases (nodules) and therefore the identification of distinct regions of the body from medical images. When both labelled and unlabelled samples are present in the training data, neither supervised nor unsupervised learning approaches are possible. Hence in such cases, semi-supervised learning algorithms can be applied.

c. **Semi-supervised Learning:** For example, semi-managed learning algorithms can be extremely useful in the case of a small amount of tagged data and a large number of untagged data.

Due to the difficulty of collecting sufficient labelled information to train a health model, semi-monitored training methods in a variety of applications can be especially efficient. [24] describes a semi-guided clustering strategy based on evidence for health care, for example.

d. **Reinforcement Learning:** Reinforcement learning (RL) approaches are those that learn a policy characteristic over time via a set of observations, behaviours, and incentives. RL has recently been employed for context-aware symptom screening for illness diagnosis [25].

16.8.2 A Look at the Healthcare Applications of ML and DL

The four main medical applications that can benefit from ML/DL methods are prediction, diagnosis, treatment, and clinical workflow; among these applications, disease diagnosis is detailed below.

1. **Uses of ML in Prognosis:** In clinical practise, prognosis is the method of determining how a disease will progress. It also involves assessing whether symptoms and signs associated with a particular illness can worsen, strengthen, or stay stable over time, as well as determining possible health issues, risks, ability to perform normal tasks, and survival chances. Multimodal patient data, such as phenotypic, genomic, proteomic, pathology test results, and medical imaging, is collected in the same way that it is in clinical settings, and this data can be used to help ML/DL models with disease prognosis, diagnosis, and therapy. For example, ML/DL models have been used extensively to identify and classify various types of cancers, such as brain tumours and lung nodules.
2. **Uses of ML in Diagnosis:**
   a. **Record-keeping in Electronic Health Care (EHRs):** On a regular basis, hospitals and medical service providers produce a large number of electronic-health-records (EHRs), which are made up of unstructured and structured data and include a patient's full medication history. ML-based approaches were utilised to extract clinical features to aid in the diagnosing process. For example, [26] discusses the use of ML for diabetes diagnosis from EHRs.
   b. **ML in Medical Image Exploration:** When it comes to medical image processing, machine learning (ML) approaches are used to extract information from images obtained using various imaging modalities such as ultrasonic, MR, CT, PET, among others. A wide range of body organs can be studied with these techniques, which provide vital functional and anatomical information as well as assistance with detecting problems, locating them, and diagnosing them. The basic goal of medical image processing is to help physicians and radiologists better detect and diagnose disorders. There are several common tasks in medical image processing. We'll discuss them in the next unit. On the horizon are fully automated intelligent medical image diagnosis systems.

- **Enhancement:** The pre-processing phase of enhancing degraded medical images has a direct impact on the diagnostic process. Different DL models, such as convolutional de-noising auto encoders and GANs, have been used in the research to de-noise medical images. GANs have also been used to successfully clean motion artefacts introduced in multi shot MRI images. Super-resolution, such as MRI de-noising [27], is another effective and impactful enhancement technique for medical images using 3D deep densely connected neural networks.
- **Detection:** The method of recognising certain disease patterns or anomalies (such as tumours or cancer) in medical imaging is known as detection. Typically, such defects are diagnosed by expert radiologists or physicians in formal clinical practise, which can take more time and effort. DL-based techniques, on the other hand, have been shown to be effective for this purpose, with multiple research for disease diagnosis published in the literature. For example, [28] proposes a locality-sensitive technique based on CNN for identifying and classifying nuclei colon carcinoma in histopathological images. Mitosis could also be diagnosed in breast cancer pathology images using a hybrid model that incorporates handcrafted and CNN features.
- **Classification:** Similar to other non-learning techniques that are at the cutting edge, DL models, particularly convolutional neural networks (CNNs), have exhibited high performance in medical picture classification tasks. CNN may be used to distinguish lung patterns in patients with lung infections and recognise multiple instances of different body organs.
- Medical image classification has also benefited from transfer learning techniques [29]. A pre-trained deep learning model (usually trained on natural images) being fine-tuned on a relatively smaller dataset of medical images in transfer learning. The results obtained using this procedure, according to the literature, are encouraging.
- **Segmentation:** First and most important step in computer-aided diagnosis (CAD) and identification systems is to extract clinically relevant information. Medical image segmentation is often solved using DL models such as CNN and recurrent neural networks (RNN). The U-net design is most commonly used for this purpose (Convolutional networks for biomedical image segmentation).
- As well as volumetric images, ML/DL architectures are being studied for segmentation of multi-modal images, such as brain [22], skin cancer, CT scans, and so on.
- **Reconstruction:** MRI and CT images are widely recreated and reconstructed in DL model models such as CNN and autoencoders. GANs (generational networks of adversaries) have recently been widely used for the recovery of medical images and produce

outstanding results. [30] Presents, for instance, a GAN-based MRI technique for the removal of moving devices.

- **Image Registration:** Existing intensity-based image registration approaches have two major drawbacks: limited capture range and poor computation. 2D and 3D image registration can be improved by using a CNN-based regression approach.
- **Retrieval:** ML/DL techniques based on deep-convolutional-neural-networks (DCNN) are used to recover medical images because traditional methods are insufficient for developing and managing multimodal medical images.

3. **Clinical Applications of ML:**

   a. **Perception of the Image:** The use of medical images is common in clinical practise, and their interpretation is carried out by specialists such as physicians and radiologists. In textual radiology reports on the body organs that were examined in the conducted analysis, they describe the results of the images being evaluated. However, preparing such reports can be extremely difficult in some situations, such as for radiologists and other healthcare professionals who are less qualified or who work in rural areas with substandard healthcare facilities. As a result of this large number of patients that attend daily, it can be very time-consuming to write high-quality reports for experienced radiologists and pathologists. So, several scientists have tried to solve the problem using NLP and ML.

   In [31] an NLP approach is proposed to interpret the clinical x-rays. The automatic labelling and definition of medical images may be used in machine learned multi-tasking systems. Boundary architecture is built with CNN and RNN is used to diagnose chest pathology in X-ray chest and report the outcomes of CNN and for the creation of a multimodal model for automated reporting, the long-term memory network (LSTM) can be used.

   b. **Real-time Health Checking with ML:** An essential and important part of treatment is an emergency resuscitation. Continual health monitoring with wearable devices, IoT cameras, and smart phones has become increasingly important for people. To collect health data, use wearable devices and smartphones. That is then uploaded to the ML/DL analytics cloud. The results are returned to the computer for further analysis (s).

4. **Workflows in Clinical Research Using ML:**

   a. **Diagnose and Disease Prediction:** One of the most promising applications of machine learning is the early detection and treatment of diseases using medical data. In numerous studies, predictive healthcare has been shown to be able to treat illnesses more effectively. In the case of cardiovascular risk prediction, [32] found that ML techniques improved prediction accuracy.

   b. **ML in Computer-Assisted Detection or Treatment:** Diagnostic computer-aided systems (CADe) and CADx systems automatically interpret images to aid clinical practise of radiologists. IBM Watson is combined into a CADx system by several methods, such as machine learning. Automatic determination, for example, of the fatty tissue of the liver by ultrasonic kurtosis [33].

c. **Reward Learning in the Clinic:** The main goal of reward learning (RL) is to have a policy mechanism for making specific decisions in an unpredictable situation in order to maximize the reward received. In order to provide the best diagnosis and treatment for patients with certain characteristics, RL can also be applied in clinical practice.
d. **ML for Clinical Time Series Analysis:** The visualisation of time series data is becoming increasingly necessary in clinical workflows. Mean arterial (BP) and intracrane (ICP) pressures, initial cerebrovascular autoregulation (CA) markers in TBI patients.
e. **Audio and Speech Handling in Clinical Practice:** These new possibilities include speech interfaces for communication-free programmes, automated transcription of patient interactions as well as clinical note synthesis. It has several advantages for each stakeholder, including patients (speech is a modern modality for assessing patient state), physicians and the healthcare industry (improve productivity and fee reduction). Speech processing is often used to diagnose both speech-related disorders, such as vocal hyper-function, and abnormalities that manifest by speech, such as dementia. Utilising linguistic features, Alzheimer's disease may be identified. Clinical speech processing seems to be notorious for its difficulties with dis-fluency and utterance segmentation. Now, we'll look at Deep Learning in disease diagnosis as well as how it can be used to save lives and reduce the cost of treatment.

16.9 DEEP LEARNING IN DISEASE DIAGNOSIS: TO SAVE LIVES AND CUTS TREATMENT COSTS

A variety of ML/DL strategies have been used to predict or diagnose a disease in its early stages so that treatment can be more straightforward and the patient's chances of healing are improved. They have been used to identify a variety of diseases with varying degrees of accuracy, depending on factors like the algorithm used, the number of features in the training dataset and other factors. This is due to a variety of factors, including:

- Increasing computing power and storage technology,
- Falling hardware costs,
- Growing healthcare costs,
- Healthcare workers are in short supply, and
- A wealth of medical data to train models

It is, however, self-evident that computers will never be able to fully replace human experts. If there are a large number of patients in the queue, DL is used to assist doctors or to pre-select and prioritise patients. A recurrent neural network (RNN) has been used to process electronic health records (EHR) for identifying heart failure onset and predicting the probability of heart failure founded on a huge amount of mixed EHR information. A NLP model has been utilised to diagnose several head disorders such as cerebral haemorrhages and cranial dislocations using a non-contrast head CT image. The Google Inception-V3 model and the transfer-learning algorithm have been used to quickly diagnose a number of eye and pulmonary diseases in children. A deep neural network decoding system was employed to recognise intra-cortical records, and the motor was subsequently regulated to aid patients in doing related acts, according to the categorisation findings.

The importance of early disease detection, as well as the ML/DL methods used to diagnose the diseases, will be discussed in this section, and the features used to make predictions.

This segment also highlights the most promising ML/DL applications in diagnosis, emphasises their potential, and identifies their existing limitations.

16.9.1 Breast Cancer

Breast cancer is the most prevalent oncology disease among women, according to the World Health Organization (WHO), with approximately 627,000 deaths each year. Many countries have implemented screening services aimed at detecting cancer at an early stage in order to save lives.

To kick off 2020, Google's artificial intelligence division DeepMind launched a deep learning model that significantly improved [34] the outcomes of an average radiologist by 11.5% while also reducing their workload by a dramatic amount. According to a recent study [35] by Korean academic hospitals, AI/DL was more sensitive than human experts in detecting cancer in fatty breasts (90% vs 78%). Using AI/DL to assist radiologists increased their efficiency by 0.881 points.

Although the research is still at an early stage, more clinical trials are needed. While models act as a second reader, they can provide a second opinion immediately. A growing shortage of skilled radiologists could be alleviated by these new technologies.

16.9.2 Early Detection of Melanoma: Skin Cancer

Globally, skin disorders are the fourth most common cause of disability. By age 70, skin cancer affects 20% of the population. 99% of cases are curable if caught early enough and treated appropriately. AI/DL will make a difference in this area. Dermatologists, like radiologists, rely heavily on visual pattern recognition to make diagnoses and diagnose patients. Using 130,000 medical images of skin pathologies, Stanford University computer scientists developed a convolutional neural network (CNN) framework [36] to detect cancer. Its accuracy impressed dermatologists, who praised the algorithm's precision.

Researchers from Seoul National University published their thesis in the Journal of Investigative Dermatology [37] in March 2020. To identify 134 skin conditions and predict malignancy, the CNN model analysed over 220,000 images. Human experts were able to distinguish between melanoma and birthmarks using AI/DL. In addition to the speed and accuracy of diagnostics, there have been proposals to run CNN algorithms on smartphones for non-professional skin examinations. Injuries that go unnoticed can be reported to the doctor.

16.9.3 Lung Cancer

About half of all cancer-related deaths are caused by a form of lung cancer. As with other types of cancer, early detection can save lives. Pneumonia and bronchitis symptoms are unfortunately very similar to those of lung cancer. The disease is therefore only discovered in advanced stages 70% of the time. According to a Google study published in 2019, a deep learning model developed in partnership with North-Western Medicine and trained on 42,000 chest CT scans performed better than radiologists with eight years of experience in diagnosing lung cancer. When it came to detecting malignant lung modes, the algorithm was 5% to 9.5% better than human experts. It had previously been shown that a different CNN algorithm [38] could identify COPD, which is a condition that often leads to cancer.

16.9.4 Testing for Diabetic Retinopathy

Ophthalmologists use AI/DL for retinal image processing, and in particular to identify diabetic retinopathy (DR) (DR). Diabetes-related retinopathy affects one in three diabetic patients, or 422 million people worldwide, and can lead to blindness. The risk of vision loss decreases with early detection. The problem with DR, however, is that it can last a long time before it becomes a problem. The deep learning methods of IBM, which were published in 2017, were 86% precise in the detection of DR and classification of its severity.

That was Google's beating. On a dataset of 128,000 retinal images the technology giant and Verily, a sister company, trained a deep convolutional neural network over a period of three years. Google's AI Eye Doctor in 2018 reached a precision of 98.6%. The algorithm is now used by doctors at India's Aravind Eye Hospital.

Early diagnosis also means less expensive treatment: the cost of drugs for serious pathology will rise by more than tenfold as compared to treatment in the early stages.

16.9.5 Assessment of Cardiac Hazard from ECG Data

In the country and around the world, heart disease remains the major cause of death among men and women. ECGs, the fastest and most basic measure of heart function, can help avoid heart attacks and reduce mortality.

Studies have shown that AI and DL can't only detect current anomalies in ECGs, but can also predict potential risks. This technology, which was developed at MIT in 2019, predicts the likelihood that a patient will die from a heart attack within 30 to 365 days after an acute coronary syndrome (ACS).

An estimated two million ECGs from a team of researchers from the Geisinger Medical Center train a deeply convolutional neural network to classify patients most likely to die during one year of diagnosis. Algorithms can detect risk trends, which are a key takeaway, which cardiologists have missed.

The use of AI/DL and misdiagnosis are expected to be saved by human specialists with inexpensive equipment.

16.9.6 Using CT Scans of the Head to Detect Strokes Early

The second cause of death is stroke, which is described as the sudden death of brain cells due to lack of oxygen. This life-threatening condition requires rapid diagnosis and treatment: according to statistics, patients seeking clinical treatment within three hours of onset, scientist Geisinger used more than 46,000 images of computed tomography of the brain to develop a model of the deep convolutional neural network (DCNN) [39]. It can show signs of intra-cerebral haemorrhage (ICH), the deadliest form of stroke with a fatality rate of 40%. 30 day rates and severe disability in most survivors.

Several studies have shown that AI/DL is also effective in the diagnosis of ischemic stroke due to large vessel occlusion (LVO). In addition, Google's machine learning tests showed that the trained algorithms correctly identified the type of stroke in 77.4% of cases.

As a result, AI/DL algorithms have the ability to tell apart haemorrhagic strokes from those caused by blood clots in the vast majority of cases When trained by neuro-radiologists, AI/DL could provide non-expert healthcare providers with a reliable "second opinion" that would allow them to make quick decisions and reduce damage. Securing and protecting personal information, on the other hand, is a different matter.

Google proposed a new method called federated learning to solve the issue of privacy. Security refers to preventing unauthorised data access, while privacy refers to safeguarding personal identity details. These methods allow hospitals to train the current algorithm on their own local datasets. So as to improve a shared model, the updates are then stored centrally. In this way, institutions share models instead of confidential data. Although the privacy-first strategy has some advantages, it also has some disadvantages, as you will see below. As an example, hospitals must have the facilities and resources to train models in order for this to be possible. Next, we'll talk about the benefits of deep learning and what it can do for you.

16.10 BENEFITS OF DEEP LEARNING

Deep learning has a number of advantages in the health-care sector. Here are a few examples:

- Deep learning recognises and tracks important relationships in your data, as well as information about previous clients, which can be used as a potential guide for patients with similar symptoms or diseases.

- When you require a risk score upon administration other than discharge, DL allows us to build a model based on whatever source of data is available.
- Deep learning generates reliable and timely risk ratings, allowing for confidence and estimated resource allocation.
- Deep learning methods result in lower costs and better results.
- Deep learning algorithms become much more precise and accurate as they communicate with training data, enabling individuals to gain unparalleled insights into patient care, variability, and diagnostics.
- GPUs, or graphics processing units, are becoming more energy efficient and faster.
- Since we can now use DL algorithms for a fraction of the cost of previous methods, innovation is booming, and algorithms are becoming more sophisticated.
- EHRs and other digitisation efforts are making health care data more available than ever before to trained algorithms.
- Deep learning, which detects patterns by linking the tools, makes diagnostics more accurate and faster.
- Deep learning, like every other board-certified dermatologist, will assess if skin lesions are cancerous.

The next topic we'll discuss is the application of DL techniques to disease diagnosis.

16.11 SCOPE OF DEEP LEARNING TECHNIQUES FOR DISEASE DIAGNOSIS

Many machine learning diagnostic applications today tend to fall into one of the following categories:

- **Chatbots:** Companies are employing AI-chatbots with speech recognition capabilities to recognise patterns in patient symptoms in order to shape a possible diagnosis, avoid disease, and/or suggest a course of action.
- **Oncology:** Deep learning is being used by researchers to train algorithms to identify cancerous tissue at a level that is equivalent to that of qualified doctors.
- **Pathology:** Pathology is a medical discipline that deals with disease diagnosis based on laboratory examination of bodily fluids including blood and urine, as well as tissues. Pathologists with microscopes have historically relied on machine vision and other machine learning tools to supplement their work.
- **Rare Diseases:** To assist clinicians in diagnosing rare diseases, facial recognition software is being combined with machine learning. Face recognition and deep learning are used to study patient images in order to find phenotypes that are related to rare genetic disorders.

Following that, we'll go through three different case studies, each of which is analysed in depth to illustrate the usefulness of DL techniques in disease diagnosis.

16.12 A DEEP LEARNING-BASED APPROACH TO DETECT NEURODEGENERATIVE DISEASES: MULTICLASS CLASSIFICATION (CASE STUDY-1)

Deep Learning (DL) is a new area that is attracting interest from researchers, especially in the fields of engineering and medicine. In this section, I discuss the applications of DL and its function in the prediction of neurodegenerative diseases such as Alzheimer's and Parkinson's disease.

The human brain is vulnerable to a wide range of disorders that can hit at any age. Autism spectrum disorder and dyslexia are two examples of developmental conditions that appear in early childhood. Psychiatric illnesses, like depression and schizophrenia, are often diagnosed in teenagers or early adulthood, but their causes can be found much earlier in life. Then, as people get older, they become more vulnerable to dementia disorders like Alzheimer's, Parkinson's, and others.

I've chosen two common brain disorders to discuss in this section: Alzheimer's disease and Parkinson's disease. Both Alzheimer's and Parkinson's disease are neurodegenerative disorders (NDD). Alzheimer's disease (AD) is the most common cause of dementia and is a psychological, permanent, progressive brain disorder.

Although the causes of AD are unknown at this time, an accurate diagnosis of AD plays a major role in patient care, especially at the early stages. ADNI, a multi-site study aimed at improving clinical trials for the prevention and treatment of AD, has the most well-known public neuroimaging dataset for the study of AD diagnosis [40].

There is a gradual interruption in the development of a chemical messenger in the brain that causes progressive deterioration and loss of neurons. Parkinson's disease (PD) is now second most common neurodegenerative syndrome after Alzheimer's disease. A clinical observational study, Parkinson's Progression Markers Initiative (PPMI), aims to confirm Parkinson's disease progression markers. A total of 400 newly diagnosed PD patients, 200 stable people, and 70 people who were clinically diagnosed with PD but did not exhibit any signs of dopaminergic deficiency are included in the PPMI database.

Alzheimer's diagnosis is made by symptoms such as trouble performing routine activities, planning difficulties, memory loss, and so on. The disorder is caused by the loss of some nerve cells, as well as the presence of plaques (neurotic) in or around the neuron and the accumulation of neurofibrillary tangles within the neuron. Since Alzheimer's disease is still an incurable disease, early detection is important for patient care. Problem solving, memory tests, concentration, and, most importantly, brain scans of a patient in the form of MRI, PET, or CT scans are some of the methods used by physicians to diagnose Alzheimer's disease. Physicians commonly use MRI scans to diagnose Alzheimer's disease. A number of deep learning-based methods that use MRI scans to automate the diagnosis and early detection of Alzheimer's disease have recently been proposed.

Muscle rigidity, tremor, and sluggish movements are the main signs of PD. Other symptoms include slurred voice, a blank face, shaky handwriting, and trouble getting out of a chair, among others. Dopamine deficiency, a neurotransmitter in the human brain, is the cause of Parkinson's disease.

The lack of dopamine in the human brain is associated to neuron depletion, a common occurrence in the elderly. Since the essence of this neurodegenerative disorder is progressive, identical to Alzheimer's, early stage diagnosis would be crucial in the treatment and care of patients.

As a result, early detection systems for these two neurodegenerative diseases are needed. Since MRI imaging offers precise neuro-anatomic biomarkers, which are essential in the diagnosis of Parkinson's disease, MRI scans are widely used to diagnose the disease. Indeed, MRI scans reveal minute anatomical information about the human brain's subcortical structures, which can be analysed to diagnose Parkinson's disease early.

A variety of deep learning-based classification methods have recently been suggested, all of which have demonstrated high classification accuracy when used to predict and classify Parkinson disease using MRI scans.

ML and DL are commonly used in the field of brain disorders to classify brain tumours, gliomas, and other brain disorders using electronic medical records and medical imaging data.

Deep convolutional neural networks (DCNN) are now very common and commonly used by researchers due to their high efficiency. Since, unlike traditional ML models, DL models do not require manual segmentation and feature extraction, they are more common and thus completely automate the task of binary or multiclass classification.

VGG 16, Inception Net, and other deep transfer learning models are commonly used in the development of CAD systems both for classification of different types of cancers and brain tumours. There is no single automated framework for the real-time classification of both AD and PD. There are a variety of deep learning-based methods for individual classification of AD or PD. The ADPP dataset, which was generated using global datasets including ADNI and PPMI, was used for training and validation in this case study [40].

In this case study, a VGG-19 architecture-based structure was used in real time to classify two of the most common neurodegenerative diseases (both Alzheimer's and Parkinson's). Since there is currently no unified framework or method for the classification of AD and PD, other common deep transfer learning models such as VGG-16, Res Net 50, and Inception Net are implemented and trained on the same ADPP dataset to provide a true comparison with the VGG-19 system.

16.12.1 Material and Methods

The method, which is built on the VGG-19 deep transfer learning architecture, is divided into two stages. The first involves downloading MRI scans of Alzheimer's and Parkinson's diseases from both the ADNI and PPMI databases. Then, since PNG (Portable Network Graphics) provides lossless compression, MRI scans in DICOM ("Digital Imaging and Communications in Medicine") format are converted to PNG (Portable Network Graphics). Only the most informative and correct MRI scans are used in the training and validation datasets, which is done manually under the supervision of a radiologist.

The VGG-19 is then optimised and trained using the ADPP dataset in the second level. The last three layers of the VGG 19 deep transfer learning architecture are updated to conform to the problem domain and perform accurate multiclass classification into the Alzheimer, healthy control ADNI, Parkinson, and healthy control PPMI classes. The conceptual classification scheme is depicted in Figure 16.1 below:

16.12.1.1 ADPP Dataset Description

The ADPP dataset, which contains 4800 MRI scans of Alzheimer's patients, healthy control scans from ADNI, Parkinson's patients, and well controls from PPMI, is utilised for training and validation/testing. Around 1200 MPRAGE MRI scans of Alzheimer's patients and healthy controls are available in the ADNI database. The PPMI database contains 1200 axial T2 weighted MRI scans of Parkinson's disease patients and healthy controls. Both the ADNI (www.adni.loni.usc.edu) and PPMI (https://www.ppmi-info.org/) datasets are freely accessible datasets that are often used by researchers especially of machine learning-based classification of neurodegenerative diseases.

Around 50 Alzheimer's and 50 stable control cases are collected in DICOM format from ADNI database. Similarly, about 50 Parkinson and 50 stable control cases are collected from PPMI dataset. Since the MRI scans are in the DICOM format, they were translated to PNG. The demographic information from the ADPP dataset used in this case study is summarised in Table 16.1.

16.12.1.2 VGG 19 Architecture

The VGG-19 architecture is part of the visual geometry group network (VGGNet) developed by Oxford University. One of the most common deep transfer learning models for image classification is VGGNet. The ImageNet database was used to train this VGGNet. The primary motivation for using a VGG-19 architecture is that it provides high accuracy, performance, and adaptability to a wide range of classification problems.

The VGG-19 architecture used here has a total of 19 layers that are divided into 5 blocks. To connect these blocks, 5 maximum pooling functions are used. In order to manage the trainable parameters, the input dimension is kept at 224*224*3 and even the filter size is kept at 3*3 in each and every layer.

Flatten, dropout, and dense are the last three layers inserted to perform multiclass classification and generate the output. The total number of parameters, trainable and non-trainable parameters, are shown in Table 16.2.

16.12.2 Results and Discussion of the Above Discussed Framework

The Google Colaboratory (colab) platform operated by the NVidia Tesla T4 GPU was used to simulate and experiment with the above discussed framework based on VGG19 architecture, as well as to compare it to the other three deep transfer learning models, namely VGG 16, ResNet50, and Inception Net. The implementation programming language was Python 3.6. The accuracy, sensitivity, specificity, and F1-score were used to assess and present the system's results. Let's

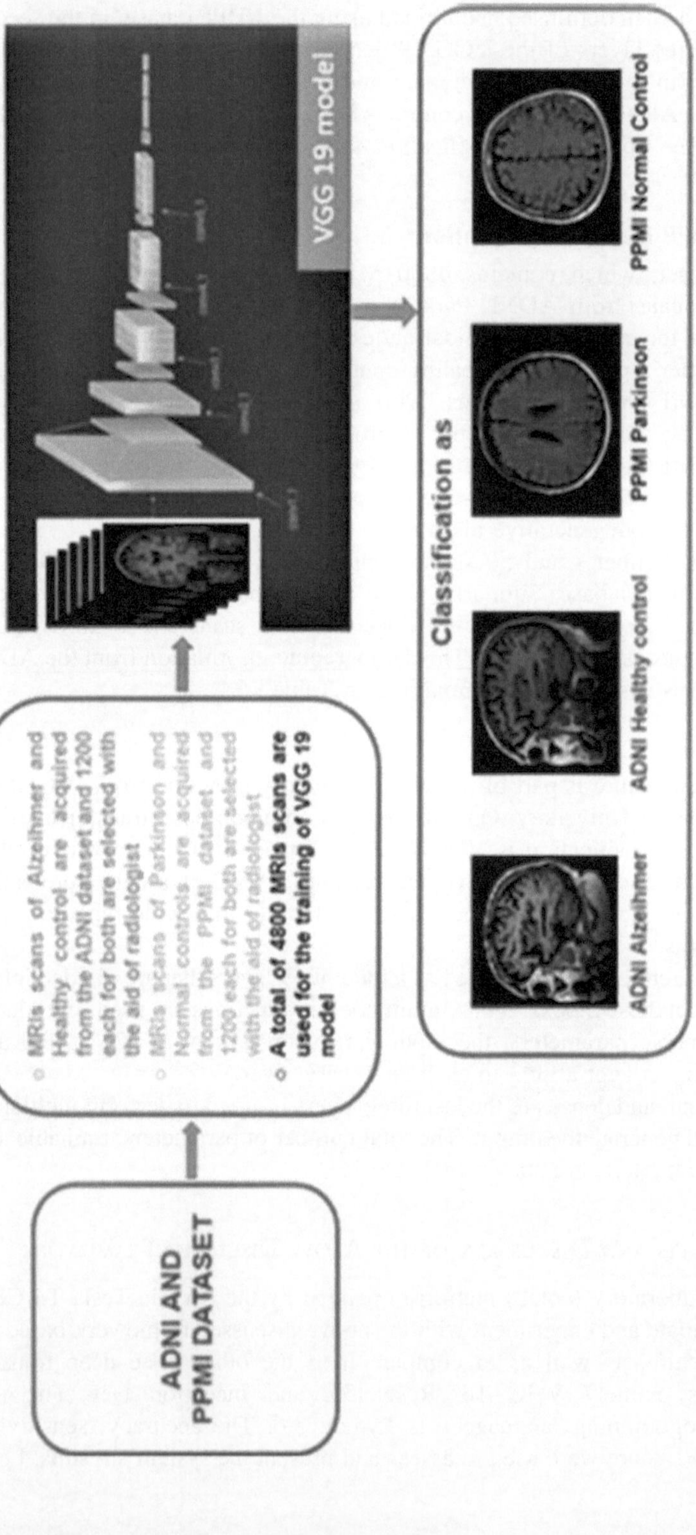

FIGURE 16.1 Automated scheme based on the VGG 19 model for the classification of Alzheimer and Parkinson neurodegenerative diseases.

TABLE 16.1
Demographic Information of the ADPP Dataset

Database	Groups	Number of Objects	Sex	Age Group	MRI Modality	Number of MRI Slices Taken
ADNI	AD	50	24 females and 26 males	65–90	MP-RAGE	1200
	HC	50	35 females and 15 males	60–93	MP-RAGE	1200
PPMI	PD	50	20 females and 30 males	39–80	T2 weighted	1200
	HC	50	26 females and 24 males	31–80	T2 weighted	1200

TABLE 16.2
Trainable and Non-trainable Parameters Information

Trainable Parameters	**4,819,972**
Non-trainable parameters	15,304,768
Total parameters	20,124,740

look at all the metrics that can be obtained from the confusion matrix as shown in Table 16.3.

1. Accuracy — Ratio of correct predictions to total predictions.
   Accuracy = (TP + TN)/(TP + FP + FN + TN)
2. Sensitivity/Recall — Ratio of true positives to total (actual) positives in the data.
   Sensitivity or Recall = TP/(TP + FN)
3. Precision — Ratio of true positives to total predicted positives.
   Precision = TP/(TP + FP)
4. F1-Score — considers both precision and recall. It's the harmonic mean of the precision and recall.

F1 Score = 2*(Recall * Precision)/(Recall + Precision)

The method is evaluated in terms of the above-mentioned classification rates employing two common training/validation splits of the ADPP dataset: 70/30 and 80/20, which means that 70, 80% of the ADPP dataset is used for training and 30, 20% for validation.

TABLE 16.3
Confusion Matrix

		Predicted Class	
		NO	**YES**
Actual Class	NO	True Negative (TN)	False Positive (FP)
	YES	False Negative (FN)	True Positive (TP)

On the ADPP dataset, this method provides the best performance with 80/20 splits. Table 16.4 summarises the classification rates.

On the same dataset, the automated framework based on VGG 19 is compared to some of the current recent deep transfer learning models such as VGG16, ResNet50, and Inception Net. Figure 16.3 display the training and validation progress graphs for VGG19, VGG16, ResNet 50, and Inception Net Model with split 70/30.

All of these models are designed with the same programming language and computational environment as the projected VGG 19 framework. Table 16.5 and Figure 16.2 show a brief comparison of their performance.

On the ADNI and PPMI datasets, the VGG19-based method is also compared to some state-of-the-art ML/DL methods for conducting Alzheimer's and Parkinson's classification. Tables 16.6 and Tables 16.7 show the results of their comparison.

Now, second case study will be discussed next.

TABLE 16.4
Performance of VGG 19 Based System on the ADPP Dataset with 70/30 and 80/20 Splits

Training and Validation Split Percentage	Neurodegenerative Diseases Type Classification	Accuracy	Precision	Sensitivity	F1 Score
70/30 split	Alzheimer	90%	100%	70%	83%
	Healthy control ADNI	90%	58%	100%	73%
	Healthy control PPMI	89%	69%	86%	76%
	Parkinson	90%	89%	74%	81%
Average Accuracy, Precision, sensitivity and F1 score		90%	80%	83%	79%
80/20 split	Alzheimer	88%	100%	67%	81%
	Healthy control ADNI	88%	52%	100%	68%
	Healthy control PPMI	98%	100%	94%	97%
	Parkinson	98%	94%	100%	97%
Average Accuracy, Precision, sensitivity and F1 score		93%	86%	91%	86%

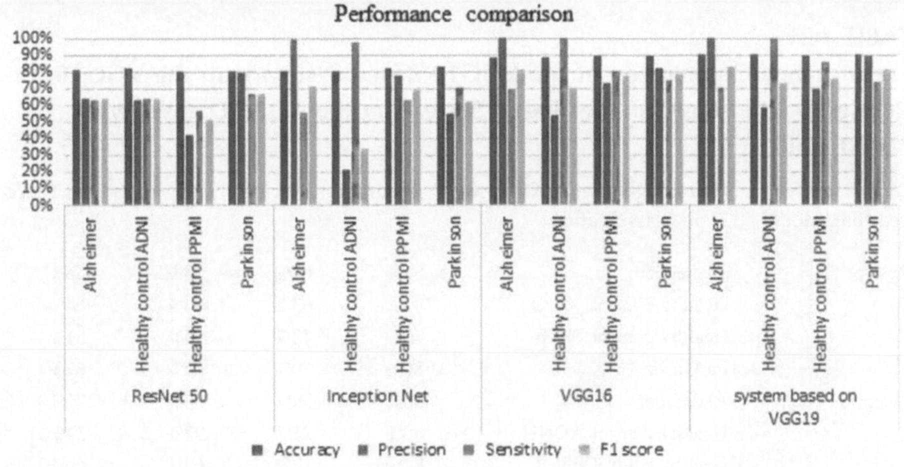

FIGURE 16.2 Performance comparison graph for comparing the performance of VGG19 based system with the VGG16, ResNet50 and Inception Net based system on the ADPP dataset with 70/30 split.

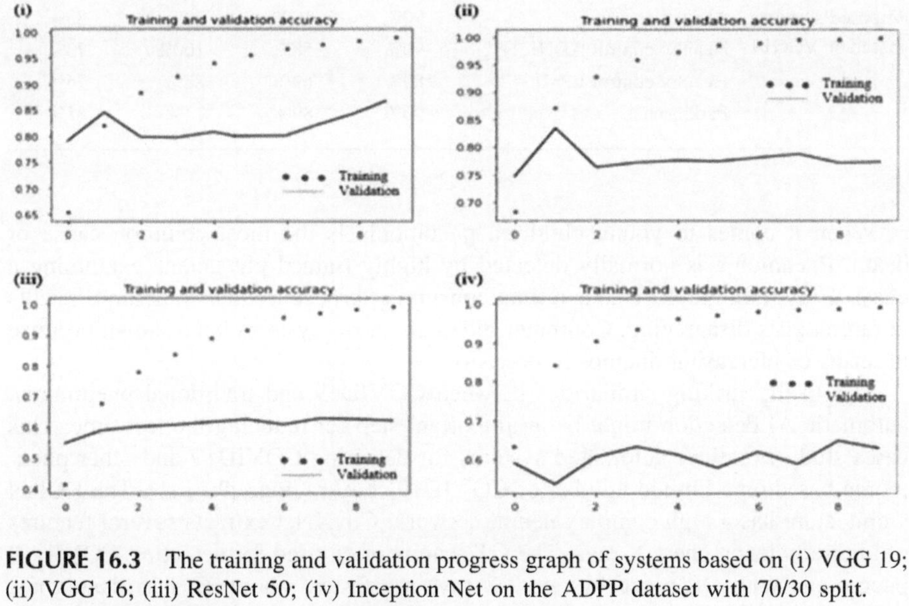

FIGURE 16.3 The training and validation progress graph of systems based on (i) VGG 19; (ii) VGG 16; (iii) ResNet 50; (iv) Inception Net on the ADPP dataset with 70/30 split.

16.13 PNEUMONIA DETECTION USING DEEP LEARNING (CASE STUDY-2)

COVID-19 outbreak has exacerbated a critical shortage of test kits, making rapid diagnostic testing one of the biggest challenges. A common COVID-19 side effect is pneumonia, which must be diagnosed as soon as possible.

TABLE 16.5
Performance Comparison of the VGG19 Based System with the VGG16, ResNet50 and Inception Net Based System on the ADPP Dataset with 70/30 Split

Deep Transfer Learning Model	Neurodegenerative Diseases Type Classification	Accuracy	Precision	Sensitivity	F1 Score
ResNet 50	Alzheimer	81%	64%	63%	64%
	Healthy control ADNI	82%	63%	64%	64%
	Healthy control PPMI	80%	42%	57%	51%
	Parkinson	80%	79%	67%	67%
Inception Net	Alzheimer	80%	99%	56%	71%
	Healthy control ADNI	80%	21%	97%	34%
	Healthy control PPMI	82%	77%	63%	69%
	Parkinson	83%	55%	70%	62%
VGG16	Alzheimer	88%	100%	69%	81%
	Healthy control ADNI	88%	54%	100%	70%
	Healthy control PPMI	89%	73%	80%	77%
	Parkinson	89%	82%	75%	78%
Proposed system based on VGG19	Alzheimer	90%	100%	70%	83%
	Healthy control ADNI	90%	58%	100%	73%
	Healthy control PPMI	89%	69%	86%	76%
	Parkinson	90%	89%	74%	81%

When it comes to young children, pneumonia is the most common cause of death. Pneumonia is normally detected by highly trained physicians examining a chest X-ray radiograph. This is a time-consuming procedure that sometimes results in radiologists disagreeing. Computer-aided diagnosis systems have shown promise in terms of increasing diagnostic precision.

Due to the striking similarities between COVID19 and traditional pneumonia, automatic AI detection might be an important step for reducing the test time. This cases study examines automated systems for detecting COVID19 and other pneumonia based on a limited number of COVID19 chest radiographs [41]. The DCNN architecture has a high complex neural network. CovXNet extracts several features of high-efficiency chest X-rays. The CT scan is often used for detecting COVID19 pneumonia with DL-based systems. X-rays are faster, smoother, less dangerous, and less cost-effective than CT scan, even if CT scan is more precise.

However, it is difficult to effectively train a very deep network because the COVID19 X-rays are scarce and therefore anticipatory training can be possible.

In place of other traditional databases, a larger radiology database was developed for patients with normal pneumonia and no COVID. To detect COVID19 with X-rays, CovXNet, a deep neural network, is used. It combines the local and global properties derived from several reception areas into an image through a

TABLE 16.6
Performance Comparison of VGG19 Based System with Other ML/DL Approaches for the Alzheimer Classification on the ADNI Dataset

Machine Learning Classifier or Deep Learning Model Used	Accuracy	Precision	Sensitivity	F1 Score
Support vector machine	83%	–	80.4%	–
Support vector machine	80.54%	–	70.59%	–
Residual Network 18 (ResNet18)	81.3%	–	–	–
VGG19 based system	90%	80%	83%	79%

TABLE 16.7
Performance Comparison of VGG19 Based System with Other ML/DL Approaches for the Parkinson's Disease Classification on the PPMI Dataset

Machine Learning Classifier or Deep Learning Model Used	Accuracy	Precision	Sensitivity	F1 Score
Multi-kernel support vector machine (SVM)	85.78%	–	87.64%	–
Alexnet	88.9%	–	89.3%	–
VGG16 and ResNet 50	82%	–	–	–
VGG19 based system	90%	80%	83%	79%

combination of depths and different propagation rates. Moreover, metallurgy is employed to optimise the predictions for various CovXNet types and thus covers multiple reception areas with the overlay technology at various x-ray resolutions. The previously learned convolutional layers can be directly translated to smaller COVID-19 X-rays and other X-rays with a few extra fine-tuning layers.

COVID-19 X-rays are analysed by this improved network using all of its prior X-ray data. By circumscribing the large X-ray sections that prompted this prediction, a gradient localisation is also integrated for future explorations.

16.13.1 Methodology

As pneumonia has clinical and physiologically similar manifestations to conventional pneumonia, it can be a successful treatment of pneumonia, the working process of the proposed method is illustrated schematically in Figure 16.4. Conveyed information from several chest x-rays from normal patients or from other traditional patients with pneumonia to further characterise the reduction in the amount of x-rays of COVID19.

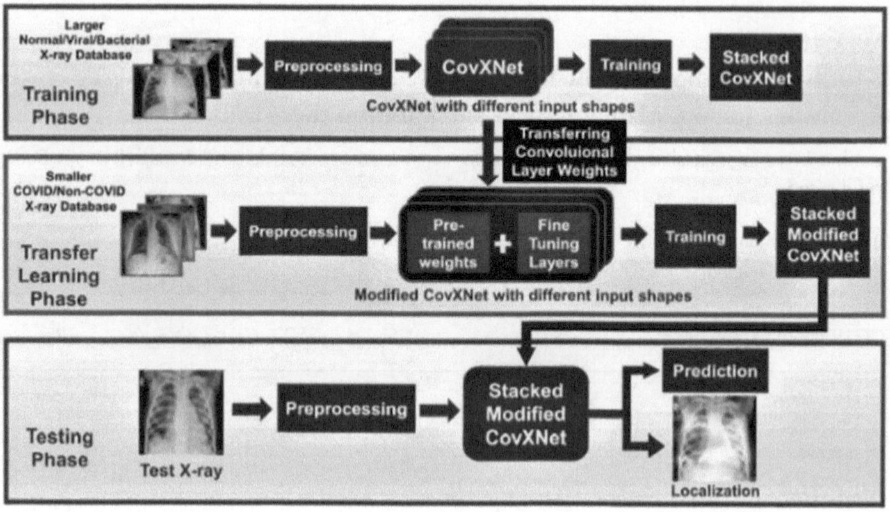

FIGURE 16.4 A diagram is shown for the entire workflow. CovXNet learns through a larger X-ray dataset during training. The summary algorithm has been used for the prediction of various CovXNet architecture X-ray resolutions. Completion with smaller COVID/non-COVID X-ray dataset of improved CovXNet capacities during transmission training. The multi-layer CovXNet modified layer and critical section localisation for X-ray inspection were provided during the testing.

In the first training process CovXNet was trained with a larger dataset containing x-rays of non-COVID bacterial/viral pneumonia patients therefore. Different resolutions were applied in the incoming X-ray following preprocessing to separately train several CovXNet models. Then every prediction of these grids is amplified by metallurgy and overlay.

Since during transmission training, the convolutionary layer weights shall be instantly transmitted as these are optimised for the extraction of major spatial functions with X-rays, additional CovXNet raffination layers with COVID19 and other pneumonia cases are carried out in less than the baseline data set. This updated, refined and qualified CovXNet pile was used in a test to predict the X-ray picture layer successfully. Localisation based on tilt was also done to identify visually the critical X-ray region to be decided on.

16.13.1.1 Structural Units

Two structural elements are the main building blocks of CovXNet architecture that are shown in Figure 16.5. In order to classification the pneumonia, these units are using depthly dilated convolutions to obtain characteristics from X-ray.

Dilated convolution is used to expand the convolution's feature map field without raising the total number of kernel parameters through increasing dilation rates.

If different characteristics from various convolutions were combined with various dilatation rates, the function extraction method would be more different.

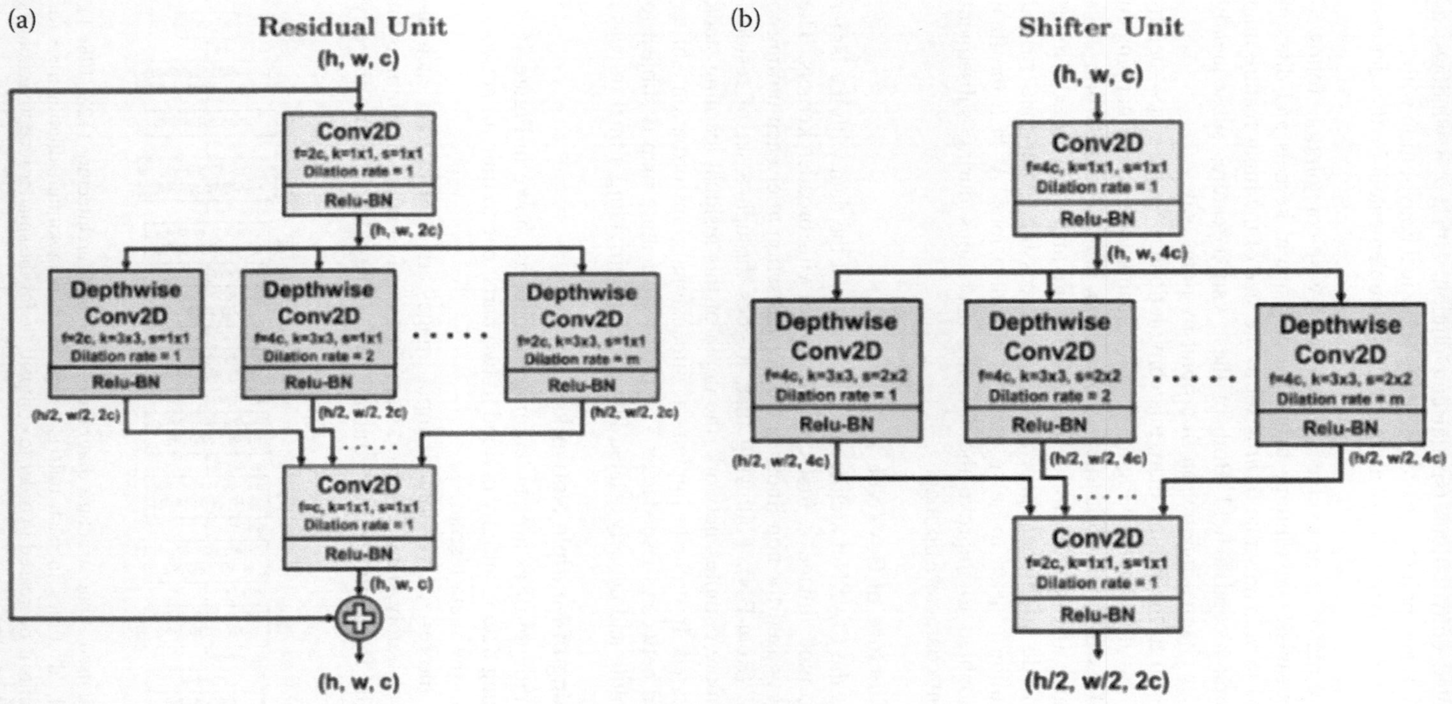

FIGURE 16.5 Units of structure discussed. The height, width, and number of channels on the characteristic map are indicated by h, w, and c, while the kernel size, steps "s" and "f" is indicated by "k" and filters are indicated by the convolution number. In a profound convolution, the dilation rate could vary from 1 to "m".

Depth-wise dilated convolutions (spatial convolution with 3 × 3 windows, as shown in Figure 16.5) and point-wise convolutions (classical convolution with 1 × 1 windows, as shown in Figure 16.5) are efficiently implemented in the defined structural units.

The input feature matrix is first subjected to a point-wise convolution, followed by a series of depth-wise convolutions using various spatial kernels and dilation rates ranging from 1 to m. The value of m is set to the size of the input feature map to cover the required receptive field. Both of these varied features subsequently undergo further inter-channel integration in a point-by-point way.

In adding the result to the feature map, this convolutionary "point-wise—depth-wise —point-wise" as illustrated in Figure 16.5(a), adapts to residual mapping in the residual map. This is for the construction of a deep, not overfit network.

As shown in Figure 16.5(b), the size of the input feature map is increased 4 times in the shift unit to add additional space reduction processing. After that, strided depth-wise convolution is used to halve the spatial dimensions. At last, the final turning point is doubled to improve the filtering operations during subsequent phases in the output characteristic map.

16.13.1.2 Architecture of CovXNet

Figure 16.6 depicts the CovXNet architecture. To interpret the data with the larger receptive field, the input image is first convolutioned with broader kernels. The rectified linear unit is used for non-linear batch normalisation after each turning to speed convergence (Relu-BN). Following that, it goes through a set of residual units. To create a more complex network, the depth of this residual learning stack (d) are being increased. In order to implement dimensional transformation, shifter units are positioned between these stacks. The processed feature map is subject to global average pooling and densely related layers before providing a final forecast.

16.13.1.3 Stacking of Multiple Networks

This stage can be thought of as a meta-learning method, as shown in Figure 16.7. The complete training data is initially divided in two parts: one to train all networks and another to train the meta learner.

Following that, the resized versions of input images are used to train each individual network separately. These networks are then used to make predictions on the remaining data for meta learner training after they have been properly

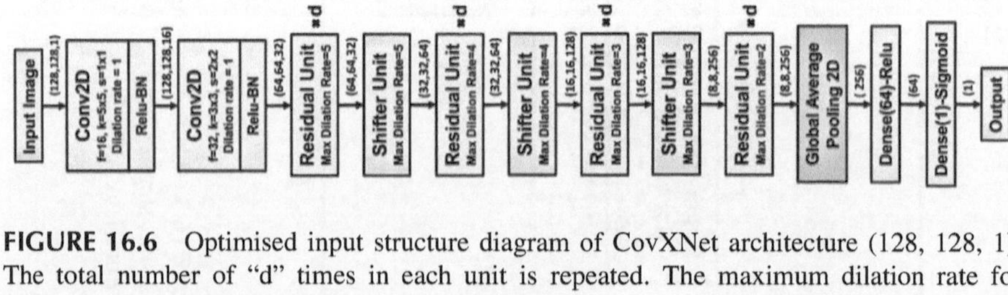

FIGURE 16.6 Optimised input structure diagram of CovXNet architecture (128, 128, 1). The total number of "d" times in each unit is repeated. The maximum dilation rate for residual and shifter units is decreased in order to compensate for the smaller receptive field as the map dimension decreases.

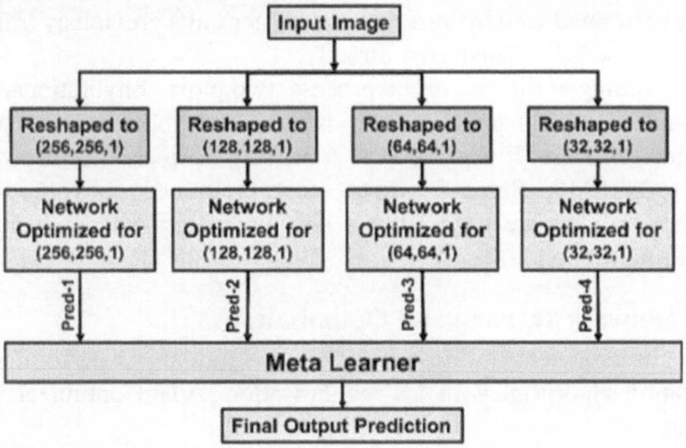

FIGURE 16.7 Individually optimised networks are stacked with the meta-learner to achieve more optimised forecasts.

optimised. Finally, to produce the final output, the meta learner is optimised by looking at all of the individual networks' predictions.

In order to achieve the best result, this meta-learner examines the forecasts for different networks.

Since the meta-learner works with forecasts from independently optimised networks it is trained by only a small portion of the samples. Therefore the meta learner can be built by means of superficial neural networks and other conventional methods.

16.13.1.4 Transfer Learning Method of CovXNet for New Corona Virus Data

Because CovXNet's purpose is to analyse X-rays with very high architectural depth and a wide variety of convolutionary layers, the representation of new COVID-19-rays can be successfully transferred. Figure 16.8 illustrates this.

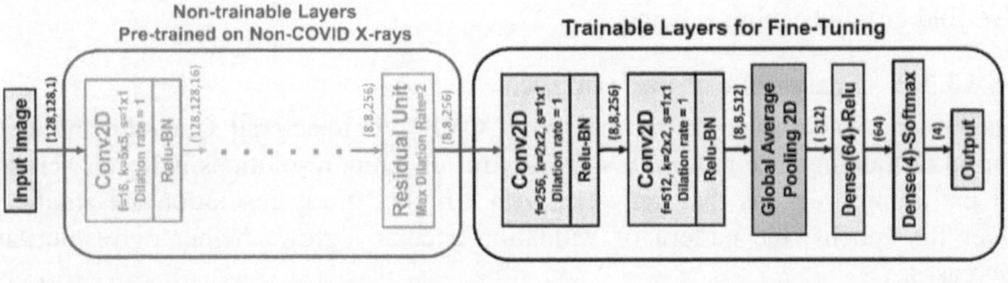

FIGURE 16.8 For fine-tuning of a limited number of images, CovXNet transfer learning framework is developed. Involving layers previously trained in non-COVID X-rays are transmitted directly. The smaller database generated by COVID-19 X-rays is finished with two additional convolutionary layers and the densely connected strata.

With their pretrained weights residual and shifter units previously trained in non-COVID radiation will be transferred directly.

For the fine-tuning at the end of the process, two more convolutionary layers are added. A standard, global pooling layer is then added for training with several densely connected layers. It is difficult to train very deep architecture with the few pictures of COVID-19. Since however most pretrained convolutionary layers without further training are used, only a few parameters for newly implemented layers need to be refined.

16.13.1.5 Network Training and Optimisation

To minimise the cross entropy loss function, the training is performed using the back propagation algorithm with L2 regularisation. Adam optimizer updates the layer's weight.

In multiple class predictions, softmax is used to normalise the probability vector for each entry, while sigmoid activation is used to normalise the binary case probability estimate.

16.13.2 Results and Discussions

The results of the above-mentioned schemes are discussed in this section. COVID-19 X-rays are used to investigate the method's robustness in various situations. Finally, some cutting-edge techniques for pneumonia diagnosis are compared to some conventional networks.

16.13.2.1 Datasets

This study analysed a dataset of 5856 images, 1583 standard radiographs, 1493 viral radiographs, and 2780 radiographs of bacterial pneumonia from Guangzhou Medical Centre, China [42].

An additional dataset of 305 X-rays from various COVID19 patients was collected and validated by a team of radiologists at Sylhet Medical School in Bangladesh and bacterial radiographs were combined (305 radiographs in each layer).

The remaining radiation (normal, infectious, and bacterial pneumonia) is used for the initial training process. The approach is tested in each of these steps with a five-fold cross-checking scheme.

16.13.2.2 Evaluation of Performance

The network is designed for normal, non-COVID viral/bacterial x-rays for the first period of training. The multi-class validity for different resolutions indicates across all the training epochs that networks with a higher X-ray resolution are smaller. Over the epochs, the pattern of validation accuracy grows higher as resolution increases.

When images of various resolutions are used by the meta-learner, the predictability is enhanced further. It significantly enhances the accuracy of all classifications. In the initial training stage, the stacking algorithm has been used. Stacking dramatically improves accuracy in relation to each network that works at various X-ray resolutions throughout all tasks.

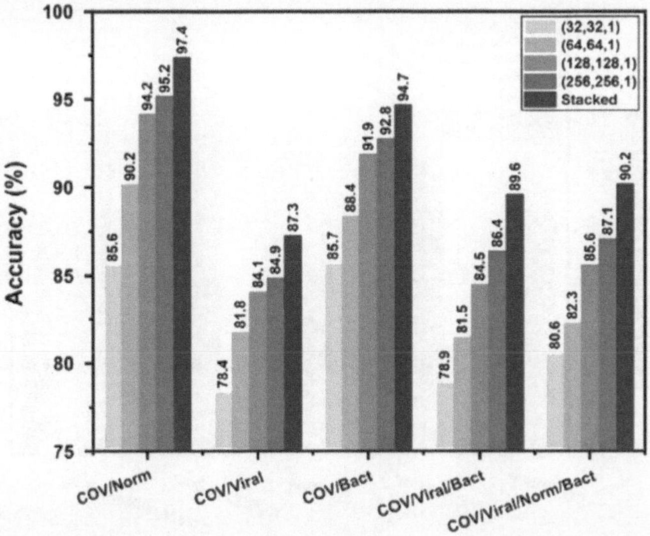

FIGURE 16.9 Despite moderate precision for the classification of COVID-19/virus pneumonia because of the overlap, a high level of efficiency has been achieved by using the stacking method in transfer learning.

These high-optimized convolution layers are moved to a smaller dataset consisting of COVID-19 x-rays for trainings after completing the initial training in non-COVID X-rays. COVID-19 X-rays have been refined for this transfer learning process in a number of normal/traditional pneumonia performance classes. Another meta-learner was trained in this procedure in a similar way to the initial training stage. Figure 16.9 shows the performance and the performance achieved after the piling up of both these individually trained networks.

Stacking with meta-learner, on the other hand, improves efficiency on all COVID-19 classification tasks. The accuracy improvement can vary, however, depending on the nature of the supervised classification used in the meta-learning process. Different DL/ML classifiers, including Xgboost, random woodlands, decision treeks, SVM, KNN, logistic regression, and Gaussian Naive Bayes algorithms are evaluated for experimentation (GaussianNB). Figure 16.10 shows the accuracy of different meta-learners for various classifying tasks. The best accuracy achieved using the Xgboost and Random Forest algorithms, which provide prediction after an additional ensemble of many boosting and bagging algorithms, respectively.

Figure 16.11 shows the multi-class confusion matrix. Due to a large degree of overlap, several COVID-19/viral cases were misclassified, as predicted. On the other hand, other classification events produce very good results. The integration of the meta-learner through the stacking of different networks will however further enhance recall of all others.

Table 16.8 compares the efficacy of CovXNet with those of other existing approaches in the initial training process for non-COVID X-rays.

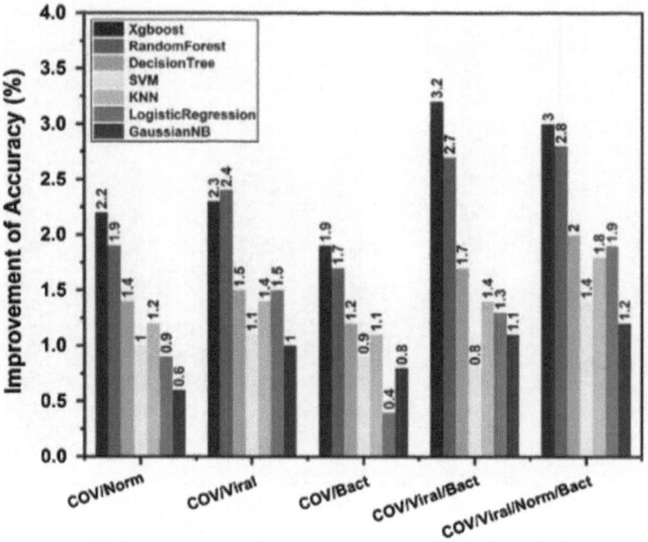

FIGURE 16.10 The impact of meta-learner selection on stacking: While each meta-learner increases performance marginally, Xgboost and Random Forest meta-learners outperform the others in most tasks.

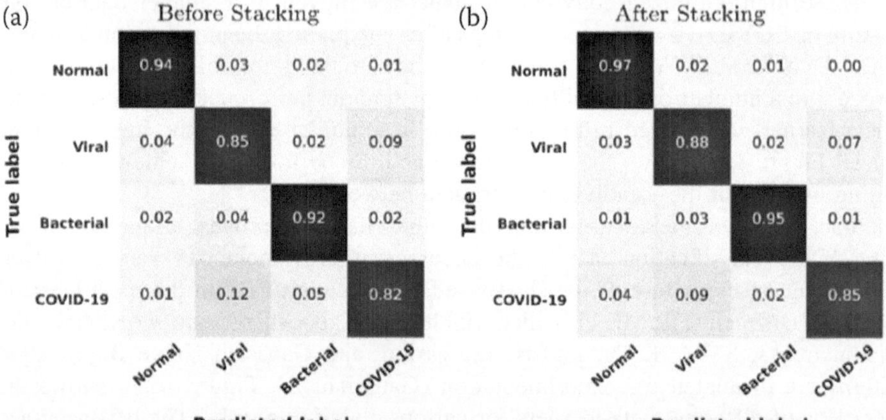

FIGURE 16.11 Before and after stacking, multi-class confusion matrices are displayed. Overlapping characteristics lead to less sensitivity for COVID-19 and virus instances than normal, bacterial pneumonia. Stacking can increase all class sensitivities.

Table 16.9 compares CovXNet to the efficacy in the detection of COVID19 and pneumonia of other traditional networks. In a number of COVID19 emission classification tasks, CovXNet Architecture provides significantly better performance than other traditional architectures.

TABLE 16.8
Comparison of CovXNet's Performance with Other Advanced Approaches for Pneumonia Detection with Non-COVID Diseases

Task	Methods	Accuracy (%)	AUC score (%)	Precision (%)	Recall (%)	Specificity (%)	F1 score (%)
Normal/Pneumonia	CovXNet	**98.1**	**99.4**	**98.0**	**98.5**	**97.9**	**98.3**
	Residual	91.2	96.4	90.7	95.9	84.1	93.4
	Inception	88.7	92.6	88.9	94.1	80.2	91.1
	VGG-19	87.2	90.7	85.6	91.1	77.9	89.3
Viral/Bacterial Pneumonia	CovXNet	**95.1**	**97.6**	**94.9**	96.1	**94.3**	**95.5**
	Residual	89.5	92.4	88.3	**96.9**	78.1	92.4
	Inception	85.8	90.6	84.5	93.8	72.1	88.9
	VGG-19	83.2	88.5	81.1	91.3	71.7	86.6
Normal/Viral/Bacterial/Pneumonia	CovXNet	**91.7**	**94.1**	**92.9**	**92.1**	**93.6**	**92.6**
	Residual	86.5	88.6	86.6	88.8	93.1	86.4
	Inception	82.1	83.6	76.4	86.9	85.2	79.9
	VGG-19	78.8	82.1	75.5	83.9	82.4	78.9

TABLE 16.9
The CovXNet Method Compares Other Conventional COVID19 Networks to Other Methods for Detecting Pneumonia

Task	Methods	Accuracy (%)	AUC score (%)	Precision (%)	Recall (%)	Specificity (%)	F1 score (%)
COVID/Normal	CovXNet	**97.4**	**96.9**	**96.3**	**97.8**	**94.7**	**97.1**
	Residual	92.1	91.2	90.4	93.4	89.2	91.9
	Inception	89.5	84.3	89.1	87.7	83.2	88.4
	VGG-19	85.3	82.7	86.3	83.9	79.9	85.1
COVID/ViralPneumonia	CovXNet	**87.3**	**92.1**	**88.1**	**87.4**	**85.5**	**87.8**
	Residual	80.4	78.9	81.1	79.3	77.1	80.2
	Inception	78.2	75.5	76.8	79	75.4	77.9
	VGG-19	72.1	67.7	70.9	74.7	69.3	72.8
COVID/BacterialPneumonia	CovXNet	**94.7**	**95.1**	**93.5**	**94.4**	**93.3**	**93.9**
	Residual	84.2	80.3	86.7	83.5	82.4	85.1
	Inception	83.1	79.9	82.2	85.2	83.6	83.7
	VGG-19	77.2	75.5	73.3	80.3	71.4	76.8
COVID/Viral/BacterialPneumonia	CovXNet	**89.6**	**90.7**	**88.5**	**90.3**	**87.6**	**89.4**
	Residual	81.1	78.8	82.5	81.3	77.5	81.9
	Inception	83.3	84.1	83.4	84.9	81.8	82.7
	VGG-19	78.1	78.5	77.5	81.7	78.2	79.6
COVID/Normal/Viral/Bacterial	CovXNet	**90.2**	**91.1**	**90.8**	**89.9**	**89.1**	**90.4**
	Residual	83.3	81.7	83.7	78.9	81.2	82.1
	Inception	83.9	78.9	81.6	85.1	83.2	83.5
	VGG-19	81.8	79.5	78.4	82.3	79.1	78.9

In conjunction with CovXNet, gradient-based class activation mapping (Grad-CAM) technique is used to find the exact area of the radiographs that activated the decision diagnosis to generate activation mapping. Such locations are further examined by overlaying the heat map with the input X-rays to view the knowledge of the network from a clinical perspective. Now, third case study will be discussed next.

16.14 EARLY DETECTION OF DEEP LEARNING-BASED DIABETIC RETINOPATHY (CASE STUDY-3)

Diabetic Retinopathy (DR) is a common complication of diabetes mellitus that causes vision-impairing lesions on the retina. It can cause blindness if not detected early. Unlike computer-aided diagnostic systems, ophthalmologists must manually diagnose DR retina fundus images, which requires time, effort, and resources and is vulnerable to error. Deep learning has recently emerged as one of the most common methods for detecting and classifying DR colour fundus images.

DR levels are five based on the incidence of these lesions: no DR (no lesions), milder non-proliferative DR (the earliest stage in which micronucleic diseases may occur only), moderate non-proliferative DR (a stage of loss of blood vessel transport capacity due to swelling and distortion), and serious, non-proliferative DR.

The goal is for the disease to be monitored automatically and information on the seriousness of the disease can be provided. We intend to do so by developing a Convolutional neural network (CNN) deep learning model which can automatically examine a patient's eye image and determine the degree of blindness [43]. This automation process will save a considerable amount of time, allowing for a large-scale examination of the diabetic retinopathy treatment process.

16.14.1 Datasets Used

Data from a number of sources used in this study:

- 35,126 images from Diabetic Retinopathy, 2015 challenge — https://www.kaggle.com/c/diabetic-retinopathy-detection/overview/timeline
  It contains 35,126 fundus images labelled with stages of DR for both the left and right eyes:
  - No retinopathic diabetes (label 0).
  - Moderate diabetic retinopathy (label 1)
  - Diabetic retinopathy moderate (label 2).
  - Serious retinopathy (label 3).
  - Diabetic retinopathy Proliferative (label 4).
- 413 images were used from the Indian Diabetic Retinopathy Image Dataset (IDRiD) (Sahasrabuddhe and Meriaudeau, 2019).
- MESSIDOR dataset (Google Brain, 2019) dataset.

The full dataset was divided into 3662 training, 1928 validation, and 13000 testing images by the organisers of the Kaggle APTOS 2019 Blindness Detection (APTOS2019) competition. https://www.kaggle.com/c/aptos2019-blindness-detection/overview

16.14.2 Metric Assessment

The basic measurement parameter is quadratic weighted kappa (Cohen's kappa). The macro F1 score, accuracy, sensitivity, and specification on holdout's dataset of 736 images obtained from the training results of APTOS2019 are other metrics considered in the Kappa score in addition.

16.14.2.1 Quadratic Weighted Kappa (QWK)

The quadratic kappa weighted factor determines the consistency between two ratings. This goes from 0 (random rating agreement) to 1 (perfect ratering agreement) (complete agreement between raters). This metric will fall below 0 if the raters have less agreement than would be predicted by chance. Between the human rater's allocated scores and the expected scores, the quadratic weighted kappa is determined.

16.14.2.2 Intuition of Cohen's Kappa

This statistic provides for the agreement that exists by chance, apart from the agreement observed in the Confusion matrix. We show what I am talking about with a simple example—suppose that we want to estimate Cohen's Kappa using Table 16.10, a confusion matrix, essentially. The raters "A" and "B" agree on 20 yes and 15 no, as is shown in the table below = 35 results, out of a total of 50. Thus P(o) = 35/50 = 0.7 was observed.

Instead of a true consensus among "A" and "B", we must find out what part of the rating is attributable to chance. As can be seen from "A" yes 25/50 = 0.5 times, "B" yes 30/50 = 0.6 times. The chance for both to say "yes" is therefore 0.5*0.6 = 0.3 at the same moment. Likewise, it is 0.5*0.4 = 0.2 that each of them will be likely to reply "no" at the same time. The probability of random agreement therefore amounts to 0.3 + 0.2 = 0.5. Let's just call it P (e).

$$K = \frac{p_0 - p_e}{1 - p_e} = \frac{0.7 - 0.5}{1 - 0.5} = 0.4 \tag{16.1}$$

Using Eqn (16.1), Cohens kappa will be 0.4. The result is 0.4, which can be defined using the Table 16.11 below.

TABLE 16.10
Agreement Table

		B	
		Yes	**No**
A	Yes	20	5
	No	10	15

TABLE 16.11
Interpretation of Kappa

	Explanation of Kappa					
	Poor	**Slight**	**Fair**	**Moderate**	**Substantial**	**Nearly perfect**
Kappa	0.0	0.20	0.40	0.60	0.80	1.0

Kappa	**Agreement**
<0	Less than chance settlement
0.01–0.20	Slight settlement
0.21–0.40	Fair settlement
0.41–0.60	Moderate settlement
0.61–0.80	Substantial settlement
0.81–0.99	Almost perfect settlement

A score of 0.4 shows that the agreement we reached is fair/moderate.

16.14.2.3 Quadratic Weight Intuition in Ordinary Classes — Quadratic Weighted Kappa (QWK)

We should use the same definition when it comes to multistage classes, while introducing the weight idea. Weights are ordinary variables, meaning that there is a greater consensus between classes "1" and "2" than classes "1" and "3" since they are closer at the ordinary level.

The performance is ordinal when the blindness is severe due to DR (this is severity of blindness, 0 not blindness, 4 the highest). Weights on a quadratic scale are used to account for this. The higher the weights of the ordinal groups, the closer they are.

$$weight = 1 - \left(\frac{distance}{maximumpossible\ \ distance}\right)^2 \tag{16.2}$$

To understand in a more logical way, let's pretend there are five shades of red: R1, R2, R3, R4, and R5. Each pair of red shades must be assigned a value between 0 and 1. To do so, let's create a variable called "Distance", which we can describe as the difference between their ordinal ranks. In our case, we'll assume a maximum distance of 4. As a result, if we use Eqn. (16.2) to calculate the weight, we get Table 16.12:

As can be seen, R1 and R4 are 0.44 by weight (since they are separate from R1 and R2 in 3 ordinal classes, which has a weight of 0.94, because they are nearer). In calculating the probabilities of observed and random chances, these weights are multiplied by the corresponding probabilities. Now we can get Quadratic weighted kappa (QWK) by Eqn. (16.3).

TABLE 16.12
Weights of Five Red Shades

Quadratic		R1	Distance
	R1	1.00	0
	R2	0.94	1
	R3	0.75	2
	R4	0.44	3
	R5	0.00	4

$$K = \frac{P_{observed} - P_{bychance}}{1 - P_{bychance}} \tag{16.3}$$

$$P_{observed} = Sum\ \ of\ \ all\ \ elements\ \ of\ \ weighted\ \ observed\ \ probabilities.$$

$$P_{bychance} = Sum\ \ of\ \ all\ \ elements\ \ of\ \ weighted\ \ bychance\ \ probabilities.$$

16.14.3 METHOD

The detection of diabetic retinopathy can be approached from multiple perspectives: classification, regression, and ordinal regression. This is probable because the disease manifests itself in stages.

16.14.3.1 Image Pre-processing and Augmentations

To bring out distinctive features from eye pictures, image pre-processing techniques such as image resizing and cropping may be used. A large number of augmentations can be used to minimise associations between image content and meta-features (for example, resolution, type of crop, zoom, or total luminosity) while also preventing the CNN model from overfitting.

Image augmentation is one of the most frequently used operations in the production of additional images from the dataset to generate new data utilising rotating flips, cutting, padding and other approaches.

Some of the image increases that are employed include optical distortion, grid distortion, piece-wise affinity transformation, horizontal tilt, vertical tilt, random rotation, random shift, random scale, random RGB value shifting, and casual brightness.

16.14.3.2 Network Architecture

We want each fundus image to be precisely identified. For the creation of neural networks, traditional profound CNN design, which comprises an extractor and a smaller decoder for a particular task (head). The neural network structure is

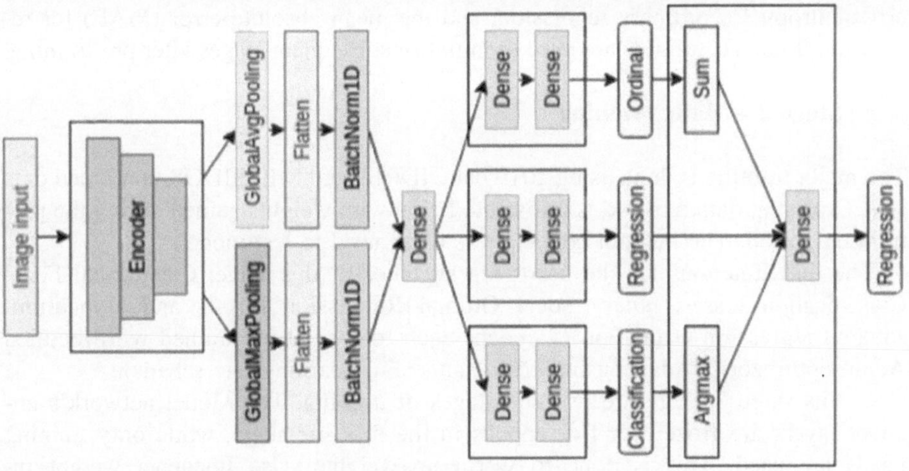

FIGURE 16.12 Three-head CNN structure.

illustrated in Figure 16.12. A multi-task learning technique can detect DR. This example uses three decoders. Everyone is trained to do his duty with the CNN backbone features:

- Head of Classification,
- Head of Regression,
- Ordinal head of Regression.

We may use any existing CNN framework for the encoder—ResNet50, EfficientNetB4, EfficientNetB5 (and ensemble these).

In this case, the classification head creates a single hot encoded vector with each stage indicated by 1. The regression head produces a real value from 0 to 4.5 and then rounds to an integer of the disease degree. The objective of the ordinary head of regression is to predict each category up to and including the objective. The final projection comes from the adjustment of a linear regression model to three head results. To minimise training time, both heads and the feature extractor are trained together. Until the post-training period, the linear regression model is kept frozen.

16.14.3.3 Training Process

- **Stage 1 - Pre Training**

Weights from Imagenet-pretrained CNN are used to initialise the feature extractor. Random weights are used to start the heads. The model is trained for 20 epochs using an SGD minibatch and a cosine-based learning rate schedule based on 2015 data.

The loss functions for each head are minimised in pre training stage. There have been uses of loss functions such as classification cross-entropy, binary cross-entropy for ordinary regression, and the mean absolute error (MAE) for regression. Encoder weights are used to initialise subsequent stages after pre-training.

- **Stage 2 - Main Training**

The major training is done using 2019 data, IDRID and MESSIDOR combined data sets. Cross-validation 5-fold is utilised to begin with weights gained during the pre-training period. The holdout collection is often used to test models.

The loss functions for the heads are switched at this stage: Categorical Focal Classification losses, binary Focal Ordinal Regression Losses and a medium-squared regression error. For 75 epochs each fold has been trained with rectified Adam optimizer (RAdam) using cosine annealing learning rate schedule

In this stage-2, there are two sub-stages of training. The Model network's encoder layers are frozen for five epochs in the first sub-stage, while only training heads are used. This is done to warm up weights (Use Imagenet weight intensification to transfer learning in tiny collections of data). The unfreezing and training of all Layers is the second sub-stage.

The 2-Dimensional integration of T-SNE is generated during the primary training in order to monitor the separation in the function space provided by the encoder. In the Figure 16.13, T-SNE is displayed of embeddings with ground truth data and predicted groups.

From Figure 16.13, photos with no DR signs can be noticed, with a wide distance from other images with any DR indicator. In addition, DR phases consecutively occur in the embedding space corresponding to genuine diagnostic sémantics.

- **Stage 3 - Post Training**

As illustrated in Figure 16.14, this involves taking the output from the three heads (classification, regression, and Ordinal Regression) and feeding it to a single dense neuron (linear activation) in order to minimise the mean square error (50 epochs).

- **Regularisation**

For improved robustness, models must be regularised at training time. Weight decay and dropout are examples of popular approaches that can be used in this situation. Regression and classification heads may also benefit from label smoothing. To discrete target marks, you can add random uniform noise. This lowers the likelihood of incorrect labelling, allowing the model to generalise more effectively and avoid overfitting.

16.14.4 Results

16.14.4.1 Model Evaluation on Test Data

Now that we know regression performance, we can utilise the closest integer rounding to determine the finale class label. We acquire the final kappa score of

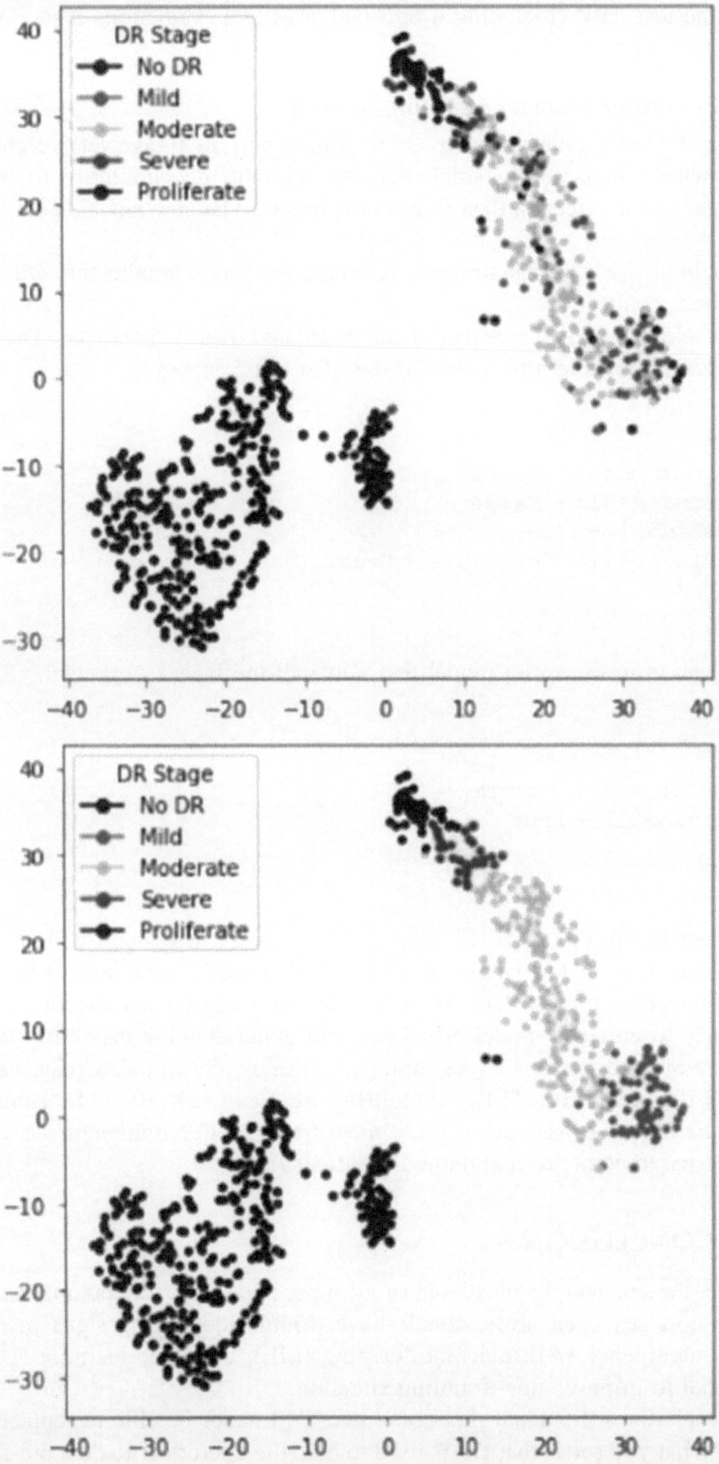

FIGURE 16.13 Feature embeddings with T-SNE. Ground truth (left) and predicted (right) classes.

0.704 in the test data. (Including a Substantial Model Predictions Agreement with Human Councillors.)

16.14.4.2 Other Transfer Learning Models

A popular Transfer Learn strategy is to utilise current ImageNet weights as initializers when encountering small datasets without any similarity to ImageNet datasets (the initials freeze), then re-train the model. The new model is the only way forward.

We could utilise a similar strategy. A simple ResNet50 architecture will likewise deliver good results.

The ResNet 50 architecture model can be trained over 2–5 epochs. (These layers are essentially trainable after resnet50 only for last 5 layers.)

```
  .........
  .........

for layer in model.layers:
  layer.trainable = False
for i in range(-5, 0):
  model.layers[i].trainable = True
  .........
  .........
```

Then we can train the entire model and make all the layers workable.

```
  .........
  .........

for layer in model.layers:
layer.trainable = True

  .........
  .........
```

As demonstrated in Figure 16.15, after only 20 epochs we obtain a high precision score—about 92% in the validation dataset. This model generates a 0.83 kappa quadratic weighted on test data. (This is a decent grade for agreement.)

Similarly to enhance model efficiency and generalisation capability with various assembly designs, we are able to employ Stratified Cross validation (5fold)—EfficientNetB4, 5EfficientNetB5, SE-Res NeXt50, etc. Table 16.13 displays the results of several of these measures. (Model architecture is modified just, other parameters are maintained identical.)

16.15 CONCLUSION

Dr. House, the greatest diagnostician of all time, once said, "Symptoms never lie". Also the most seasoned professionals have trouble identifying signs in real life. Artificial intelligence (AI), machine learning (ML), and deep learning (DL) have the potential to improve this troubling situation.

However, it is self-evident that computers will never be able to replace human experts. "What you see is that DL is used to help the doctors or to do a pre-selection

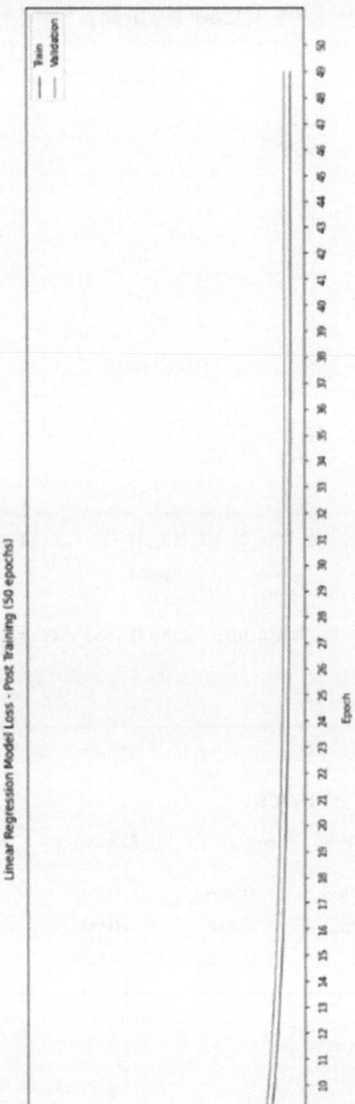

FIGURE 16.14 Post training—Epochs (vs) loss.

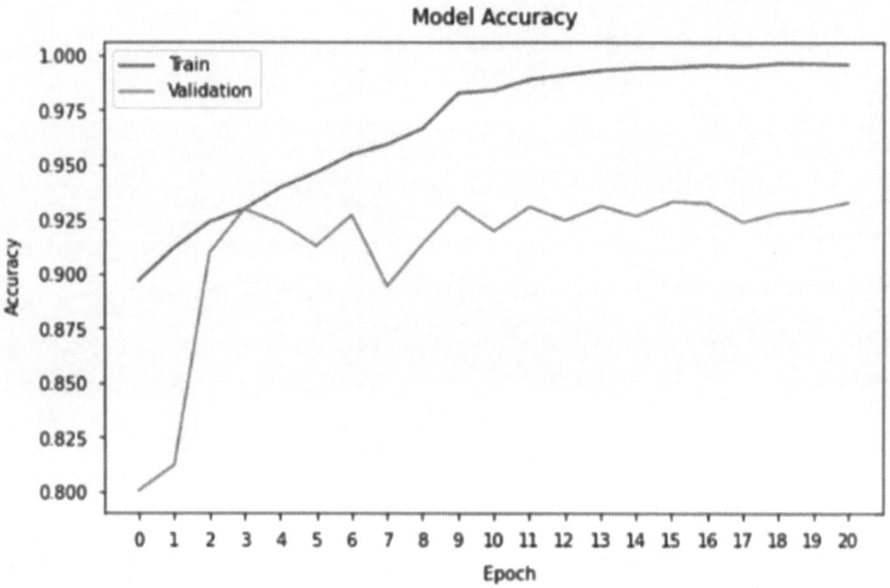

FIGURE 16.15 ResNet50 (transfer learning)—Epoch (vs) Accuracy

TABLE 16.13
Results of Experiments and Metrics

Model	QWK	Macro F1	Accuracy	Sensitivity	Specificity
EfficientNet-B4	0.966	0.806	0.902	0.809	0.977
EfficientNet-B5	0.963	0.812	0.902	0.807	0.976
SE-ResNeXt50 (512 × 512)	0.971	0.853	0.928	0.868	0.983

and prioritise cases if there are several patients in the queue", Erwin Bretscher, a healthcare specialist, explains the current scenario.

A DL system that can assist in disease detection can help to solve the issue of unequal medical resource distribution and increase medical quality in areas where medical services are limited. At the same time, the auxiliary diagnostic system will increase the patient's care experience by speeding up the treatment process.

DL could be used even more extensively in diagnostic workflows if it weren't for certain constraints. What prevents the wider use of DL in medical diagnosis?

Money, first of all: ML projects are costly, work-intensive, and require a great many computer resources. In the absence of documented usage cases, health facilities are generally subject to restrictive budgets and potential investors can be careful about future profitability.

But there are a number of other challenges apart from money worries. There are just a few examples: regulatory obstacles, lack of information about emerging diseases, the data silos and regulations on privacy, lack of standardisation, and loss of faith.

DL algorithms are frequently black boxes, which means they don't explain why these results are reached. Although in many circumstances there are no problems with lack of interpretability, it is important in healthcare, where the lives of people are at stake.

Hospitals and their patients need to know how and whether it's judged by the system. Otherwise, the diagnostics of the IT system cannot be relied on. Ultimately, with the explanatory AI (XAI) the confidence problem must be resolved, an emerging area in which machine learning attempts to provide domain experts with simple modelling reasons. The XAI solutions developed are very simple and are of little application. Since however, these algorithms help to make decisions more transparent, they are expected to eventually determine healthcare.

However, intelligent DL algorithms allow medical practitioners to "second pair of eyes", which can otherwise be neglected as a result of exhaustion, diversions, lack of expertise, and other human factors. We will have additional diagnostic solutions in the near future which leverage deep learning algorithm to greatly increase patient care. But who will decide and be held accountable? A live professional apparently: for that, the AI/DL is yet too young.

REFERENCES

[1] Hussain, B., Du, Q., Zhang, S., Imran, A., Imran, M.A. Mobile edge computing based data-driven deep learning framework for anomaly detection. *IEEE Access* 2019, 7, 137656–137667.

[2] Debnath S., Barnaby D.P., Coppa K. et al., Machine learning to assist clinical decision-making during the COVID-19 pandemic. *BioMed Central* 2020, 6, 2332–8886.

[3] Hathaliya, J.J., Tanwar S., Evans R. Securing electronic healthcare records: A mobile-based biometric authentication approach. *Journal of Information Security and Applications* 2020, 53, 102528.

[4] Wang M., Zhu T., Zhang T., Zhang J., Yu S., Zhou W. Security and privacy in 6G networks: New areas and new challenges, *Digital Communications and Networks* 2020, 6, 3, 281–291, 10.1016/j.dcan.2020.07.003.

[5] Liu, C., Wang, Z., Wu, S., Wu, S., Xiao, K. Regression Task on Big Data with Convolutional Neural Network. In Proceedings of the International Conference on Advanced Machine Learning Technologies and Applications, Cairo, Egypt, 28–30 March 2019; pp. 52–58.

[6] Luo, J., Tang, J., So, D.K., Chen, G., Cumanan, K., Chambers, J.A. A deep learning-based approach to power minimization in multi-carrier NOMA with SWIPT. *IEEE Access* 2019, 7, 17450–17460.

[7] Yu, A., Yang, H., Yao, Q., Li, Y., Guo, H., Peng, T., Li, H., Zhang, J. Accurate fault location using deep belief network for optical fronthaul networks in 5G and beyond. *IEEE Access* 2019, 7, 77932–77943.

[8] Xue, S., Ma, Y., Yi, N., Tafazolli, R. Unsupervised deep learning for MU-SIMO joint transmitter and noncoherent receiver design. *IEEE Wireless Communications Letters* 2018, 8, 177–180.

[9] Dong, R., She, C., Hardjawana, W., Li, Y., Vucetic, B. Deep learning for hybrid 5G services in mobile edge computing systems: Learn from a digital twin. *IEEE Transactions on Wireless Communications* 2019, 18, 4692–4707.

[10] Chien, W.C., Weng, H.Y., Lai, C.F. Q-learning based collaborative cache allocation in mobile edge computing. *Future Generation Computer Systems* 2020, 102, 603–610.

[11] Qing, C., Cai, B., Yang, Q., Wang, J., Huang, C. Deep learning for CSI feedback based on superimposed coding. *IEEE Access* 2019, 7, 93723–93733.

[12] Jiang, Z., Chen, S., Molisch, A.F., Vannithamby, R., Zhou, S., Niu, Z. Exploiting wireless channel state information structures beyond linear correlations: A deep learning approach. *IEEE Communications Magazine* 2019, 57, 28–34.

[13] Jiang, Z., Chen, S., Molisch, A.F., Vannithamby, R., Zhou, S., Niu, Z. Exploiting wireless channel state information structures beyond linear correlations: A deep learning approach. *IEEE Communications Magazine* 2019, 57, 28–34.

[14] Niu, D., Liu, Y., Cai, T., Zheng, X., Liu, T., Zhou, S. A Novel Distributed Duration-Aware LSTM for Large Scale Sequential Data Analysis. In Proceedings of the CCF Conference on Big Data, Wuhan, China, 26–28 September 2019; pp. 120–134.

[15] Gante, J., Falcão, G., Sousa, L. Deep learning architectures for accurate millimeter wave positioning in 5G. *Neural Processing Letters*2020, 51, 487–514. 10.1007/s11 063-019-10073-1.

[16] Kim, M., Kim, N.I., Lee, W., Cho, D.H. Deep learning-aided SCMA. *IEEE Communications Letters* 2018, 22, 720–723.

[17] Ozturk, M., et al. A novel deep learning driven, low-cost mobility prediction approach for 5G cellular networks: The case of the control/data separation Architecture (CDSA). *Neurocomputing* 2019, 358, 479–489.

[18] Yan, M., et al. "Intelligent resource scheduling for 5G radio access network slicing. *IEEE Transactions on Vehicular Technology* 2019, *68*, 7691–7703.

[19] Dong, R., et al. Deep learning for hybrid 5G services in mobile edge computing systems: Learn from a digital twin. *IEEE Transactions on Wireless Communications* 2019, 18, 4692–4707.

[20] Gu, R., Zhang J. "Ganslicing: A GAN-Based Software defined mobile network Slicing scheme for IOT Applications. IEEE International Conference on Communications, IEEE, 2019.

[21] Tanwar S., Parekh K., Evans R. Blockchain-based electronic healthcare record system for healthcare 4.0 applications. *Journal of Information Security and Applications*, 2020, 50, 102407.

[22] Partha G., Mali K., Das S.K. Chaotic firefly algorithm-based fuzzy C-means algorithm for segmentation of brain tissues in magnetic resonance images. *Journal of Visual Communication and Image Representation* 2018, 54, 63–79.

[23] Ghosh, P., Mali, K., Das, S.K. Use of spectral clustering combined with normalized cuts (N-Cuts) in an Iterative k-Means clustering framework (NKSC) for superpixel segmentation with contour adherence. *Pattern Recognition and Image Analysis* 2018, 28, 400–409. 10.1134/S1054661818030161.

[24] Sohail, M.N., Ren J., Muhammad M.U. A euclidean group assessment on semi-supervised clustering for healthcare clinical implications based on real-life data. *International Journal of Environmental Research and Public Health*2019 16.9, 1581.

[25] Kao, H.-C., Tang K.-F., Chang E. Context-aware Symptom Checking for Disease Diagnosis Using Hierarchical Reinforcement Learning. *Proceedings of the AAAI Conference on Artificial Intelligence*, 2018, 102407.

[26] Zheng, T., et al. A machine learning-based framework to identify type 2 diabetes through electronic health records. *International Journal of Medical Informatics* 2017, 97, 120–127.

[27] Chen, Y., et al. "Brain MRI super resolution using 3D deep densely connected neural networks. IEEE 15th International Symposium on Biomedical Imaging (ISBI 2018), IEEE, 2018.
[28] Sirinukunwattana, K., et al. Locality sensitive deep learning for detection and classification of nuclei in routine colon cancer histology images. *IEEE Transactions on Medical Imaging* 2016, 35.5, 1196–1206.
[29] Yu, Y., et al. Deep transfer learning for modality classification of medical images. *Information* 2017, 8.3, 91.
[30] Usman, M., et al. Motion corrected multishot MRI reconstruction using generative networks with sensitivity encoding. arXiv preprint arXiv:1902.07430 2019.
[31] Zech, J., et al. Natural language–based machine learning models for the annotation of clinical radiology reports. *Radiology* 2018, 287.2, 570–580.
[32] Weng, S.F., et al. Can machine-learning improve cardiovascular risk prediction using routine clinical data? *PloS one* 2017, 12.4, e0174944.
[33] Ma, H.-Y., et al. A computer-aided diagnosis scheme for detection of fatty liver in vivo based on ultrasound kurtosis imaging. *Journal of Medical Systems* 2016, 40.1, 1–9.
[34] McKinney, S.M., Sieniek, M., Godbole, V. et al. International evaluation of an AI system for breast cancer screening. *Nature*2020,577, 89–94. 10.1038/s41586-019-1799-6
[35] Kim, H.-E., et al. Changes in cancer detection and false-positive recall in mammography using artificial intelligence: A retrospective, multireader study. *The Lancet Digital Health* 2020, 2.3, e138–e148.
[36] Kubota, T. Deep learning algorithm does as well as dermatologists in identifying skin cancer. Online, Jan 2017.
[37] Han, S.S., et al. Augmented intelligence dermatology: Deep neural networks empower medical professionals in diagnosing skin cancer and predicting treatment options for 134 skin disorders. *Journal of Investigative Dermatology* 2020, 140.9, 1753–1761.
[38] González, G., et al. Disease staging and prognosis in smokers using deep learning in chest computed tomography. *American Journal of Respiratory and Critical Care Medicine* 2018, 197.2, 193–203.
[39] Arbabshirani, M.R., et al. "Advanced machine learning in action: Identification of intracranial haemorrhage on computed tomography scans of the head with clinical workflow integration." *NPJ Digital Medicine* 2018, 1.1, 1–7.
[40] Bhatele K.R., Bhadauria S.S. Classification of neurodegenerative diseases based on VGG 19 deep transfer learning architecture: A deep learning approach. *Bioscience Biotechnology Research Communications* 2020, 13.4.
[41] Kermany D., Zhang K., Goldbaum M., Labeled optical coherence tomography (OCT) and chest X-ray images for classification 2018, *Mendeley Data* 2.2.
[42] Mahmud, T., Rahman M.A., Fattah S.A. CovXNet: A multi-dilation convolutional neural network for automatic COVID-19 and other pneumonia detection from chest X-ray images with transferable multi-receptive feature optimization. *Computers in Biology and Medicine* 2020, 122, 103869.
[43] Tymchenko, B., Marchenko P., Spodarets D. "Deep learning approach to diabetic retinopathy detection. arXiv preprint arXiv:2003.02261 2020.

17 New Approaches in Machine-based Image Analysis for Medical Oncology

E. Francy Irudaya Rani
Assistant Professor, Department of Electronics and Communication Engineering, Francis Xavier Engineering College, Tamil Nadu, India

T. LurthuPushparaj
Assistant Professor, Department of Chemistry (PG), TDMNS College, Tamil Nadu, India

E. Fantin Irudaya Raj
Assistant Professor, Department of Electrical and Electronics Engineering, Dr. Sivanthi Aditanar College of Engineering, Tamil Nadu, India

M. Appadurai
Assistant Professor, Department of Mechanical Engineering, Dr. Sivanthi Aditanar College of Engineering, Tamil Nadu, India

CONTENTS

17.1 Introduction....334
17.2 Classical Methods....335
17.3 Machine Learning Methods in Oncology....336
17.3.1 Supervised Learning....337
17.3.1.1 Support Vector Machine....337
17.3.1.2 Logistic or Linear Regression (LR)....338
17.3.1.3 Decision Tree....338
17.3.1.4 Random Forest Algorithm (RF)....339
17.3.1.5 Naive Bayes....340
17.3.1.6 K-Nearest Neighbour....340
17.3.1.7 Artificial Neural Network....341
17.3.2 Unsupervised Learning....341
17.3.2.1 K-means Clustering....342

DOI: 10.1201/9781003217497-17

17.3.2.2 Principle Component Analysis....343
17.3.2.3 Independent Component Analysis....344
17.3.2.4 Autoencoders....344
17.3.2.5 Singular Value Decomposition....345
17.3.3 Reinforcement Learning (RL)....345
17.4 Application of ML in Oncology....345
17.4.1 Brain Oncology....346
17.4.2 Skin Oncology....347
17.4.3 Breast Cancer Prognosis Prediction....348
17.4.4 ML in Lung Oncology....349
17.4.5 Gastric Oncology....350
17.5 Discussion....351
17.5.1 ML Program Performance Analysis....351
17.5.2 Pros and Cons of ML Algorithm....353
17.5.3 ML in Cancer Staging....354
17.5.4 Predicting and Evaluating Treatment Response....354
17.6 Conclusion....355
References....355

17.1 INTRODUCTION

Nobody can deny the importance of detecting cancer at an early stage. Most tumors have no screening or diagnosing methods in finding them at an earlier stage. Even those who are checked for cancer today may fall through the holes in the treatment process. Cancer diseases are integrated with numerous gene components that impact tissue signaling. Also, its biological connections with external surroundings may affect the genetic response to treatment, and modify susceptibility to therapeutic interventions is crucial. The detection of such changes necessitates the simultaneous examination of several features using sensitive and precise methods. Because most biological traits are continuous variables, and these must be reduced to categorical variables before being used in clinical decision-making. Difference of opinion among many physicians while picking over whether or not to perform a medical procedure when adapting medicine to an affected person is a massive issue. Because health care professionals acquire massive amounts of information, containing incredible signals and information at a rate what 'conventional' analysis methods can handle. These are some of the challenges with oncology investigation aside from being a tumor and requiring a substantial amount of infected tissues for evaluation, is indeed the progressively well-recognized intra- carcinoma and inter- carcinoma diversity all over cancer category, whereby diverse characteristic spots can generate a different extrapolative assessment. Henceforth, the official outcome of such investigation is based on the unique site of the tumor wherein the tissue was collected. AI-powered execution tools could help enhance the solubility by allowing the study of all individual tumor slides to produce an integrated precise signature representative of the complete lesion. Image analyzes showed to be one of the most effective ways that AI has influenced society. The use of ML algorithms is in a large percentage of AI applications in healthcare.

McCarthy and his team established machine learning-based methodologies in cancer in the 1950s to predict the various phases of the disease, the area where it spreads, the depth to which the disease has infiltrated, and other factors that clinicians consider. ML enables computers to execute tasks other than those for which they were initially programmed [1]. ML is used to discover analytical similarities among information to make inferences based on the previous instance. It is heavily influenced by cognitive psychology, neuroscience, computing, statistical principles, data mining, and performance forecasting. ML algorithms for general medical oncology research have countless times recently. A dynamic system tunes machine learning models to make correct estimates for the training data by providing them with experiences inside the provisions of training data. The model must generalize their learning expertise and make them an accurate prediction of future unknown data which is to be used. During training, a model's generalization ability will be evaluated using a second data set, the validating set, and are used as reinforcement for further model tweaking. The finished model is tested in a testing dataset, that can be used to demonstrate how the whole system would perform while presented with challenging, different data after numerous iterations of training and tuning. Machine learning algorithms are subjected to more training samples. It can recognize underlying patterns in the data to accomplish tasks without the need for human interference. Incorporating ML strategies throughout routine medical practice may be easier, least expensive, and a little less disruptive even than conducting genomic investigations.

There are knowledge gaps, that must be addressed to successfully blend machine learning with clinical oncology and maximize its effectiveness. Physicians now receive limited data science and machine learning training, which limits their capacity to comprehend mechanisms, apply algorithms effectively, and support research. Furthermore, most data analysts are unfamiliar with oncologic workup and care. This limits the capacity to discover essential and appropriate clinical use cases. Clinical oncology sections and bioinformatics and machine learning divisions should work together more, and strategic relationships with technology companies should be developed where it is possible. ML expert systems can indeed serve as effective supporting resources for accurate inpatient techniques, in contrast to their usefulness as decision assistance platforms. As a result, machine learning enters the picture soon, as it was among the most effective methods for integrating, analyzing, and making predictions based on vast, heterogeneous data sources. It is confirmed by the findings of multiple studies indicating that ML-based techniques are as accurate as expert pathologists and can increase the human reader's performance in detection and diagnostic contexts when used in conjunction with conventional protocols.

17.2 CLASSICAL METHODS

Traditionally, malignancies were classified based on their anatomical site and patient characteristics, and they were handled with one-size-fits-all medicines that ignored the person's biological history. In the biomedical sciences, mathematical models can be used to explain biological premises based on laboratory findings, physical examination, and theoretical interpretations of biological processes. Because of a lack of sufficient biological data, statistical tools, and computing capacity, mathematical modeling of biological systems has been difficult to produce. During the 1960s and 1980s, perspective medicine was phased out in favor of an evidence-based, patient-centered strategy that relied on diagnostic pathology conducted by microscope of tumor tissue or specimens on a microscopic slide, which did not necessarily yield the most accurate results. This process was taken to another level by incorporating a computerized system for slide image processing and storage. The procedure of scanning histopathology slides using whole-slide scanners (WSI), which has since been presented in 1999 [2], is included in this computerized diagnosis. However, the origins of computer vision can be traced back to the 1980s, when researchers developed a method for scanning simple images from a microscope. Here information from the blood sample has been converted into a piece of optic information, then this optic density informations was stored as a matrix form. This form was useful for determining the existence of various transcription factors using the details in the scanned image. The digitization of microscopic pictures enables quantifiable machine-based image recognition, which could be clinically useful in detecting illness and predicting patient outcomes. A detailed review comprising Sixteen clinical examiners and samples from 1,992 patients with a variety of human cancers was the important massive multicenter examination of clinical outcome among diagnostic imaging and traditional microscopy. The standard diagnostic effectiveness of digitized WSIs was found to be comparable to that of conventional microscopy-based techniques in this investigation.

In 1995, the term ‘genomic medicine’ was used to describe a method of diagnosing the disease at the molecular level [3]. Genomic medicine has produced significant biological discoveries at an unparalleled rate, thanks to breakthroughs in genotyping and sequencing technology, bioinformatics, systems biology, and computational biology. Personalized medicine is the ultimate goal of genomic medicine, which strives to build on this foundation by transferring these discoveries into clinical practice. Artificial neurons were first presented in 1943 as a framework for the processing of data by neurons in the biological brain, which led to the development of machine learning. As we acquire conviction in computer models’ ability to forecast human biological processes, they will aid us in navigating the complicated environment of disease, eventually resulting in better and trustworthy disease diagnosis, risk assessment, and therapy strategies. Some unsupervised machine learning approaches are so similar to statistical methods that they could be mistaken for a high-powered version of the very same thing.

17.3 MACHINE LEARNING METHODS IN ONCOLOGY

Computational models are influencing cancer diagnosis and treatment. ML tasks are often broadly dichotomized into supervised or unsupervised learning [4]. In classic machine learning tasks, raw input data are generally pre-engineered into characteristics, then they were interpreted to collect information that impacts growth. More digitized, multimodality testing data sets with information over various time points are needed to limit the estimation methods and diagnostic procedures on a per-patient basis. Because machine learning is a driven approach, its initial process is taken out to choose significant attributes from raw input data. These quantitative

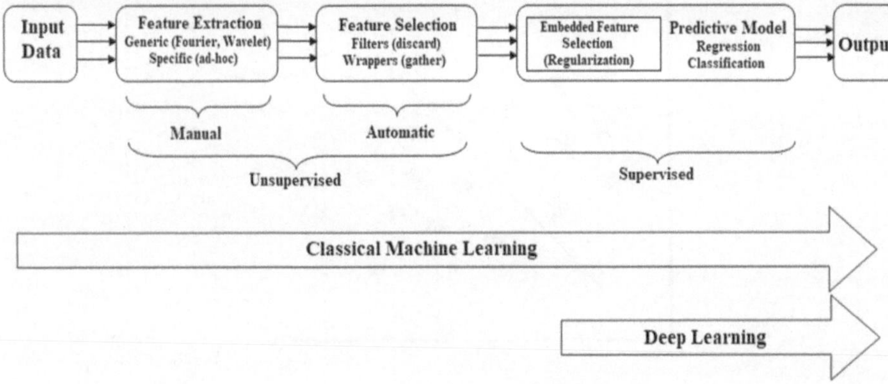

FIGURE 17.1 General ML pipeline sequences in oncology.

qualities of data summarise the information communicated by the data and are stored in arrays or matrices. The data is then fed into generic forecasting analytics, such as classifiers and support vectors, which train to execute a specific task. Figure 17.1 shows the main blocks utilized throughout most ML-based diagnostic systems.

17.3.1 Supervised Learning

In its most basic form, supervised learning seeks to match mathematical function labels to a known dataset that really can map incoming data sets to output categories. These known data are then utilized to build a software programming algorithm that can forecast health outcomes based on unknown variables despite recognizing the disease status [5]. This type of machine training relies on human input to label the various stages of the process of learning. In classifier and predictive tasks, supervised learning algorithms have proven to be successful [6]. Two categories of problems benefit from supervised learning algorithms: regression and classification problems. The primary predicted outcome in classification tasks is discrete. This parameter is divided into many groups and categories, like 'affected' and 'not affected', or 'cancer' and 'noncancer'. In regression issues, like the risk of acquiring coronary heart disease for a person [7], the appropriate output variable is a real value. The foregoing are the most well-known supervised algorithms with good reproducibility and precision: Support Vector Machines (SVMs), Naive Bayes (NB), Decision Tree (DT), Random Forests (RF), Logistic or Linear Regression (LR), K-nearest neighbor (KNN), and Artificial Neural Network (ANN).

17.3.1.1 Support Vector Machine

The SVM algorithm is capable of classifying both linearity and non-linearity input. It begins by mapping every data point through an n-dimensional attribute vector, whereby 'n' indicates the total number of attributes. The hyperplane that splits these data elements into two groups is then identified, with the minimum separation for both categories being maximized and classifying errors being minimized [8]. The

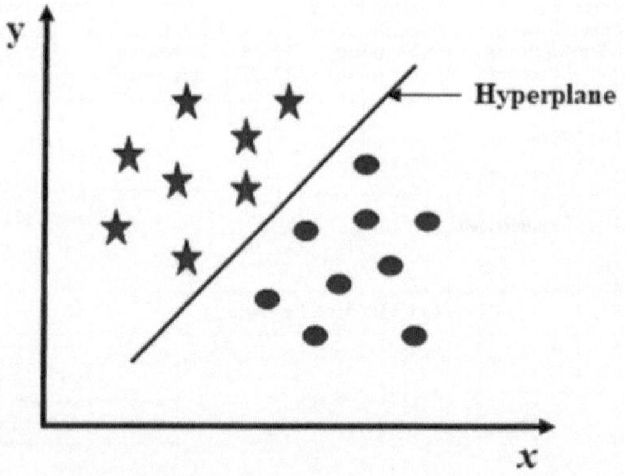

FIGURE 17.2 Illustration of SVM work. Here hyperplane maximizes the separation of two different classes ('star' and 'circle').

minimal proximity for a grouped class is defined by the length of both the selection hyperplane and the class's adjacent occurrence. In more technical terms, each feature vector is first plotted as a point in an 'n' dimensional space, from each feature's value becoming the value of a given coordinate. To complete the categorization, we must first locate the hyperplane that separates the two categories by the greatest margin. An SVM classifier is seen in Figure 17.2 in a basic workflow with a hyperplane.

17.3.1.2 Logistic or Linear Regression (LR)

It is always a reliable and well-used supervised learning methodology that elaboration of conformist regression. This model may concentrate only on a binary value which commonly reflects the frequency of occurrence of an event that does not occur. The procedure can be used to determine the likelihood that a particular event relates to a specific class group and the result will be marked in between from zero to one. To utilize the LR as a base predictor, a minimum threshold limit must be set to distinguish between two classes. In this scenario, an incoming event will be classified as class A if the probability value is more than 0.50; else, it will be classified as class B [7]. Multinomial logistic regression is the name given to this extended variant of LR.

17.3.1.3 Decision Tree

The decision tree (DT) is one of the first and most widely used ML-based cataloging techniques. It is based on logical making decisions, i.e., testing and results for categorizing data items into the treelike structure. A DT tree trunk nodes usually have numerous layers, with the root node being the first or upper node. Testing on input parameters or characteristics is represented by all root nodes. The classification algorithm forks towards the optimal offspring node depending on the tryout outcome, and the procedure of testing and branching goes on until everything achieves the terminal node. The choice outcomes are represented by the leaf or terminating nodes. DTs have been proven to be simple to read and acquire, and they

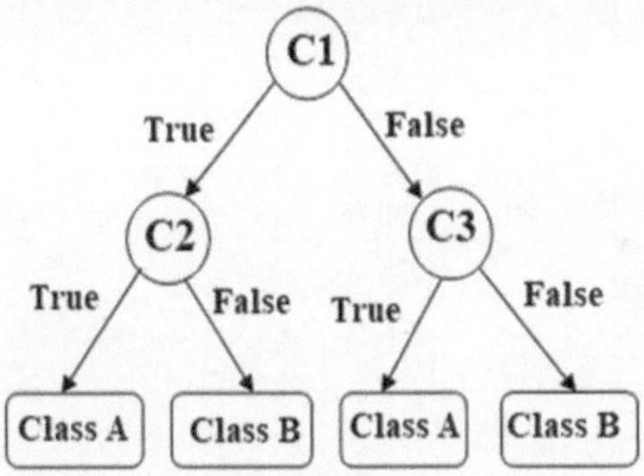

FIGURE 17.3 Workflow of decision tree. For successful classification of decision outcome class A & B each sample C1, C2 & C3's branch is labeled by 'True' and 'False' from their ancestor node.

are used in so many other clinical imaging techniques [9]. When navigating a tree for such a sample's categorization, the outcome of all checks for each vertex, all along paths will provide enough knowledge to decide a guess about both the sample's classes. Figure 17.3 shows a diagram of a complete DT, with its components and rules.

17.3.1.4 Random Forest Algorithm (RF)

A random forest is a collection of multiple description-based classifiers made up of numerous DTs just like a forest [10]. Overfitting of something like the training samples is common with deep DTs, resulting in a massive fluctuation in classification outcomes for tiny changes in the input data. This algorithm seems acutely susceptible to their training data, rendering them vulnerable to errors while dealing with the test dataset. Different sections of the training dataset are used to train the various DTs of an RF. Each DT of the forest must transmit down the input vector of the new sample size to categorize it. The classification conclusion is subsequently determined by each DT considering a separate section of the input vector. After that, the forest determines whether to employ the class with the most 'votes' (for distinct categorization decisions) or the total among all forest trees (for numeric classification outcome). The RF algorithm can minimize the issues produced by only evaluating one DT for the same dataset because it takes into account the results of numerous separate DTs. The RF method is illustrated in Figure 17.4.

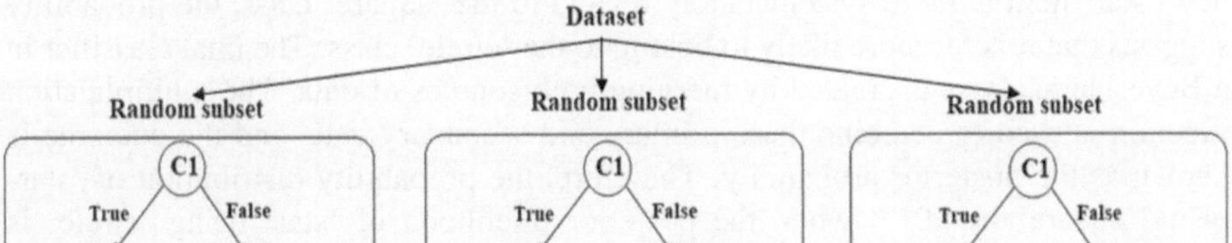

FIGURE 17.4 Pictorial representation of random forest with multiple decision trees. Each random trees were trained using subset's training data.

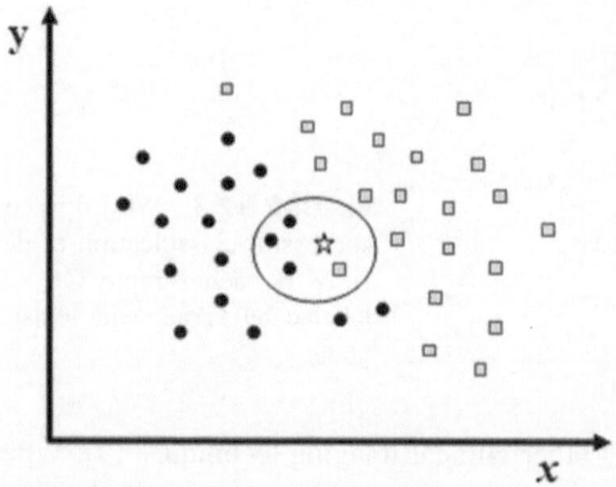

FIGURE 17.5 Illustration of Naïve Bayesian approach workflow. Here there are two classes of 'circle' and 'square'. New instance 'star' needs to be classified either to 'circle' or 'square'class.

17.3.1.5 Naive Bayes

The Bayes theorem [11] is the basis for the Naïve Bayesian approach. This theorem can be used to define the likelihood of an occurrence depending on foreknowledge of the event's circumstances. This predictor implies that a character in a class is not directly connected to any other property, even though variables in that class may be interdependent. Figure 17.5 illustrates how the NB technique works by addressing the task for classifying a new instance into either the 'square' or 'circle' class. Because there are twice as many 'square' objects as 'circle', it's reasonable to assume that every new observation would have a 'square' membership instead of a 'circle' membership. This belief is referred to as the prior probability in Bayesian analysis. As a result, 'square' and 'circle' have a previous likelihood of 0.62 and 0.38, respectively. To categorize the 'star' piece, we must first construct a big circle around it that contains several points, regardless of their class designations. This diagram considered four points (three 'circle' and one 'square'). As a result, the probability of 'star' being given 'square' is 0.025, and the probability of 'star' being given 'circle' is 0.15. Although the probability distribution suggests that perhaps the new 'star' item is more systematically related to the 'square' class, the probability suggests that it is far more likely to belong to the 'circle' class. The final classifier in a Bayesian analysis is created by merging both sources of data. The multiplication function is used to combine these primary and secondary data, and the outcome is known as the posterior probability. Therefore, the probability distribution of 'star' being 'square' is 0.017, while the posterior likelihood of 'star' being 'circle' is 0.049. The additional 'star' item must be classified as a component of a 'circle' category, according to the NB approach (Figure 17.5).

17.3.1.6 K-Nearest Neighbour

One among the simplest and earliest classification method is the K-nearest neighbor (KNN) technique [12]. It is like a simplified form of an NB classifier. The KNN algorithm, unlike the NB method, does not require the use of probability values. In

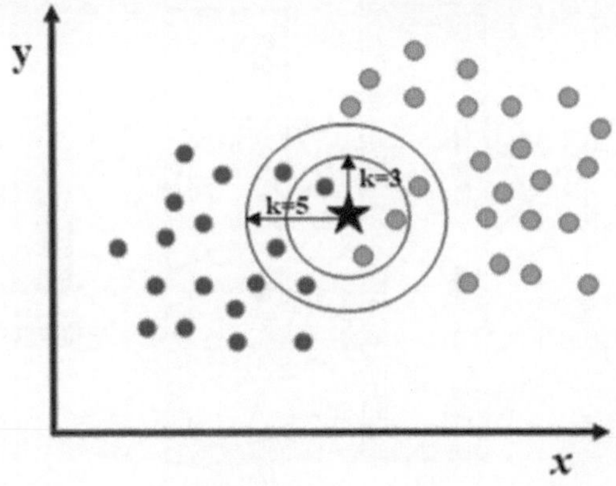

FIGURE 17.6 Illustration of K- nearest neighbor approach workflow.

the KNN algorithm, K is referred to as the amount of nearest neighbors allowed to take a vote. For the same sample object, selecting different values for 'K' can result in different classification accuracy. The KNN's classification process for a new image set is given in Figure 17.6. When K=3, the new 'star' item is classed as 'grey circle', but when K= 5, it is labeled as 'black circle'.

17.3.1.7 Artificial Neural Network

Artificial neural network (ANNs) is an important class of machine learning algorithms influenced by the way the human brain's neural networks work. Nerve cells in the biological brain are interconnected to one another by many axon connections, which form a graph-like design. These connections can indeed be reconfigured to aid in the adaptation, processing, and storage of data. ANN methods can also be depicted as several distributed nodes. As per the interconnectivity, one node's output becomes the input for yet another node's future processing. Based on changes they execute, nodes are usually organized into a layered array. An ANN architecture can have one or more hidden layers in addition to the source and destination nodes. Weights are assigned to nodes and edges to allow for the adjustment of communication signal qualities, which can then be boosted or reduced via repeated training. ANNs can give easy and early decisions for the given patient's test data and subsequent adaptation of the matrix, node, and edge values. An ANN including its interlinked large number of nodes is depicted in Figure 17.7.

17.3.2 Unsupervised Learning

It's a variant of machine learning wherein algorithms are educated on an unlabeled dataset and afterward left alone to operate on it. Because, unlike supervised learning, we have the input data, but no associated output data, this learning technique cannot be applied directly to a regression or classification problem. The key benefits of this strategy include obtaining significant information from unlisted data then thinking from their expertise like actual AI, and solving cancer problems even when there is no comparable data for input. This machine learning approach

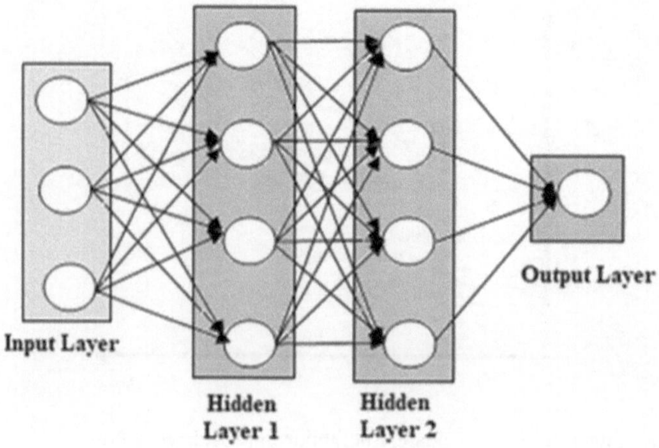

FIGURE 17.7 Structure of artificial neural network with two hidden layer.

can classify the image dataset into subgroups based on image similarity. (Clustering is a mechanism of gathering objects into groups so that things with some of the most similarities stay in one group and have far less or even no similarities with objects from another group; Association is a means of evaluating the number of attributes that take place together through a large database by determining the relationships between the variables.) Independent Component Analysis (ICA), K-Means Clustering (K-MC), Principle Component Analysis (PCA), Autoencoders, and Singular Value Decomposition (SVD) are some of the common clustering methods utilized in this ML [13].

17.3.2.1 K-means Clustering

K-means is a conservative unsupervised classification algorithm (Figure 17.8) that sheds light on some good clustering problems [14]. The concept is based on a clear and uncomplicated strategy to grouping a given collection of data into a certain number of groups (expect k groupings). The basic concept is to define k centroids, one for each group. The distance between each pixel and each cluster focus is calculated. The separation may be of simple Euclidean capacity. Using the segregation algorithm, a single pixel is contrasted to all associated targets. The pixel was assigned to a certain group with the shortest separation between them all. The center is re-evaluated at this moment. Every pixel is compared including all cluster centers once more. The method for each pixel proceeded again until the interior brain area was reached. As a result, the centroids within each bunch are also the sites at which the intervals between each element in that cluster are constrained. As a result, the K-means technique reduces the total differences between each item and its cluster centroids for each cluster Ck [15]. The four major phases of the k-means algorithm are: (stage i) place k elements randomly within a space and represent its co-ordinates clusters, (stage ii) assign each item throughout space to a group dedicated to all of that, (stage iii) recalculate k centroids and adjust their positions, and (stage ii) Repeat (ii) and (iii) until center the k centroid components.

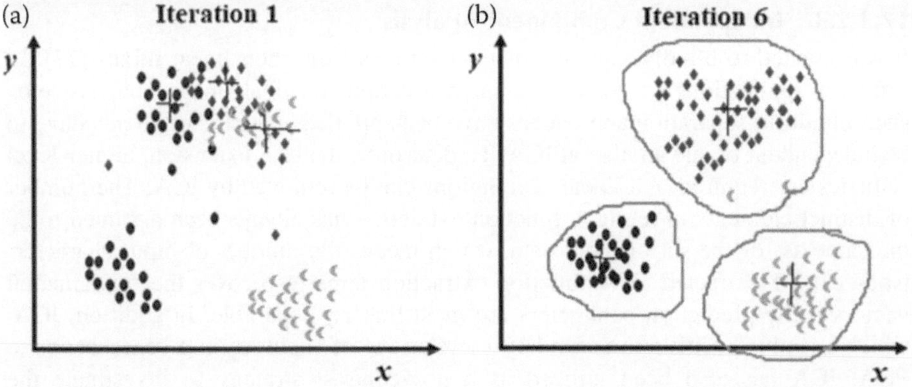

FIGURE 17.8 K-means clustering (a) Initial centroids representation (b) k-means coverage.

17.3.2.2 Principle Component Analysis

The extraction and selection of features are crucial procedures to diagnose and classify a malignancy. An optimum set of functions should have efficient, discriminatory functions, while mainly reducing the redundancy of characteristics to prevent the problem of 'dimension degradation' [16]. The principal components analysis (Figure 17.9) has been the most popular dimensionality reduction technique (PCA). PCA works with an asymmetrical matrix or a symmetric matrix of correlation, and resolution of the props and props of the matrix. It is a sort of algorithm for dimension reduction that is used to minimize redundancy and compress data sets by extracting features. This process uses a linear process to build a new depiction of data that gives a collection of 'main components'. The first key element is the direction that maximizes the set of data variance. While the second primary element similarly finds the greatest variability of the data, this is entirely unrelated to the primary component and gives the first element a direction that is orthogonal, or perpendicular. This procedure is repeated based on the number of dimensions, where the next major component is the most variant direction to the previous components.

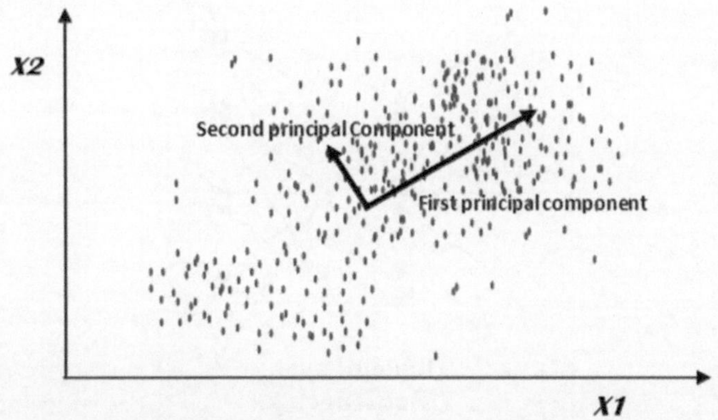

FIGURE 17.9 Principle component analysis.

17.3.2.3 Independent Component Analysis

It was created to blindly separate, distinct sources from their linear mixes [17]. In different applications of hearing signal distinction, medical image analysis, etc., such blindfold separation approaches have been applied. These coefficients have to be independent of one another at ICA. To determine the ICA extension, higher-level statistics are required. All linear correlations can be removed by ICA. The number of distinct elements in the ICA function extraction has always been assumed to be the same as for the set of input data, which means the number of input characteristics can be extracted. ICA function extraction aims to recover the fundamental vectors if the prediction parameters are most linearly separable. In addition, ICA, which is only sensitive to secondary correlations of input, is in a sense better to PCA. ICA has also been utilized as a non-contrast strategy to investigate the characteristics of expression of genes in people with cancer and to identify new genomic samples underneath enormous quantities of micro-array data [18].

17.3.2.4 Autoencoders

After making the outcome value equal to the input value, autoencoders may automatically identify nonlinear features from unlabeled data. An autoencoder (Figure 17.10) builts by connecting the basic neurons in which the result of one layer of the network is the input to another neuron network layer. This network forms by a 'butterfly' topology. Here the number of inputs corresponding to the outputs comprises the hidden units of bottlenecks in the center. 'Encoding' is the stage from the input to the hidden layer. The stage from the hidden units to the output nodes is decoding. This design leads the database to find a compressed display of the information while maintaining the main elements of the data (Figure 17.1). Cancer type identifications using omics data is an application of this approach. Discovering the subtype is a difficult challenge and often involves the integration of many heterogeneous datasets. Because cancer involves various oncogenes and is disturbed by several pathways [19]. Autoencoders is adopted in the recent fusion of three heterogeneous data sets for subtype detection of liver disease.

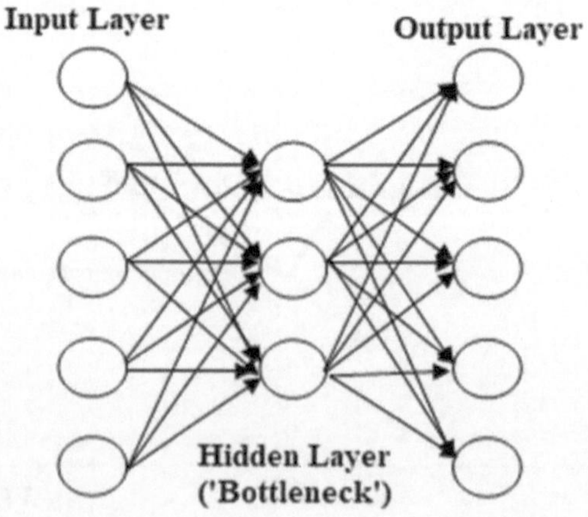

FIGURE 17.10 Simple autoencoder structure.

17.3.2.5 Singular Value Decomposition

It is a way of transforming the image data into three USV matrices. SVD is yet another way for reducing the dimension of matrix A into three independent variables matrices. $A=USV^T$, where U and V are orthogonal matrices, is termed as SVD by equation. S is a diagonal matrix. S values are a singular matrix of A values, which can be used to represent images [20]. The use of a single restructuring value enables us to describe an image with only a reduced collection of values. It can retain the greatest elements of the picture named SV. These singular values are diagonally arranged and have values bigger than zero. Even in matrix S, all those other elements are zero. This suggests that the first SVs are the key elements of the picture. It can be used to detect various MRI brain images. To categorize the MR brain images first the new image is loaded. Next, the SV value is calculated for the systems. Now the values are compared with the standard New V with baseline. The brain MRI is abnormal if there is a difference in the threshold value. The brain MRI also calculates the differences in the brain value, if this value is not the tumor.

17.3.3 Reinforcement Learning (RL)

This strategy doesn't tell the researcher the steps to be taken, but rather which acts give a greater reward after trying them. Trial and error search and backpropagation are the most distinctive elements of enhancement. ML is utilized to solve numerous complex tasks that are generally regarded as fairly cognitive in reinforcement learning. RL is a training procedure that uses a positive or negative hint or indication. The successful adoption of the RL approach (Figure 17.11) had led to an enormous transformation in the healthcare setting and had provided an opportunity to streamline and strengthen the work of medical specialists. This RL was subsequently utilized to determine the suitable local threshold and structured element values and also to separate the ultrasound pictures of the prostate.

17.4 APPLICATION OF ML IN ONCOLOGY

For the early and accurate prediction of cancer in patients, more and more precise algorithms were constructed by eminent researchers based on ML and qualitative

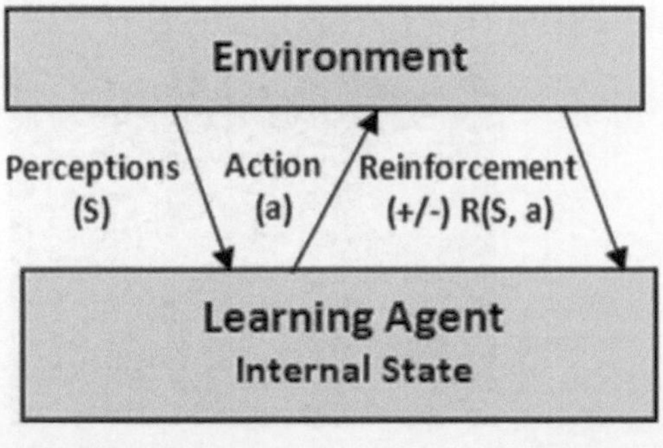

FIGURE 17.11 Reinforcement learning.

imaging platforms. ML-based methods are developed from a variety of unstructured and structured data sources. This approach consolidates the previous decision with that of the current decision. It assists the physician as a highly efficient practitioner who has thorough knowledge in oncology and helps them to take flawless decisions to treat cancer patients. This raise in role ranges from diagnostic computer-aided identification to decision-making, helping to greatly minimize strain and burnout due to misinterpretation and human failure.

17.4.1 Brain Oncology

Progress in ML imagery capacity has strengthened brain cancer's forecasting capability. For the brain and other major essential organs, solutions of individualized physiological models are accessible in medicine [21,22]. Amin and his co-worker have suggested a new way to separate and classify brain tumors [23]. Different causes of SVM classification are utilized to categorize the multiple stages of Carcinogenic or Non-cancerous images after segregating area of interest (ROI), comprising brightness, contour, and texture. Based on AUC (Area Under Curve) and ACC (accurate) measurement performance, the suggested technique was cross-validated by three different data sources. The results show the effectiveness of the technique proposed (Figure 17.12).

In another report, Deepak et al., [24] concentrated on the classifications of different brain cancers, primary tumor, malignant tumors, and pituitary. The suggested model employed a preexisting GoogleNet with changes at the frequency maximum for various sorts of tumor categorization. The GoogleNet deep neural network based on CNN achieves an increase in the precision of 92.25% which also improved the multiclass SVM to 97.82%. A supervised technique to identify brain malformation in MRI was present in three main steps. The first objective is a formulation of the CNN model. The second is to divide the image set by the k-mean algorithm. The third is the classification of brain components as normal or abnormal classes as per a developed CNN model [25]. A deep-learning model is adopted by Ren and his co-workers [26]. The author constructs a histogram equalization for the relevant data in earlier studies.

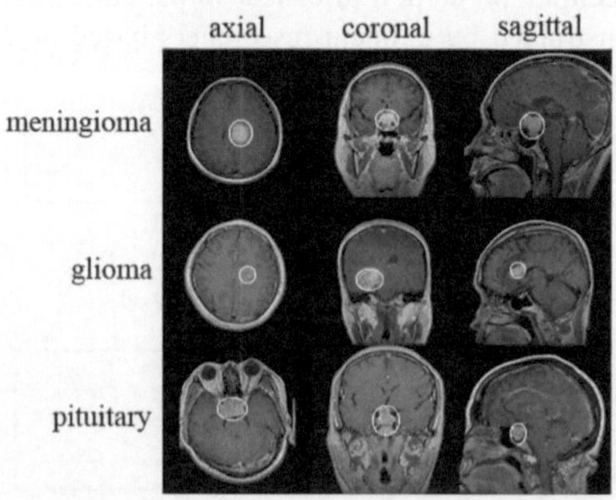

FIGURE 17.12 Different stages of brain tumor output for axial, coronal, and sagittal plane.

The hybrid approach was adopted by combining Weighed fuzzy kernel clustering (WKFCOM) and the Fuzzy Cmean kernel method (KFRCOM). The research showed that with 2,36% lower error rates, WKFCOM performs better than KFCOM. A novel method using Template-based K-mean clustering, as opposed to C-mean algorithms from FUZZY [27]. This procedure divides the MRI pictures into three separate clusters: White Matter, Gray Matter, and brain fluid. The technology claims that the Fuzzy C-mean method is quantitatively and qualitatively better.

17.4.2 Skin Oncology

Machine-assisted methods that use dermoscopic pictures have been provided to outperform dermatologists in making clinical decisions and detecting highly suspicious situations [28]. Class I used medical procedures to autonomously extract the relevant medical traits such as symmetry, multiple hues, and abnormal differential structures. Artificial intelligence is used exclusively in Class II to recognize data patterns in texture and color data [29]. The ABCD rule and a three-point checklist were utilized to create ML programs for extracting the features in the majority of the work (Figure 17.13). Paniagua et al. [30] took a dermoscopy image as an input and suggested a methodology that consisted of four modules: image preprocessing, lesion segmentation, ABCD extraction and classification from a lesion, and SVM classification.

On a collection of 129 Dermoscopy images, test results demonstrated that perhaps the approach has an efficiency of 90.83%, a sensitivity of 95.26%, and a specificity of 83.39%. Ramya et al. [31] employed an adaptive histogram equalization approach with a Wiener filter in yet another research. They employed GLCM for extracting features and SVM as a tumor image predictor, and they achieved a sensitivity of 90%, precision of 95%, and specificity of 85%. For skin cancer diagnosis and detection, Premaladha and Ravichandran [32] presented the Median filter and Limited Adaptive Histogram Equalization approaches. Standardized Otsu's Segmentation, a unique technique that decreased the changeable lighting issue for segmentation, was utilized to separate skin lesions. Aima and Sharma [33] used CNN to treat acute melanoma

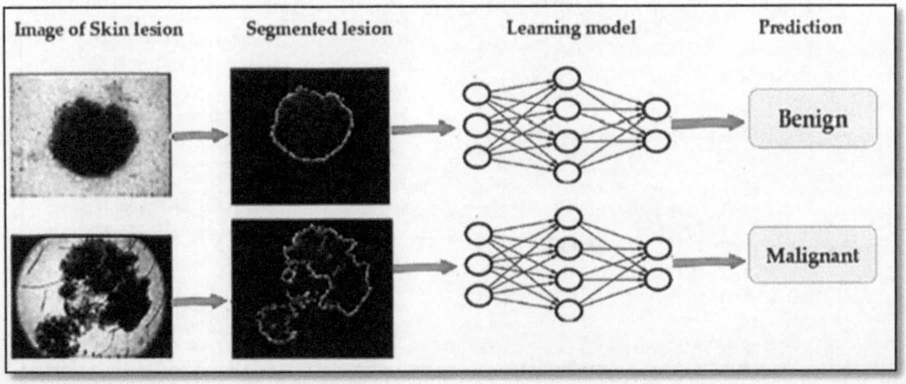

FIGURE 17.13 Skin melanoma prediction output.

skin cancer in 514 dermoscopic pictures from the ISIC dataset. They had a 74.76% accuracy and a 57.56% validation loss. Similarly, Fan X et al. [34] developed a CNN model and used a mobile phone to pretrained 10,115 photos of melanoma for the implementation method. With 75.28% model accuracy, their strategy reduced latency, saved electricity, and boosted privacy. Saba et al., [35] used a deep convolutional neural network to develop an automated method for skin lesion identification and recognition. An entropy technique was used to select discriminative information. They double-checked their work upon on PH2 and ISIC 2017 datasets, claiming that their approach outperformed previous methods by 98.42% on the PH2 dataset, 95.10% on the ISBI dataset, and 94.89% on the ISBI 2017 dataset.

17.4.3 Breast Cancer Prognosis Prediction

Deep learning-trained medical images can boost malignancy restaging accuracy even further. By effectively identifying data instances into important categories depending on tumor intensity, integrating distinct information types and a Deep Neurol Network (DNN) learning approach can provide a successful foundation for breast cancer research (Figure 17.14). Sun et al. [36] developed a multifunctional DNN for breast cancer prognostic prediction using high-dimensional data. The design of the approach's architecture, as well as the merging of multi-dimensional data, are both innovative aspects of their system. Jhajharia et al. [37] used principal component analysis (PCA) to train ANNs to discover patterns and relationships of data for categorization of new instances by preprocessing the data and obtaining attributes in its most relevant manner. Ching et al. [38] propose Cox-nnet, a new ANN-based technology for predicting patient diagnoses utilizing high-throughput transcriptomics data. By examining properties represented in Coxnnet's hidden state nodes, Cox-nnet exposes substantially deeper biological evidence at both the

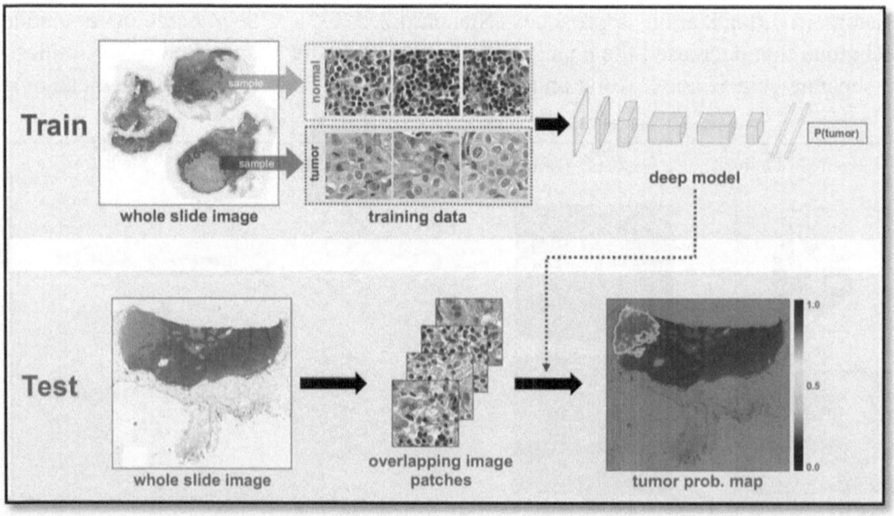

FIGURE 17.14 Brest cancer sample output.

pathway and gene layers. For optimizing paclitaxel therapy in clinical practice, Bomane et al. [39] used three classifier variables that were separately linked to the cytotoxic-drug sensitivities and mortality of patients with breast cancer.

In another study, the researcher used ANNs to perform a survival comparison between two separate breast cancer samples with nuclear morphometric characteristics in each [40]. The findings revealed that ANNs can accurately estimate recurrence probability and distinguish between patients who have a favorable and bad prognosis. Delen et al. [41] develop a forecasting framework based on ANN and decision tree (DT) and a logistic regression approach, employing over 150,000 examples. They confirmed that the DT is the best estimator with 93.68% accuracy. Followed by Autoencoders has 91.28% accurateness and LR classification methods with the lowest precision on the validation data set (89.24%). Sepehri et al. [42] examined two ML processes for constructing prognostic models in women with breast cancer using medical and 18F-FDG PET/CT radiomics data. The findings revealed that the proposed system has significant predictive value in predicting the progression of the illness and death.

17.4.4 ML in Lung Oncology

ML gains attraction in speeding up the development of pattern detection and image processing techniques. In particular for lung cancer recognition and prevention, which is attracting more attention [43]. Chabat et al. [44] developed a multidimensional local texture vector for surface analysis information that includes empirical values of Computer Tomography signal attenuate dispersion, procurement variables, and co-occurrence identifiers. An automated Bayesian identifier is adopted to separate pieces of information. Using five different scale metrics derived from co-occurrence matrix accuracy, entropy, contrast, homogeneity, and energy dimension of both feature extraction was reduced and it is given in Figure 17.15. Zhi-Hua et al. [45] introduced Neuronal Ensemble-based Diagnosis (NED), which

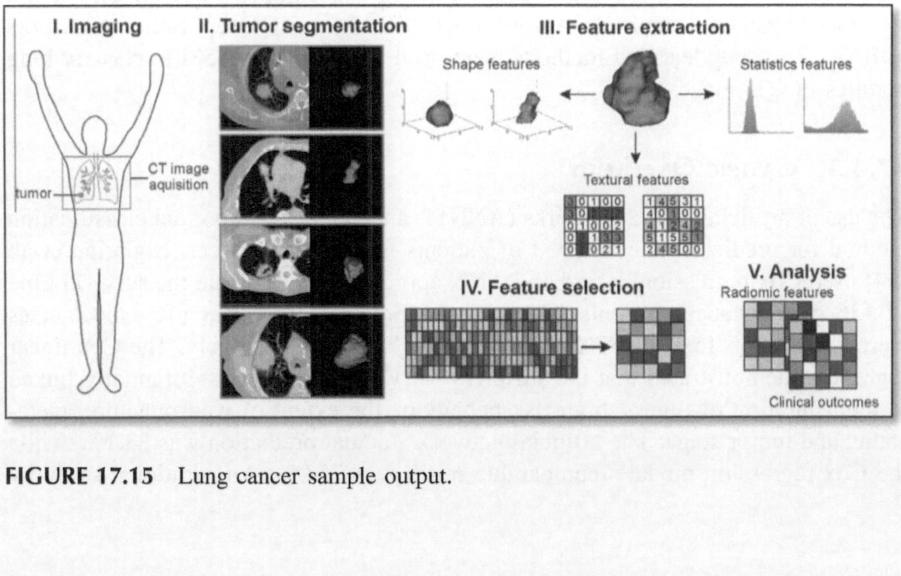

FIGURE 17.15 Lung cancer sample output.

used a convolutional neural network outfit to distinguish pulmonary cancerous cells when it comes to recognizing cancer cells, this method is extremely accurate.

Roy and his co-workers [46] developed a system that uses a fuzzy reasoning technique to detect lung cancer nodules. For image contrast improvement, this technique involves grey conversion. Adaptive threshold models are used to divide the resulting image. To improve classification performance, variables like; area, entropy, mean, correlation, minor axis length, and main axis length are extracted. It gives the system's overall accuracy at 94.16%. The method's drawback is that it does not identify malignancy as cancerous, which would be the suggested model's successful development. Sangamithraa and his co-worker [47] used the Fuzzy K-Means clustering method to segment the lung. Also, a statistical Gray Level Co-occurrence Matrix (GLCM) is used to take out attributes. The Backpropagation Neural Network (BPN) is a supervised neural net used for categorization. The author pre-processed CT images with median and Wiener filters to remove undesirable artifacts. The Fuzzy K - nearest neighbor segmented image is then used to extract the features using entropy, contrast, correlation, homogeneous, and area. With an accuracy of 90.79%, the result tells whether the CT image is affected by cancer or not. Makaju et al. [48] used watershed segmentation to separate the image representation. The image with tumor nodules is a highlight in the segmentation findings. Afterward, attributes for the segmented malignancy nodules were recovered utilizing various GLCM parameters. Finally, an SVM was used to classify cancer nodules. To detect lung cancer Gopi Kasinathan et al. [49] use Convolution Neural Network (CNN) classifier. The accuracy was 97%, the sensitivity was 89%, and the specificity was 91%. Wafaa Alakwaa et al. [50] use a threshold strategy for image identification. The computed tomography images are classified into positive and negative for lung cancer using 3D CNN. This yielded an accuracy rate of 86.6%. To improve the classification performance, Manickavasagam and Selvam [51] used the Gaussian filter. Watershed separation is adopted for segmentation. The accuracy of the results is 97.89%, which is higher than that of the neuro-fuzzy controller and the neighborhood increasing approach. For lung cancer classification, Sun et al. [52] employed three deep learning algorithms: Convolution Neural Network, Stacked Denoising Autoencoder (SDAE), and Deep Belief Networks (DBNs). The deep learning methods were used by Song et al. [53] to classify lung nodules in CT images.

17.4.5 Gastric Oncology

The use of artificial neural networks (ANN) is an even more important classification method for predicting the survival of patients with gastric cancer. Biglarian et al. [54] used Cox regression hazard and ANN approaches to estimate the survival time of 436 gastric cancer patients. The patients' predicted five-year life expectancies were 77.98%, 53.15%, 40.82%, 32.05%, and 17.49%, respectively. The Cox linear regression demonstrated that the sufferers' survival rates were substantially linked to their duration of illness, high-risk behaviors, the extent of wall puncture, metastatic, and tumor stage. The artificial network's actual prediction was 83.1%, while the Cox regression model's comparable result was 75.0%. An additional study by

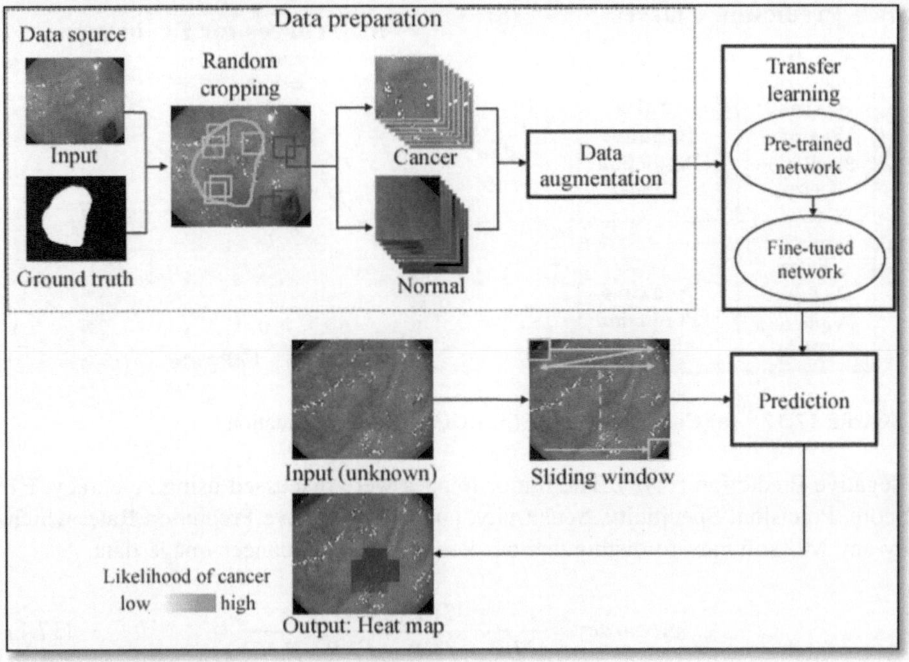

FIGURE 17.16 Gastric cancer sample output.

Karhade et al. [55] found that perhaps the ANN model is a much more strong method for investigating important prognostic indicators for gastric cancer patients, that are suggested for identifying possible risks. Maroufizadeh et al. [56,57] demonstrated that the artificial neural network is much more effective than the traditional inferential statistics (Weibull regression model) in detecting significant variables for stomach cancer patients [58,59]. In comparison to the Kaplan–Meier and Cox multivariable logistic regression models, we evaluated the use of machine learning in survival analysis (Figure 17.16).

17.5 DISCUSSION

17.5.1 ML Program Performance Analysis

The confusion matrix and the region operating characteristic (ROC) curve have traditionally been used to evaluate the therapeutic efficacy of classification models using the ML approach. Figure 17.17(a), explains the confusion matrix's basic structure and ROC curve.

If the ML model accurately diagnoses a malignancy appearance, it would be labeled as True Positive Prediction (TPP). If it appropriately predicts a non-cancerous picture, it will be tagged as True Negative Prediction (TNP). If the program incorrectly predicts a non-cancerous image as malignancies, it would be labeled as False Positive Prediction (FPP) and vise - versa and marked as False

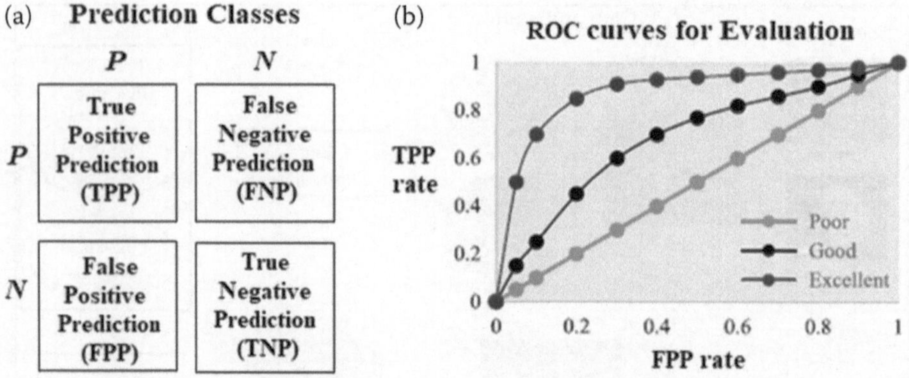

FIGURE 17.17 (a) Confusion matrix (b) ROC curve for evaluation.

Negative Prediction (FNP). The tumor images were discussed using Accuracy, F1 Score, Precision, Specificity, Sensitivity, and False Positive Prediction Rate, which by any ML software to distinguish cancerous from non-cancer image data.

$$Accuracy = \frac{TPP + TNP}{TPP + TNP + FPP + FNP} \tag{17.1}$$

$$False\ positive\ prediction\ rate = \frac{FPP}{FPP + TNP} \tag{17.2}$$

$$Precision = \frac{TPP}{TPP + FPP} \tag{17.3}$$

$$F1\ score = \frac{2_{*}TPP}{2_{*}TPP + FNP + FPP} \tag{17.4}$$

$$Sensitivity = \frac{TPP}{TPP + FNP} \tag{17.5}$$

$$Specificity = \frac{TNP}{TNP + FPP} \tag{17.6}$$

The positive result predicting rate is plotted against the misdiagnosis predicting the rate at varying levels of intensity to construct a ROC [60,61], which is an underlying and potential core for diagnostic test examination. The area under the Curve (AUC) is another method for determining a classifier's trustworthiness. Figure 17.17(b) exemplifies the predictive efficiency of the classifiers; the classifier that formed the red ROC curve has a greater forecasting ability than that of the other classification models that derived the blue and black ROC curves.

17.5.2 Pros and Cons of ML Algorithm

We have listed the various benefits and drawbacks of supervised machine learning algorithms based on their decision-making capabilities. Many machine learning applications employ Artificial Neural Networks because they can discover complicated nonlinear correlations between dependent and independent variables, need less traditional test modeling, and are excellent for both regression and classification issues. High-performing ANN also has some drawbacks, such as being a 'black box' implementation wherein the user does not have direct exposure to the correct supervisory process. Being algorithmically exclusive to prepare the set-up for a complicated categorization task and requiring pre-processing of the independent factors. The Naive Bayes classifier is a widely used framework, with features such as being simple and useful for huge datasets. Being applicable both in single and multiple class categorization issues. It only requires a small quantity of grounding image database for this. It also can create probabilistic estimates and work with both discrete and continuous picture data. The constrain includes the requirement that data classification will be mutually exclusive. However, the fact that classification accuracy is largely dependent on the parameters may provide negative outcomes. The Decision Tree program has several benefits, including being simple to grasp and analyze the outcome report, being simple to utilize different data in various types such as numerical, conventional, and categorical, and being able to be examined using statistical analysis. This procedure can't split if a non-leaf single node characteristic or parameter value is missing, and it requires jointly exclusive classes. When compared with DT, the Random forest approach will also have advantages and disadvantages. The advantages are, it has a lower probability of variance, overfitting of the training phase, it grows well for big picture databases, and can provide predictions of which variables or characteristics are significant in categorization. The downsides are it is highly complicated and computationally intensive, then it requires the definition of a large number of the classification algorithm, that it is easy to overfit, and that it favors variables that could take a while a large number of possible options when calculating the importance of a variable. The following are some of the benefits of the K-nearest neighbor (KNN) method. This program can handle noisy examples with enough feature values for categorization or predictive applications [62–66]. KNN is a basic technique that can quickly classify instances. The disadvantages are, as the number of qualities grows, it becomes computationally intensive. Here the KNN features are taken into account, which can lead to poor categorization. We have discovered the merits of logistic regression (LR). It is a simple process that can be done quickly as well as, it is possible to update models. Quickly and it is not based on any considerations about the underlying of independent variables (s). The disadvantages are, LR does not provide acceptable accuracy when inputs have complex associations. It does not take into account the two variables have a linear connection. The main aspects of LR are subject to overconfidence, and thus generic LR is dichotomous. Similarly, the Support vector machine, SVM, offers certain advantages. It is more robust than other programs in handling multiple features. There's less chance of overfitting, and it's good at identifying unstructured material like texts and photographs. This program also has some drawbacks, such as being computationally intensive for huge datasets, performing poorly when the data contains noise. As a result, the relevance and influence of parameters in the resulting model are hard to grasp, and this basic SVM can only categorize two groups until otherwise enhanced.

17.5.3 ML in Cancer Staging

The most common method for cancer staging is to use a supervised classification method to forecast lifespan and then examine the predictors to determine staging criteria [67]. Unsupervised classification, on the other hand, is beneficial in distinguishing the normal gene from the abnormal one in the cancer types. Regarding this, a clustering procedure on the lung and breast cancer image sets was performed [68]. It confirms that the resulting groupings were clinically distinct, although the algorithm does not explicitly evaluate survival. Given the noise and complexity of assessing survival, it can be useful to derive subgroups without a stated outcome. Clustering is a new approach to malignancy identification that divides sufferers into clinical categories more broadly. Unsupervised learning has been used to discover cancer gene signatures. This has been used by experts to learn about different cancer characteristics. The discovery of such cohorts opens the door to a better knowledge of disease and a more customized strategy to treatment options.

17.5.4 Predicting and Evaluating Treatment Response

Machine learning algorithms will give an accurate result based on evidence-based insight in the image data set of any patient. The decision taken in selecting an appropriate treatment and monitoring methods for a particular patient will be decided by the ML program. The personalized drug reaction to alternative medicine and their potential side effect will decide the above decision. Currently, more databases on genetic profiles for human cells are added to the online data server. This new data will help the researcher to evaluate the disease correctly. For colorectal oncology studies, the cancer gene sequence data will be more useful. It is also used for colorectal tissue, Pancreatitis cancer, leucovorin, fluorouracil, and oxaliplatin tissue infection. Most of the ML procedures are designed to get an accurate decision for the patient, who undergoes radiation therapy or chemotherapy. For non–small-cell lung cancer and breast cancer, the ML program radiomics, and a combination of clinical and imaging data have been used, respectively [69]. Not limiting to the advanced applications of ML in cancer treatment, it is surprising that the ML programs are used to predict the possible side-effects of the medicine given to cancer patients [70]. Because of the MLS superiority in decision and evaluation making the classical two-dimension decision-making procedure –RECIST has been ruled out. The modern ML predicts that the classical decision given by the RECIST program on the outcome changes track for NSCLE patients is not accurate. For instance, ML can do the same performance in NSCLC patients like diagnostic imaging. Recently brain images from MRI and CT scans are also evaluated with ML procedure rather than RECIST one.

17.6 CONCLUSION

Image processing techniques can provide superior, extremely precise healthcare services for people with cancer. Also, it discloses fundamental psychological abnormalities with the help of different machine learning techniques. Although the application of ML classification algorithms in cancer is beneficial, there are still numerous obstacles to overcome before they can fully fulfill their potential in everyday clinical oncology practice. Most importantly, they have the potential to enhance patient outcomes by allowing for early identification. The purpose of this chapter is to provide additional insight into the ML-based algorithms that are developed for, and perhaps to comprehend the performance of various strategies for machine learning for decision making and stage prediction in oncology. We examined more numbers of the machine learning process with supervised methodologies that appeared in different literature surveys from 1950 to 2021. We discovered that 16.38% of the publications used upwards of one supervised machine learning model for disease diagnosis. Only 55.6% of the remaining 83.79% of articles employed any one of the supervised machine learning algorithms described here, with ANN (33.22%) and Naive Bayes (29.51%) being the most popular. The remaining 28.18% of articles used unsupervised, semi-supervised, or non-machine learning data mining methods.

We saw a huge increase in machine learning (ML) applications in oncology, including disease diagnostic prediction, treatment response prediction, process automation, and decision support automation. Though the ML can provide a more precise decision on location, depth, and stages, each method has its own set of advantages and disadvantages. The availability of high-quality input data and the translation technique used to extract clinical features are both critical factors in any ML's conclusion. More digital and multimodal diagnostic imaging data sets derived from MRI, CT, dermoscopy, mammography, biopsy, X-ray, and test models on a per-patient basis are required to overcome this. Also, real-time approaches can help us better understand cancer and how it affects people, owing to the quantity of clinical data available. The machine learning procedure is adopted to determine the presence of carcinoma in the breast. It is done on mammography and breast density analysis, lung cancer using CT scans, cancer vulnerability using genetic data, and pancreas carcinoma susceptibility using EMR data within an elevated sample. The way patients receive treatments and clinicians make clinical decisions is predicted to change as a result of ML. Diagnostics will be faster, less expensive, and more precise than ever before. Cancer screening policy and practice will be influenced by this early warning system. As machine learning becomes more widely used in oncology research, more medical pictures will become available, allowing researchers to develop more robust and advanced algorithms.

REFERENCES

[1] Chellappa R., Theodoridis S., Schaik, A. V. 'Advances in machine learning and deep neural networks'. *Proceedings of the IEEE*. 2021; 109(5):607–611.

[2] Bera K., Schalper K. A., Rimm D. L., et al. 'Artificial intelligence in digital pathology — new tools for diagnosis and precision oncology'. *Nature Reviews-Clinical Oncology*. 2019; 16(11):703–715.

[3] Malebary S. J., Khan, Y. D. 'Evaluating machine learning methodologies for identification of cancer driver genes'. *Scientific Report.* 2021;11:12281.

[4] Rauschert S., Raubenheimer K., Melton P. E., Huang, R. C. 'Machine learning and clinical epigenetics: A review of challenges for diagnosis and classification'. *Clinical Epigenetics*. 2020; 12(51):1–11.

[5] Tseng H.-H., Wei L., Cui S., Luo., Ten Haken R. K., El Naqa I., 'Machine learning and imaging informatics in oncology'. *Oncology and Informatics*, Published online: November 23, 2018, 10.1159/000493575.

[6] McCarthy J. J., McLeod H. L., Ginsburg, G. S. 'Genomic medicine: A decade of successes, challenges, and opportunities'. *Science Translational Medicine*. 2013; 5 (189):1–17.

[7] Uddin S., Khan A., Hossain M. E., Moni, M. A. 'Comparing different supervised machine learning algorithms for disease prediction'. *BMC Medical Informatics and Decision Making*. 2019; 19(281):1–16.

[8] Joachims, T. 'Making large-scale SVM learning practical'. Technische Universität Dortmund, Sonderforschungsbereich 475: *Komplexitätsreduktion in multivariaten Datenstrukturen*. 1998; 28.

[9] Cruz J. A., Wishart, D. S. 'Applications of machine learning in cancer prediction and prognosis'. *Cancer Informatics*. 2006; 2:59–77.

[10] Breiman, L. 'Random forests'. *Machine Learning*. 2001; 45(1):5–32.

[11] Lindley, D. V. 'Fiducial distributions and Bayes' theorem *Journal of the Royal Statistical Society: Series B (Methodological)*. 1958; 1:102–107.

[12] Cover T. M., Hart, P. E. 'Nearest neighbor pattern classification'. *IEEE Transactions on Information Theory*. 1967; 13(1):21–27.

[13] Ciompi F., De Hoop, B. et al. 'Automatic classification of pulmonary peri-fissural nodules in computed tomography using an ensemble of 2D views and a convolutional neural network out-of-the-box'. *Medical Image Analysis*. 2015; 26:195–202.

[14] Haraty R. A., Dimishkieh M., Masud, M. 'An enhanced k-Means clustering algorithm for pattern discovery in healthcare data'. *International Journal of Distributed Sensor Networks*. 2015; 11(6):615740.

[15] Arunkumar, N. et al. 'K-Means clustering and neural network for object detecting and identifying abnormality of brain tumor'. *Soft Computing*. 2019; 23:9083–9096.

[16] Chaurasia V., Pal, S. 'Applications of machine learning techniques to predict diagnostic breast cancer'. *SN Computer Science*. 2020; 1(5):1–11.

[17] Zheng C. H., Chen Y., Li, X. X. 'Tumor classification based on independent component analysis'. *International Journal of Pattern Recognition and Artificial Intelligence*. 2006; 20(2):297–310.

[18] Wei K., Vanderburg C. R., Gunshin H., Rogers J. T., Huang, X. 'A review of independent component analysis application to microarray gene expression data'. *BioTechniques*. 2008; 45(5):501–520.

[19] Franco, E. F. et al. 'Performance comparison of deep learning autoencoders for cancer subtype detection using multi-omics data'. *Cancers*. 2021; 13(9): 2013.

[20] Abbadi N K El., Kadhim, N. E. 'Brain tumor classification based on singular value decomposition'. *International Journal of Advanced Research in Computer and Communication Engineering*. 2016; 5(8):1–5.

[21] Sharma A., Rani, R. 'A systematic review of applications of machine learning in cancer prediction and diagnosis'. *Archives of Computational Methods in Engineering*. 2021; 28:4875–4896.

[22] Tiwari A., Srivastava S., Pant, M. 'Brain tumor segmentation and classification from magnetic resonance images: Review of selected methods from 2014 to 2019'. *Pattern Recognition Letters*. 2019; 131:244–260.

[23] Amin J., Sharif M., Yasmin M., Fernandes, S. L. 'A distinctive approach in brain tumor detection and classification using MRI'. *Pattern Recognition Letters*. 2017; 139:1–10.
[24] Deepak S., Ameer, P.M. 'Brain tumor classification using deep CNN features via transfer learning'. *Computers in Biology and Medicine*. 2019; 111:103345.
[25] Hashemzehia R., Mahdavi S. J. S., Kheirabadi M., Kamel, S. R. 'Detection of brain tumors from MRI images base on deep learning using hybrid model CNN and NADE'. *Biocybernetics and Biomedical Engineering*. 2020; 40(3):1225–1232.
[26] Ren T., Wang H., Feng H., Xu C., Liu G., Ding, P. 'Study on the improved fuzzy clustering algorithm and its application in brain image segmentation'. *Applied Soft Computing*. 2019; 81(11):105503.
[27] Alam, Md S. et al. 'Automatic human brain tumor detection in MRI Image using template-based K Means and improved fuzzy C means clustering algorithm'. *Big Data and Cognitive Computing*. 2019; 3(2):1–18.
[28] Huang S., Yang J., Fong S., Zhao, Q. 'Artificial intelligence in cancer diagnosis and prognosis: Opportunities and challenges'. *Cancer letters*. 2020; 471:61–71.
[29] Saba, T. 'Recent advancement in cancer detection using machine learning: Systematic survey of decades, comparisons and challenges'. *Journal of Infection and Public Health*. 2020; 13(9):1274–1289.
[30] Paniagua, L. R. B. et al. 'Computerized medical diagnosis of melanocytic lesions based on the ABCD approach'. *CLEI Electronic Journal*. 2016; 19(2):1–6.
[31] Ramya V., Navarajan J., Prathipa R., Kumar, L. A. 'Detection of melanoma skin-cancer using digital camera images'. *ARPN Journal of Engineering and Applied Sciences*. 2015; 10:3082–3085.
[32] Premaladha J., Ravichandran, K. 'Novel approaches for diagnosing melanoma skin lesions through supervised and deep learning algorithms'. *Journal of Medical Systems*. 2016; 40:96.
[33] Aima A., Sharma, A. K. 'Predictive approach for melanoma skin cancer detection using CNN'. *SSRN Electronic Journal*. 2019: 28-29:546.
[34] Fan, X. et al. 'Effect of image noise on the classification of skin lesions using deep convolutional neural networks'. *Tsinghua Science and Technology*. 2020; 25(3):425–434.
[35] Saba T., Khan M. A., Rehman, A. et al. 'Region extraction and classification of skin cancer: A heterogeneous framework of deep CNN features fusion and reduction'. *Journal of Medical Systems*. 2019; 43:289.
[36] Sun D., Wang M., Li, A. 'A multimodal deep neural network for human breast cancer prognosis prediction by integrating multi-dimensional data'. *IEEE/ACM Transactions on Computational Biology and Bioinformatics*. 2019; 16(3):841–850.
[37] Guptaa P., Garg, S. 'Breast cancer prediction using varying parameters of machine learning models'. *Procedia Computer Science*. 2020; 171:593–601.
[38] Ching T., Zhu X., Garmire, L. X. 'Cox-nnet: An artificial neural network method for prognosis prediction of high-throughput omics data'. *PLOS Computational Biology*. 2018; 14:e1006076.
[39] Bomane A., Goncalves A., Ballester, P. J. 'Paclitaxel response can be predicted with interpretable multi-variate classifiers exploiting DNA-methylation and miRNA data'. *Frontiers in Genetics*. 2019; 10:1041.
[40] Park K., Ali A., Kim D., An Y., Kim M., Shin, H. 'Robust predictive model for evaluating breast cancer survivability'. *Engineering Applications of Artificial Intelligence*. 2013; 26:2194–2205.
[41] Delen D., Walker G., Kadam, A. 'Predicting breast cancer survivability: A comparison of three data mining methods'. *Artificial Intelligence in Medicine*. 2005; 34:113–127.

[42] Sepehri S., Upadhaya T., Desseroit M.-C., Visvikis D., Le Rest C. C., Hatt, M. 'Comparison of machine learning algorithms for building prognostic models in nonsmall cell lung cancer using clinical and radiomics features from 18F-FDG PET/CT images'. *Journal of Nuclear Medicine*. 2018; 59(S1):328.
[43] Asuntha A., Srinivasan, A. 'Deep learning for lung cancer detection and classification'. *Multimedia Tools and Applications*. 2020; 79:7731–7762.
[44] Chabat F., Yang G.-Z., Hansell, D. M. 'Obstructive lung diseases: Texture classification for differentiation at CT1'. *Radiology*. 2003; 228(3):871–877.
[45] Zhou Z.-H., Jiang Y., Yang Y.-B., Chen, S.-F. 'Lung cancer cell identification based on artificial neural network ensembles'. *Elsevier Artificial Intelligence in Medicine*. 2002; 24: 25–36.
[46] Sujitha R., Seenivasagam, V. 'Classification of lung cancer stages with machine learning over big data healthcare framework'. *Journal of Ambient Intelligence and Humanized Computing volume*. 2021; 12:5639–5649.
[47] Singh G. A. P., Gupta, P. K. 'Performance analysis of various machine learning based approaches for detection and classification of lung cancer in humans'. *Neural Computing and Applications*. 2019; 31:6863–6877.
[48] Makaju S., Prasad A. A., Elchouemi, S. 'Lung cancer detection using CT scan images'. *Elsevier, Procedia Computer Science*. 2018; 125:107–114.
[49] Kasinathan, G. et al. 'Automated 3-D lung tumor detection and classification by an active contour model and CNN classifier'. *Expert Systems With Applications*. 2019; 134:112–119.
[50] Alakwaa W., Nassef M., Badr, A. 'Lung Cancer detection and classification with 3D convolutional neural network (3D-CNN)'. *International Journal of Advanced Computer Science and Applications*. 2017; 8(8):409–417.
[51] Manickavasagam R., Selvan, S. 'Automatic detection and classification of lung nodules in CT image using optimized neuro fuzzy classifier with cuckoo search algorithm'. *Journal of Medical Systems*. 2019; 43:77.
[52] Sun W., Zheng B., Qian, W. 'computer aided lung cancer diagnosis with deep learning algorithms' Proc. SPIE. 2016; 9785:1–8.
[53] Song Q. Z., Zhao L., Luo X. K., Dou, X. C. 'Using deep learning for classification of lung nodules on computed tomography images'. *Journal of Healthcare Engineering*. 2017:1–7.
[54] Biglarian, H. E. et al., 'Application of artificial neural network in predicting the survival rate of gastric cancer patients'. *Iranian Journal of Public Health*. 2011; 40(2):80–86.
[55] Karhade A. V., Thio Q., Ogink P., Kim J., Lozano-Calderon S., Raskin K., Schwab, J. H. 'Development of machine learning algorithms for prediction of 5-year spinal chordoma survival'. *World Neurosurgery*. 2018; 119:e842–e847.
[56] Ha E. J., Baek J. H., Na, D. G. 'Deep convolutional neural network models for the diagnosis of thyroid cancer'. *The Lancet Oncology*. 2019; 20:193–201.
[57] Mori Y., Berzin T. M., Kudo, S. E. 'Artificial intelligence for early gastric cancer: early promise and the path ahead'. *Gastrointestinal Endoscopy*. 2019; 89:816–817.
[58] Ichimasa, K. et al. 'Artificial intelligence may help in predicting the need for additional surgery after endoscopic resection of T1 colorectal cancer'. *Endoscopy*. 2018; 50:230–240.
[59] Zhu Y., Wang, Q. C., et al. 'Application of convolutional neural network in the diagnosis of the invasion depth of gastric cancer based on conventional endoscopy'. *Gastrointestinal Endoscopy*. 2019; 89:806–815.
[60] Fawcett, T. 'An introduction to ROC analysis'. *Pattern Recognition Letters*. 2006; 27(8):861–874.

[61] Bertsimas D., Wiberg, H. 'Machine learning in oncology: Methods, applications, and challenges'. *JCO Clinical Cancer Informatics*. 2020; 4:885–894.
[62] Raj, E. F. I., Balaji, M. 'Analysis and classification of faults in switched reluctance motors using deep learning neural networks'. *Arabian Journal for Science and Engineering*. 2021; 46(2):1313–1332.
[63] Ch, G., Jana, S., Majji, S., Kuncha, P. E. F. I. R., Tigadi, A. 'Diagnosis of COVID-19 using 3D CT scans and vaccination for COVID-19'. *World Journal of Engineering*. 2021. 10.1108/wje-03-2021-0161.
[64] Gampala, V., Sunil Kumar, M., Sushama, C., Fantin Irudaya Raj, E. 'Deep learning based image processing approaches for image deblurring'. *Materials Today: Proceedings*. 2021. 10.1016/j.matpr.2020.11.076.
[65] Agarwal, P., Ch, M. A., Kharate, D. S., Raj, E. F. I., Balamuralitharan, S. 'Parameter estimation of COVID-19 second wave BHRP transmission model by using principle component analysis'. *Annals of the Romanian Society for Cell Biology*. 2021; 25(5):446–457.
[66] Priyadarsini, K., Raj, E. F. I., Begum, A. Y., Shanmugasundaram, V. Comparing DevOps procedures from the context of a systems engineer. 2020. *Materials Today: Proceedings*. 10.1016/j.matpr.2020.09.624.
[67] Niranjana, R., Ravi, A., Vedhapriyavadhana, R., Francy Irudaya Rani, E., Narayanan Prasanth, N. 'Breast cancer detection using deep learning neural network with image processing techniques'. *Solid State Technology*. 2020; 63(5) 2020.
[68] Francy Irudaya Rani, E., Niranjana, R., Abirami, M., Grace Priya, A., Indiranatchiyar, A. 'Brain tumor detection using ANN classifier'. *International Journal of Emerging Technology and Innovative Engineering*. 2019; 5(9):670–678.
[69] Lu W., Fu D., Kong, X., et al. 'FOLFOX treatment response prediction in metastatic or recurrent colorectal cancer patients via machine learning algorithms'. *Cancer Medicine*. 2020; 9:1419–1429.
[70] Bloomingdale P., Mager, D. E. 'Machine learning models for the prediction of chemotherapy-induced peripheral neuropathy'. *Pharmaceutical Research*. 2019; 36:35.

18 Performance Analysis of Deep Convolutional Neural Networks for Diagnosing COVID-19: Data to Deployment

K. Deepti
Assistant Professor, Dept of ECE, Vasavi College of Engineering(A), Osmania University, Hyderabad, India

CONTENTS

18.1 Introduction....361
18.2 Literature Review....363
18.3 The Attributes of the Dataset and Visualizations to Interpret the Data....363
18.4 The Model Formulation to Classify the Data to Diagnose COVID-19....368
18.4.1 InceptionResNetV2....371
18.4.2 ResNet152V2....371
18.4.3 Xception....372
18.4.4 DenseNet201....372
18.5 Loss Function: Categorical Cross Entropy....372
18.6 Evaluation Metrics and Results....376
18.7 Model Deployment....380
18.7.1 Designing the Website....380
18.7.2 An Overview of Deployment....380
18.7.3 Working of Website....383
18.8 Conclusion....384
References....384

18.1 INTRODUCTION

Recent progress in machine learning algorithms that have resulted in better performance can be attributed to the use of convolution layers, which can correctly identify despite variations in the image. Neural Networks are the types of machine

DOI: 10.1201/9781003217497-18

learning algorithms that don't need to be programmed with a clear set of distinct rules describing what to do with the input data. The neural network instead learns from processing many labeled examples that are provided to it during training to learn, what attributes of the input are necessary to provide the correct output [1]. Once a sufficient number of examples have been processed, the neural network can initiate to process new, unobserved inputs and successfully return precise results. Convolutional Neural Network (CNN) is a feature-based machine learning algorithm that is mainly used in classification problems [2]. Since CNN requires minimum pre-processing, it is widely preferred over other classification algorithms. By applying proper filters, spatial and temporal dependencies in the image can be captured which results in an efficient classification. The performance analysis of machine learning algorithms to diagnose COVID-19 is discussed in this chapter.

COVID-19 (Corona Virus Disease 2019) disease declared as a pandemic by WHO has caused millions of deaths and has adversely affected the livelihood of people across the globe. Scientists in the last decade have worked on viruses like SARS (Severe Acute Respiratory Syndrome), MERS (Middle East Respiratory Syndrome), etc. and the world has been able to contain these viruses since the vaccines were prepared and administered to people in a lucid manner without a considerable delay [3]. In the interim, several methods of prediction have been proposed by researchers such as Plasma Therapy but an exact proven alternative solution is not found till date. Even today, people are losing lives due to COVID-19 and the diagnosis cost is also high in the context of country and individuals [4]. Diagnosing COVID-19 against other diseases which have a similar effect on lungs is quite challenging and rigorous procedures are required to reduce the risk for patients unaffected with COVID-19.

Diagnosing COVID-19 against other diseases which have a similar effect on lungs is quite challenging and rigorous procedures are required to reduce the risk for patients unaffected with COVID-19 [5]. One of the critical observations pertaining to this COVID-19 is that it affects the throat of the patient in the initial phases followed by difficulty in breathing. On the other hand, it has been reported in many cases that this disease has no effect in the initial phases [6]. So naive diagnosis is clearly not the solution for screening the infected ones. Besides, allegedly infected patients are required to be in isolation and take adequate medication so that healthy people might not be infected. New strains of the virus have been detected in several countries and have already spread to many countries [7]. Subsequently, there has been a rapid rise in cases in recent days proving that the infection is following a chain process. Fortunately, Lung X-ray images of healthy people and COVID-19 affected patients have been made available for analysis on online repositories like Kaggle and GitHub from March 2020. Hence medical imaging is a promising method of analyzing and diagnosing COVID-19 and can also aid in screening COVID-19 infected patients against those infected by other diseases like Lung Opacity and Viral Pneumonia which have a similar effect on lungs as that of COVID-19 with help of chest X-Ray images.

Having understood the significance of radiography-based diagnosis, the Lung X-ray images of patients infected with COVID-19 are collected. Ground Glass Opacity or Lung Opacity and Viral Pneumonia along with those of healthy patients from Kaggle repository and applied Deep Learning to classify these appropriately. The collected data set is analyzed using a CNN based on VGG16 (Visual Geometry

Group) based architecture for the initial layers of the network adopting the approach of transfer learning.

18.2 LITERATURE REVIEW

Researchers across the world have proposed several frameworks and models to diagnose COVID-19 over the last 12 months. Extensive research is going on determining the role of Artificial Intelligence (AI) and Machine Learning (ML) in healthcare and medicine and challenges in implementing ML models. This section presents the related works which proposed different frameworks and methods for analyzing and diagnosing COVID-19. The advantages and anomalies in each of these methods are also discussed. A frame work named COVID-CAAPS based on capsule networks to detect COVID-19 disease using X-ray images was proposed that have overcome class imbalance using convolution layers and capsules [8]. The model constraint was a smaller number of trainable parameters were considered. A CNN based on ResNet and inception with 6432 chest X-ray images was considered that has given an accuracy of 97.97% in predicting COVID-19 [9]. But the drawback was it was unable to distinguish COVID-19 from other diseases which have a similar effect on lungs of a patient. A Local Binary Pattern (LBP) to find out the characteristics of chest X-ray images is used where in a SVM (Support Vector Machine) technique to diagnose Pneumothorax is adopted [10]. A multi-scale texture segmentation is used to remove the impurities present in the chest X-ray images and segmented the abnormal regions of lungs [11]. A rid boundary with Sobel Edge Detection is used to find the whole abnormal region of the disease in the images. But the drawback was it is difficult to predict that COVID-19 causes Pneumonia in addition to other symptoms. The research is also been continuing to the use of Sieve Neural Network Architecture in diagnosing COVID-19 [12].

18.3 THE ATTRIBUTES OF THE DATASET AND VISUALIZATIONS TO INTERPRET THE DATA

The dataset for training, development and testing the model has been obtained from Kaggle repository which comprises lung X-ray images. All the images are in Portable Network Graphics file format with a resolution of 299*299 pixels of patients infected with COVID-19, Ground Glass Opacity or Lung Opacity, Viral Pneumonia along with those of healthy people. The data set consists of 21170 lung X-ray images out of which 3616 images are of COVID-19, 6012 images are of Ground Glass Opacity, 1345 images are of Viral Pneumonia and 10200 lung X-ray images of healthy people. This dataset is further divided into training, validation and testing sets each consisting of 16500, 3130 and 1540 images respectively so that the training set comprises 80% of the data obtained. It should be noted that no data cleansing is required in this case. As per the bar graph presented in Figure 18.1, healthy and Ground Glass Opacity samples compose 80% of the dataset. So, an interesting challenge for the model is plausible difficulty in identifying COVID-19 and Pneumonia samples.

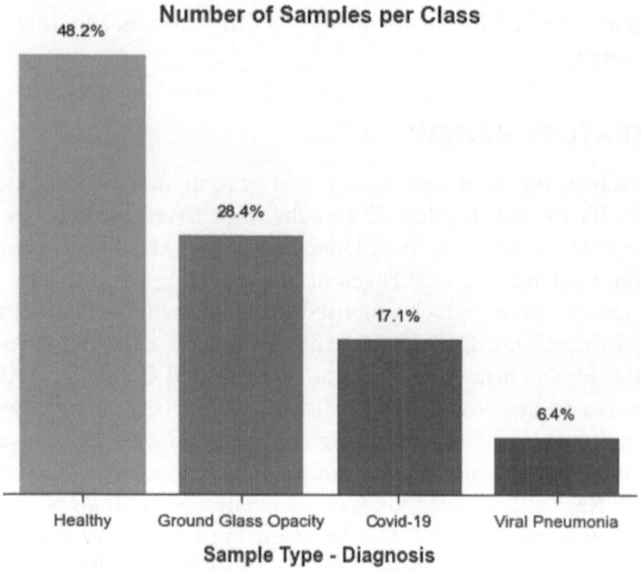

FIGURE 18.1 Percentage of samples in each class of dataset.

To examine the patterns between image color values and their class, it is imperative to plot the distribution of mean and standard deviation of pixel values for each class in the dataset. Figure 18.2. represents the sample random radiography images from each class. Figure 18.3 is a scatter plot that analyses the relationship between the mean value and standard deviation of images in the dataset wherein each class is distinguished by a different color for the corresponding dots. Most of the images occupy the central region of the scatter plot and hence there is not much contrast in their pixel values. Most of the images occupy the central region of the scatter plot and hence there is not much contrast in their pixel values. This sets a right context for leveraging Deep Learning to classify the images accurately.

From Figure 18.3. COVID-19 is the only class whose samples form a small cluster towards the bottom-left of the plot where the values of mean and standard deviation are low. Since the dots of all the classes are on top of each other, an individual scatter plot is necessary for each class to obtain some important details. Figure 18.4 presents the scatter plots of mean and standard deviation for each of the classes individually. The figure shows that the normal and Ground Glass Opacity samples have a similar scatter with outliers having higher standard deviation and lower mean values. However, samples of Viral Pneumonia present a concentrated plot which shows that these images have higher correlation with each other. COVID-19 scatter is peculiar in the sense that unlike any other class, the points are scattered across the entire plot even though they are less in number compared to Normal and Lung Opacity images. This shows that there is a clear distinction among the samples of COVID-19.

The visualization in Figure 18.5 presents the obtained samples from repository in a chart format. In the chart, the crescent brightness of the images increases as their

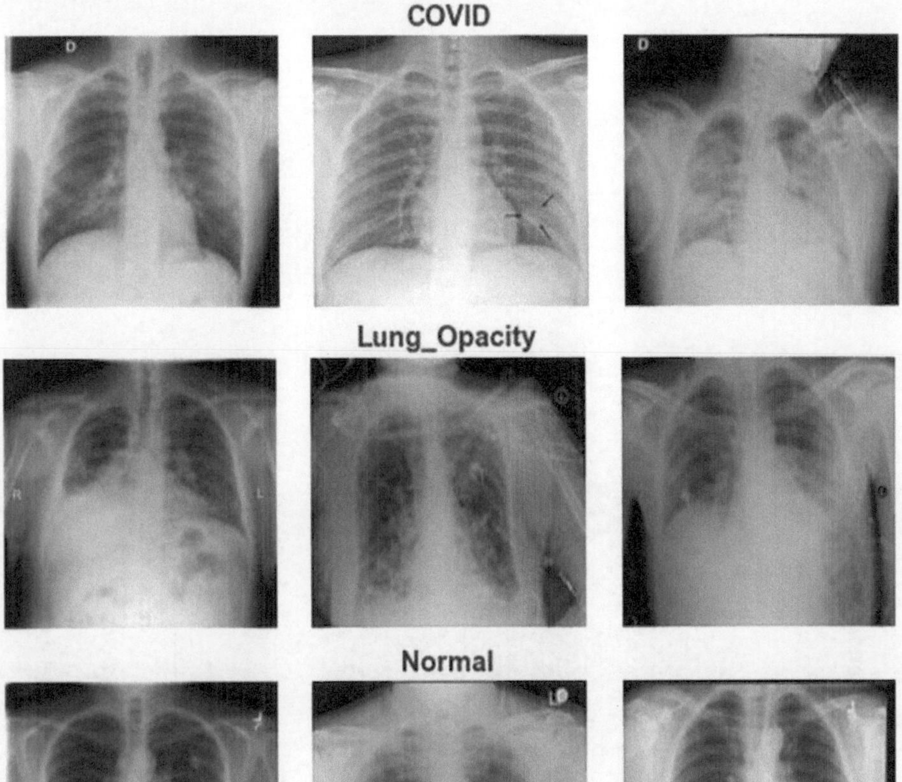

FIGURE 18.2 Random images from each class.

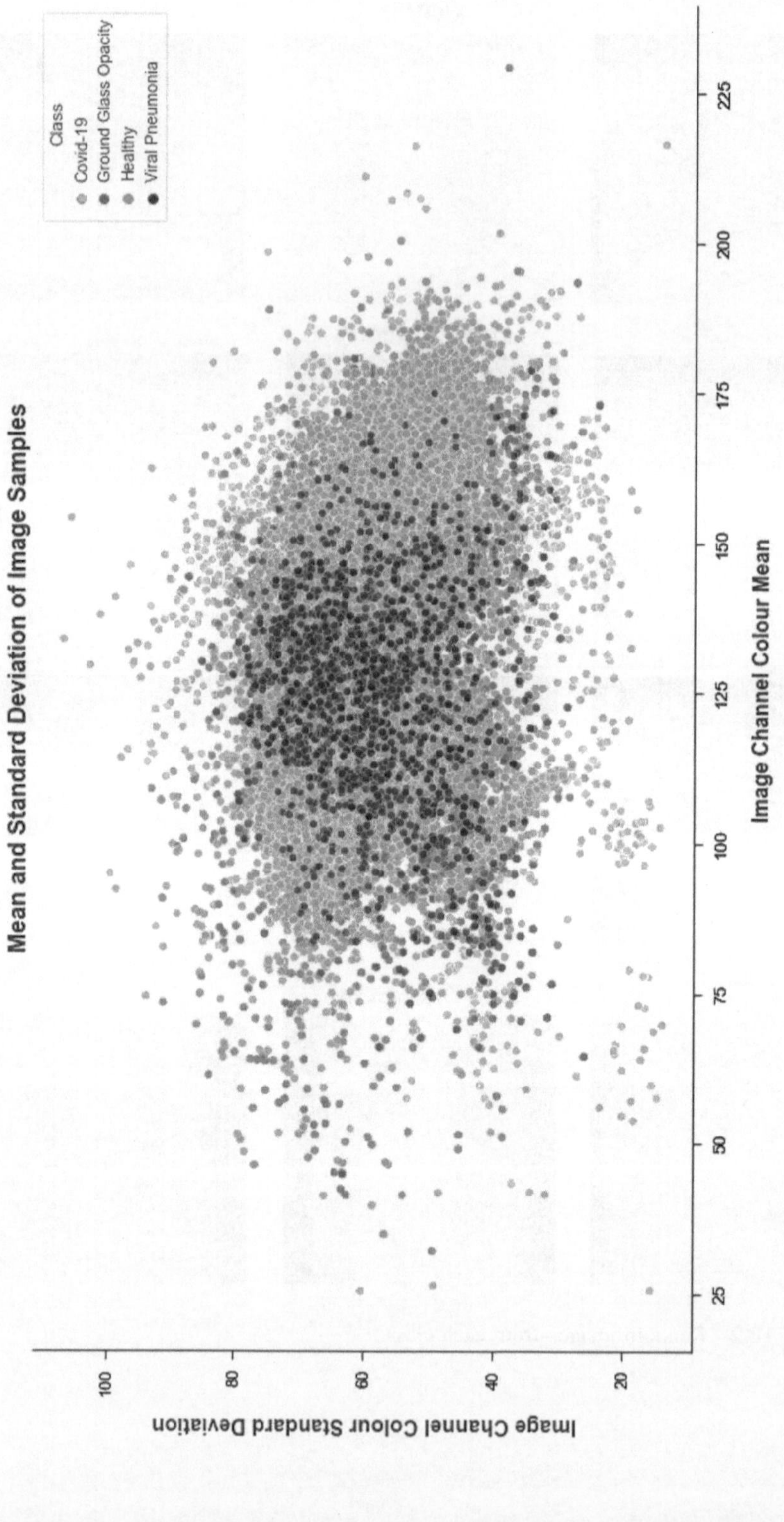

FIGURE 18.3 Scatter plot showing the distribution of mean and standard deviation of pixel values.

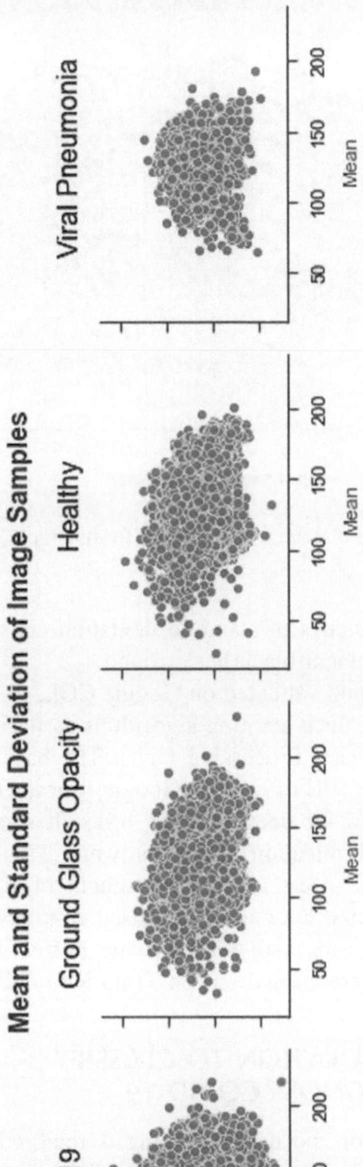

FIGURE 18.4 Scatter plots for mean and standard deviation of pixel values in images of each class.

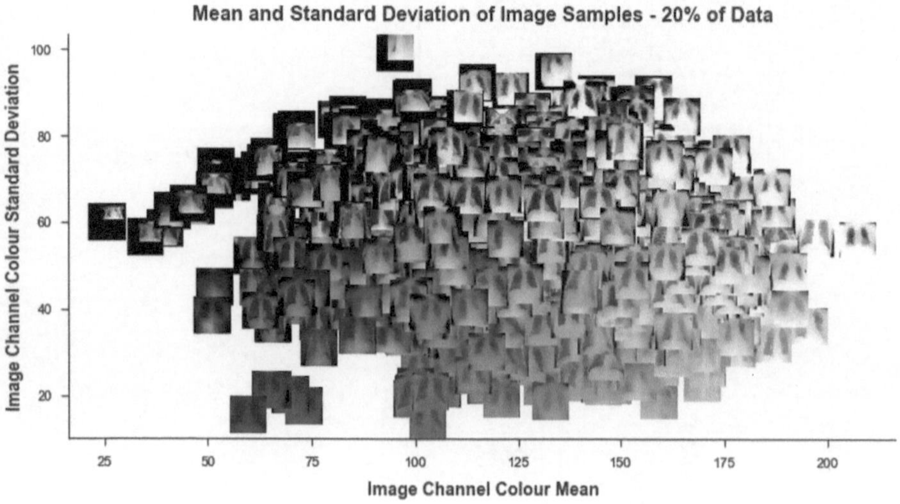

FIGURE 18.5 Obtained lung X-ray images in a chart format replacing the dots in the scatter plot.

mean value increases. Higher values of standard deviation constitute images that have higher contrast and a dominant black background.

The model has been trained and validated on Google COLAB platform which is a very useful tool for executing deep learning algorithms as it gives free access to dedicated GPUs and TPUs (Tensor Processing Unit). The base hardware for the training face of the model is the TPU offered by Google over the cloud. A TPU is a hardware accelerator specialized for deep learning tasks. It shortens the training time by performing matrix multiplication in the hardware. TPU is a 65,536 8-bit MAC matrix multiply unit that offers a peak throughput of 92 TeraOps/second (TOPS). According to the authors, the matrix unit uses systolic execution to save energy and time by reducing reads and writes of the buffer. Subsequently, the validation and testing phases were carried out on Tesla K80 GPU over the cloud.

18.4 THE MODEL FORMULATION TO CLASSIFY THE DATA TO DIAGNOSE COVID-19

As stated in the previous section, no data cleansing is required for the obtained dataset. The model has been built using the approach of Transfer Learning. This is a popular method where a model or network built for some task is reused for initial layers of a new model built for a specific purpose. The process model for classification of X-rays is shown in Figure 18.6. Note that this process works only when the features are general and suitable to both the base and target tasks, instead of being specific to the base task. To be more specific, the model uses the Pre-trained model approach which includes the steps of selecting a source model, reusing the source model and tuning the model.

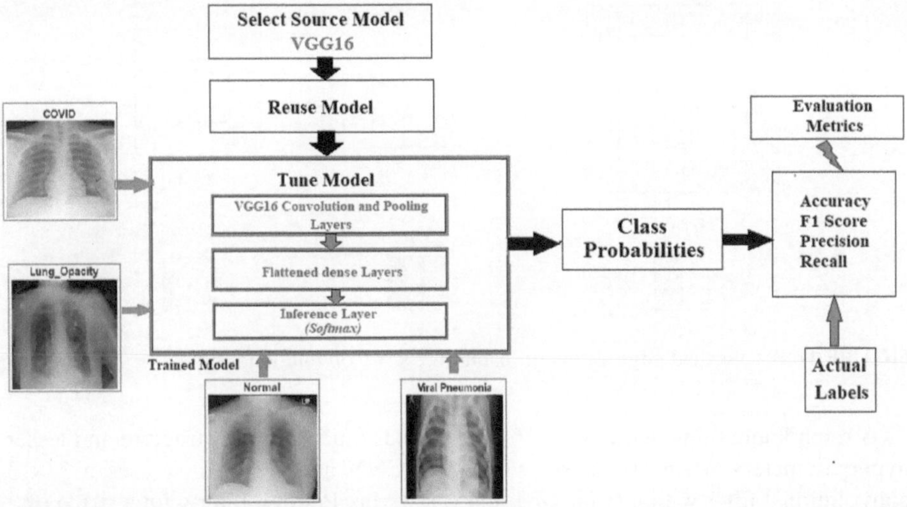

FIGURE 18.6 Model for classification of X-ray images.

The biggest benefit of this approach. The biggest benefit of this approach is that a concrete model need not be trained from scratch for a given target task given the large number of weights in each CNN layer which in turn span across multiple layers. This reduces the training time significantly and hence offers a good amount of time to validate and analyze the results. Additionally, transfer learning and fine-tuning with custom fully connected layers often lead to better performance than training from scratch on the target dataset. One of the challenges of Computer Vision problems is that the number of inputs to layers of a Neural Network can get really big. For example, the number of input parameters from a 1MP image is 3 million and if the first hidden layer of the neural network has 1000 neurons, the weight matrix of this layer has the dimensions, $1000 \times 3M$ summing up to 3 billion weights. So, the computation cost and memory requirements are huge if a normal neural network is trained with images. Convolutional Neural Networks solve this problem by employing 'Convolution' as their key operation. Figure 18.7 shows the edge detection performed by a convolution layer in a CNN. The input is one of the three color channel matrices (dimensions are 6×6) of an image whose vertical edges are to be detected. It is then convolved with another matrix called as a filter which is of dimensions 3×3. The filter is applied to each of the 3×3 sub-matrices of the input matrix. The result of this 3×3 convolution is the first element of the output matrix indicated by the same color as that of the corresponding sub-matrix. Thereafter, an activation function such as ReLU (Rectified Linear Unit) is applied to the output matrix before passing this matrix as input to the next layer. In practice, the input image consists of three channels and hence the filters are also three-dimensional instead of being two-dimensional. There exists another layer apart from the convolutional layer called as Max pooling layer. In such layer, the filter when convolved with sub-matrices of the same dimensions, outputs the maximum value in each of the sub-matrices.

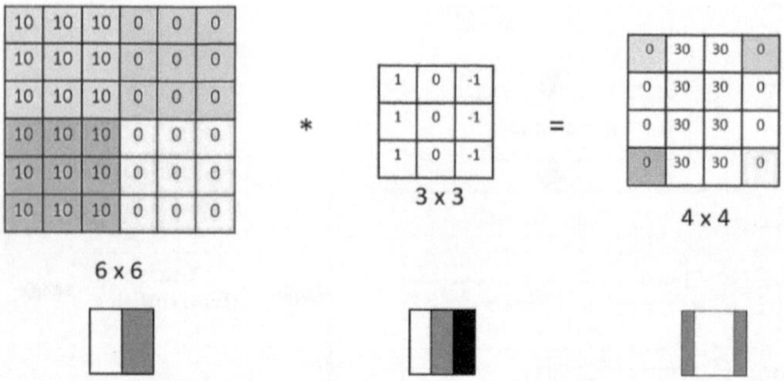

FIGURE 18.7 Vertical edge detection using a 3 × 3 Convolutional filter.

A remarkable thing about VGG16 is that it has much simpler structure and lesser hyperparameters when compared with other CNN architectures. It uses a 3 × 3 convolutional filter with a stride of 1 and 2 × 2 Max Pooling filter with a stride of 2 in all the layers. The padding is also same for all the layers. The relative uniformity of the architecture made VGG16 a quite attractive choice to researchers. Figure 18.8 shows the architecture of VGG16 with all the convolutional and pooling layers. The network has 13 convolutional layers and five max-pooling layers. It comes with three fully connected layers towards the end followed by a Softmax layer that was originally intended to classify 1000 different classes from the ImageNet database. The number 16 in the title signifies 13 convolutional + 3 fully connected layers. The initial 13 Conv layers and pooling layers together act as feature extractors for the obtained dataset of X-ray images.

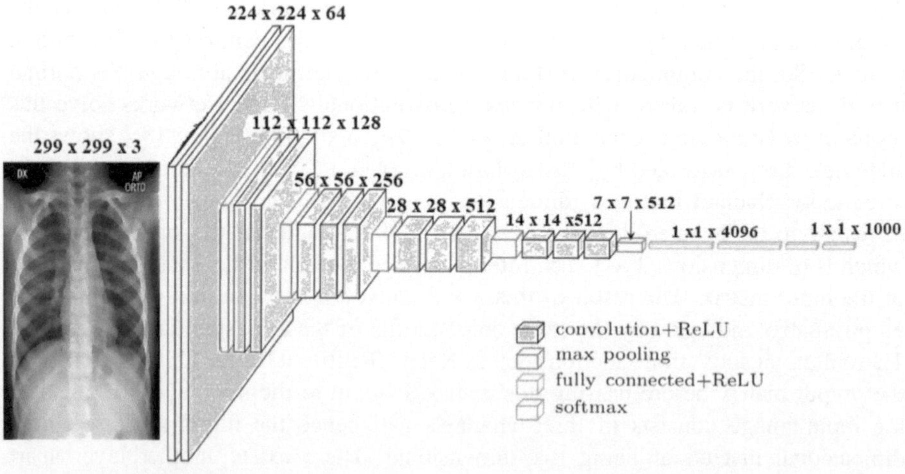

FIGURE 18.8 VGG16 architecture.

18.4.1 InceptionResNetV2

InceptionResNetV2 combines the Inception and Residual network architectures having good performance at a relatively lower computational cost. It is comprised of Residual Inception blocks where a filter expansion layer follows each Inception block. This filtering layer is a 1 × 1 convolutional layer without activation as shown in Figure 18.9. In this network, batch normalization is done on top of the convolutional layers instead of summations. This network consists of 572 layers with 55,873,736 parameters. As per Keras documentation, this network has a Top-1 accuracy of 0.803.

18.4.2 ResNet152V2

Residual networks are a family of deep convolutional neural networks which are comprised of residual blocks aimed at alleviating parameter degradation in deep neural networks. The residual block consists of a small feedforward network alongside a shortcut connection which transfers the inputs of the block directly to the output of the block and gets added to the feedforward network as shown in Figure 18.10. This network provides better accuracy without much complexity. ResNet152 has the best Top-1 accuracy of 0.780 among the ResNet family as per Keras documentation with a total of 60,380,648 parameters.

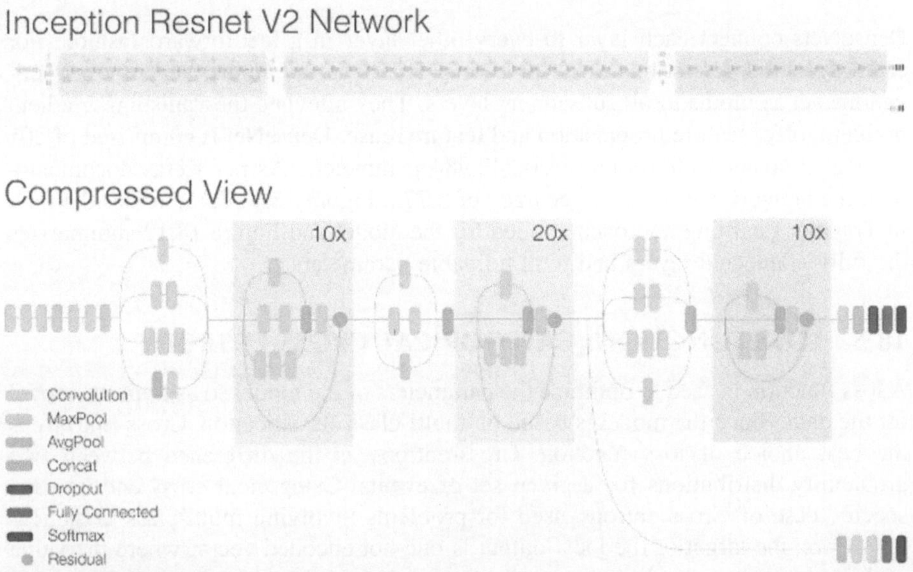

FIGURE 18.9 Compressed view of InceptionResNetV2.

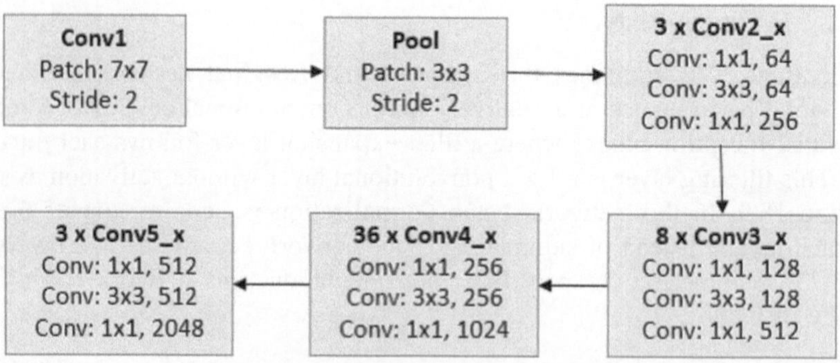

FIGURE 18.10 Basic architecture of ResNet152V2.

18.4.3 Xception

Xception network is a modification to the Inception family of CNNs. It performs better than InceptionV3 for both ImageNet and JFT datasets with a modified depthwise separable convolution. This is a pointwise convolution followed by a depthwise convolution. Due to this, In Xception, there is no intermediate ReLU non-linearity as present in InceptionV3. The network consists of 126 layers with a total of 22,910,480 layers. As per Keras documentation, it has a Top-1 accuracy of 0.790. Features transferred from distant tasks often perform better than random initial weights.

18.4.4 DenseNet201

DenseNets connect each layer to every other layer in a feedforward fashion. For each layer, the activations of all preceding layers act as inputs, and its own activations act as inputs to all subsequent layers. They alleviate the vanishing-gradient problem, offer feature propagation and feature reuse. DenseNet is comprised of 201 connected layers with a total of 20,242,984 parameters. As per Keras documentation, the network has a Top-1 accuracy of 0.773. Figure 18.11 summarizes the flow of Transfer Learning approach applied for the model and Figure 18.12 summarizes the fully connected layers and total trainable parameters

18.5 LOSS FUNCTION: CATEGORICAL CROSS ENTROPY

A loss function is used to optimize the parameters of the model so as to fit the model for the data. Since the model is based on multi-class classification, Cross Entropy is the best choice of loss function. Cross-entropy is the difference between two probability distributions for a given set of events. Categorical cross entropy is a specific case of Cross entropy used for problems involving multi-class classification. Here, the target or the ideal output is one-hot encoded vector where the value of the output corresponding the correct class is 1 and all others are zeros. The value of the loss function decreases with each epoch through the dataset. The training and validation for accuracy and loss for Inception ResNetV2 is shown in Figure 18.13

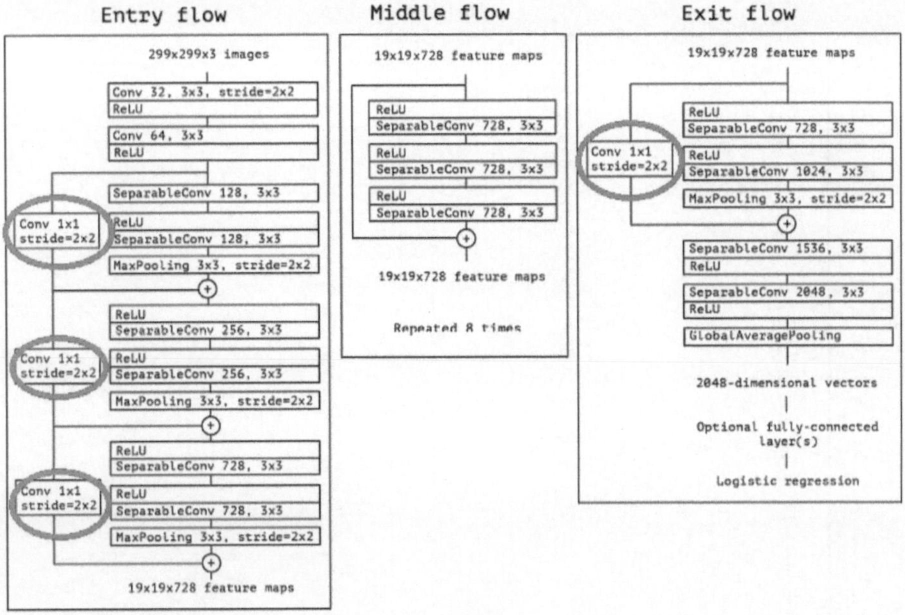

FIGURE 18.11 Overall architecture of Xception.

Layers	Output Size	DenseNet-121	DenseNet-169	DenseNet-201	DenseNet-264
Convolution	112 × 112	7 × 7 conv, stride 2			
Pooling	56 × 56	3 × 3 max pool, stride 2			
Dense Block (1)	56 × 56	[1 × 1 conv, 3 × 3 conv] × 6	[1 × 1 conv, 3 × 3 conv] × 6	[1 × 1 conv, 3 × 3 conv] × 6	[1 × 1 conv, 3 × 3 conv] × 6
Transition Layer (1)	56 × 56	1 × 1 conv			
	28 × 28	2 × 2 average pool, stride 2			
Dense Block (2)	28 × 28	[1 × 1 conv, 3 × 3 conv] × 12	[1 × 1 conv, 3 × 3 conv] × 12	[1 × 1 conv, 3 × 3 conv] × 12	[1 × 1 conv, 3 × 3 conv] × 12
Transition Layer (2)	28 × 28	1 × 1 conv			
	14 × 14	2 × 2 average pool, stride 2			
Dense Block (3)	14 × 14	[1 × 1 conv, 3 × 3 conv] × 24	[1 × 1 conv, 3 × 3 conv] × 32	[1 × 1 conv, 3 × 3 conv] × 48	[1 × 1 conv, 3 × 3 conv] × 64
Transition Layer (3)	14 × 14	1 × 1 conv			
	7 × 7	2 × 2 average pool, stride 2			
Dense Block (4)	7 × 7	[1 × 1 conv, 3 × 3 conv] × 16	[1 × 1 conv, 3 × 3 conv] × 32	[1 × 1 conv, 3 × 3 conv] × 32	[1 × 1 conv, 3 × 3 conv] × 48
Classification Layer	1 × 1	7 × 7 global average pool			
		1000D fully-connected, softmax			

FIGURE 18.12 DenseNet architectures.

and 14 respectively. The model is trained using the Adam Optimizer with a learning rate of 0.001 and Categorical Cross entropy as the loss function.

$$L(Y, \hat{Y}) = -(\sum Y * \log(\hat{Y}) + (1 - Y) * log(1 - \hat{Y}))$$

Where Y = True Label, $\hat{Y}$ = Predicted Label $L(Y, \hat{Y})$ is the Loss Function.

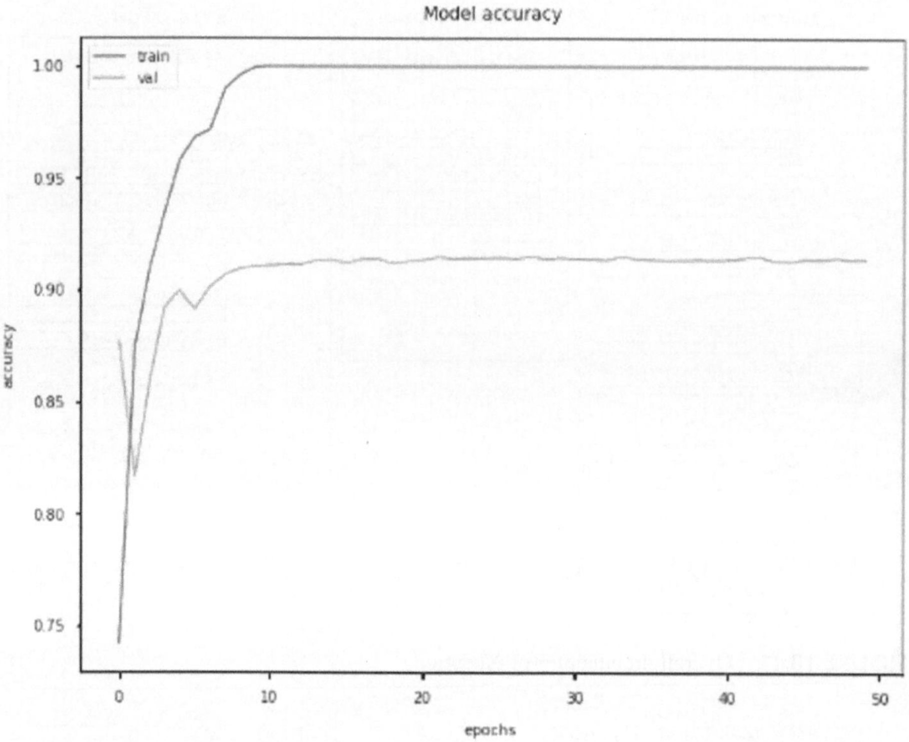

FIGURE 18.13 Training and validation accuracy for InceptionResNetV2 model.

Steps to train the model:

1. Preprocessing the X-ray Images

   The images need to be stored in a directory where each sub-directory contains images of a specific class. So the model uses ImageDataGenerator() function of Keras API (Application Program Interface) which accepts the images as per their corresponding sub-directories and generates input and output labels automatically. In addition it also performs data augmentation as follows:

   a. *Reshaping the images:* It reshapes an image to dimensions (299, 299, 3) as per the dataset for better performance.
   b. *Random Rotation Range: 5°*
   c. *Zoom Range:* 0.2 (in proportion with the image size)
   d. *Width Shift Range:* 0.2 (In proportion with the image size)
   e. *Height Shift Range:* 0.2 (In proportion with the image size)

2. Applying the X-ray images as input parameters to the input layer of pre-trained model.

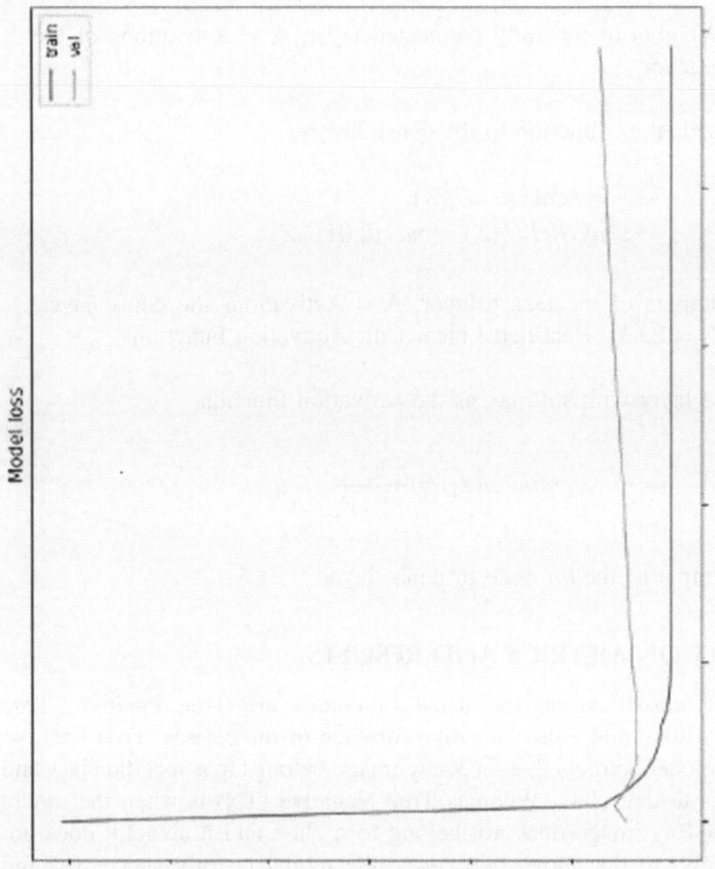

FIGURE 18.14 Training and validation loss for InceptionResNetV2 model.

3. Capture the outputs of the ultimate convolutional layer of the pre-trained model. Apply these as inputs to a Global Average Pooling layer.
4. Flatten the dimensions of the outputs to n × 1.
5. Add the dense layers or Fully Connected layers with a number of hidden units = 256. Without activation, the outputs of the dense layers are of the form:

$$Z = W * A + b$$

Where W = Weights of the fully connected layer, A = Activations of the previous dense layer

6. Apply the activation function to the dense layers.

$$A = LeakyReLU\,(Z)$$
$$LeakyReLU\,(Z) = max\,(0.01,\ \ Z)$$

Where Z = Outputs of the Dense layer, A = Activations the dense layer, LeakyReLU(Z) = Leaky Rectified Linear Unit Activation Function

7. Add a dense layer with softmax as the activation function.

$$softmax\,(Z_i) = \frac{e^{Z_i}}{\sum_{j=1}^{k} Z_j}$$

Where Z_i = Output of the *ith* node of dense layer

18.6 EVALUATION METRICS AND RESULTS

When performing classification, the usual outcomes are True Positive, True Negative, False Positive and False Negative for each of the classes. True Positive (TP) is when the model predicts that an X-ray image belongs to a specific class and it actually belongs to that class. Whereas True Negative (TN) is when the model predicts that an X-Ray image does not belong to a class and it actually does not belong to that class. In the above two cases, the model is truly successful and accurate. On the other hand, False Positive (FP) and False Negative (FN) result when the model is not accurate. False Positive is when the model predicts that a given X-ray image belongs to a class but it actually does not belong to that class. Finally, False Negative is when the model predicts that a given X-ray image does not belong to a class but it actually belongs to that class.

Hence for a better understanding and evaluation of a trained model, a confusion matrix is plotted with four of these outcomes for each class on testing data in Figure 18.15. It basically shows the number of TPs, TNs, FPs and FNs that resulted when test data are passed as inputs to the validated model. The diagonal elements

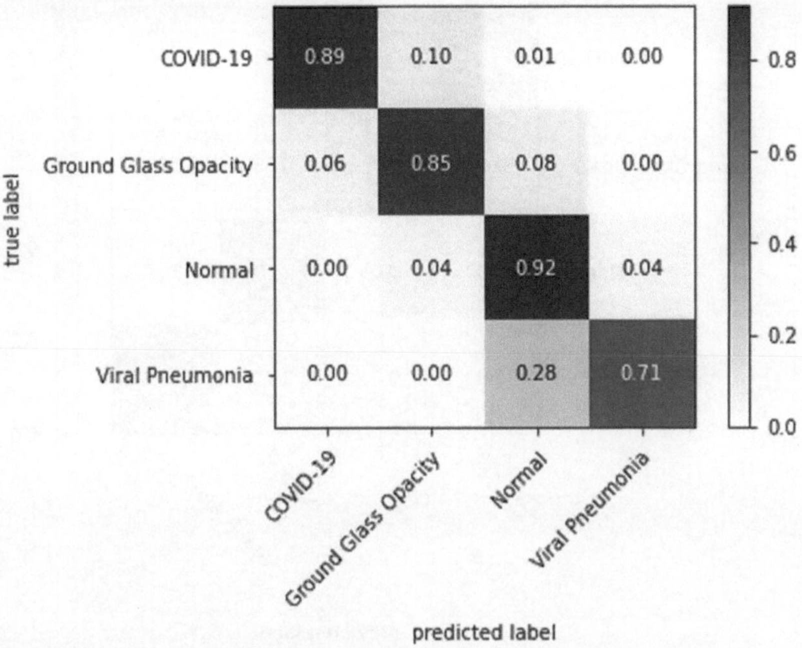

FIGURE 18.15 Confusion matrix of test data of InceptionResNetV2 model.

represent the number of True Positives for each class. The number of False Negatives for each class is the sum of the values in the corresponding row excluding the True Positives. Whereas the total number of False Positives for each class is the sum of the values in the corresponding column excluding the number of True Positives. The confusion matrix generated from test data in ResNet152V2 model, Xception model and DenseNet201 model is represented in Figures 18.15, 18.16 and 18.17 respectively. Finally, the total number of True Negatives for a class is the sum of the elements in all the rows and columns excluding the row and column of that class. Based on these four outcomes, several evaluation metrics are defined as

a. Accuracy:

$$\text{Accuracy} = \frac{\text{True Positives} + \text{True Negatives}}{\text{True Positives} + \text{True Negatives} + \text{False Positives} + \text{False Negatives}}$$

b. Precision:

$$Precision = \frac{True\ Positives}{True\ Positives + False\ Positives}$$

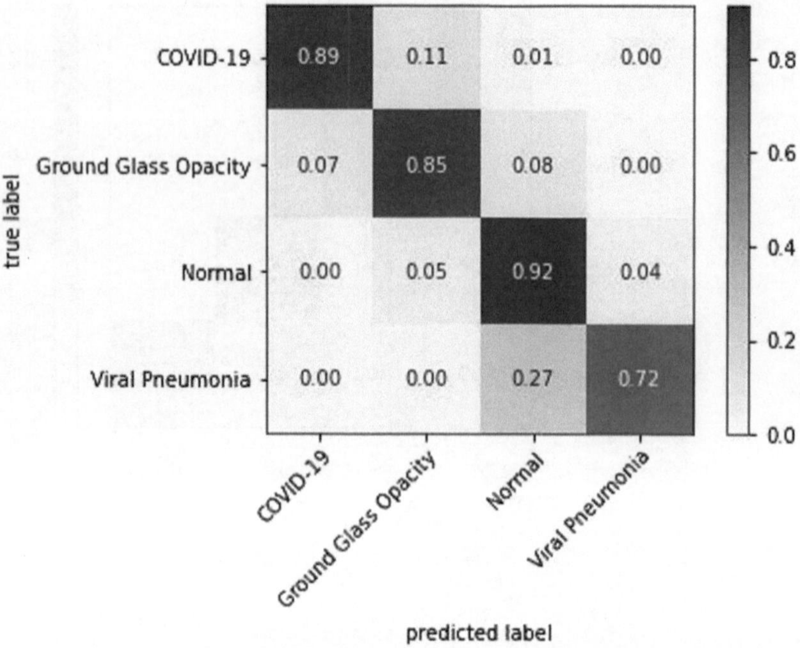

FIGURE 18.16 Confusion matrix of test data of ResNet152V2 model.

c. Recall:

$$Recall = \frac{True\ Positives}{True\ Positives + False\ Negatives}$$

d. *F1 Score:* This metric performs well on an imbalanced dataset as it takes into account both the False Positives and False negatives. It is defined as the harmonic mean of Precision and Recall and hence gives the same weightage to both of these.

$$F1\ \ Score = \frac{2 * Precision * Recall}{Precision + Recall}$$

(Figure 18.18)

Table 18.1 lists the values of evaluation metrics obtained for the trained model with test set images as inputs. Note that accuracy is not a monotonically increasing function with each epoch since the model uses Adam optimizer. The comparison of evaluation metrics of the four deep learning models is represented as bar graph in Figure 18.19. It can be noticed that InceptionResNetV2 outperforms the other models in terms of accuracy, precision, recall and F1 score. Being a 572 layered network, it is comprised of residual inception blocks where a filter

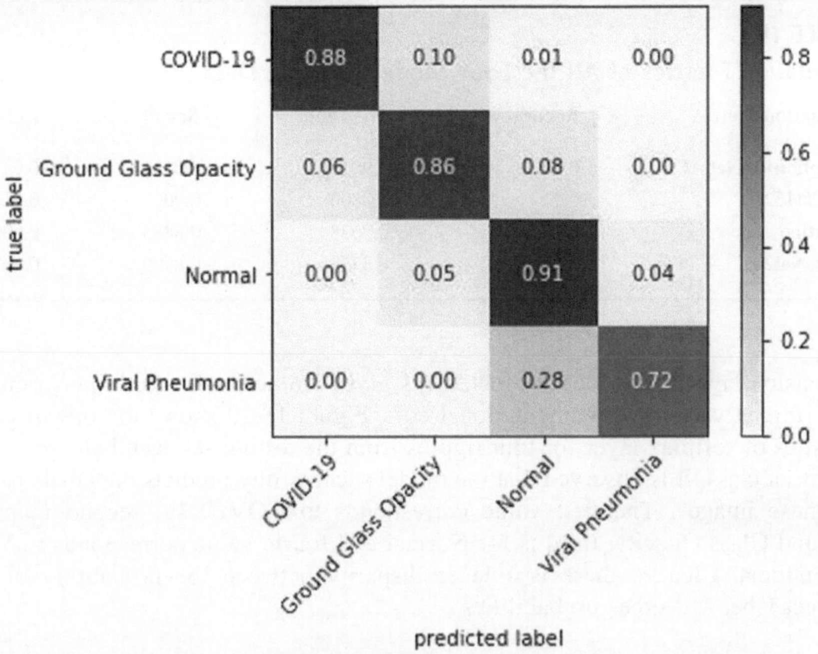

FIGURE 18.17 Confusion matrix of test data of Xception model.

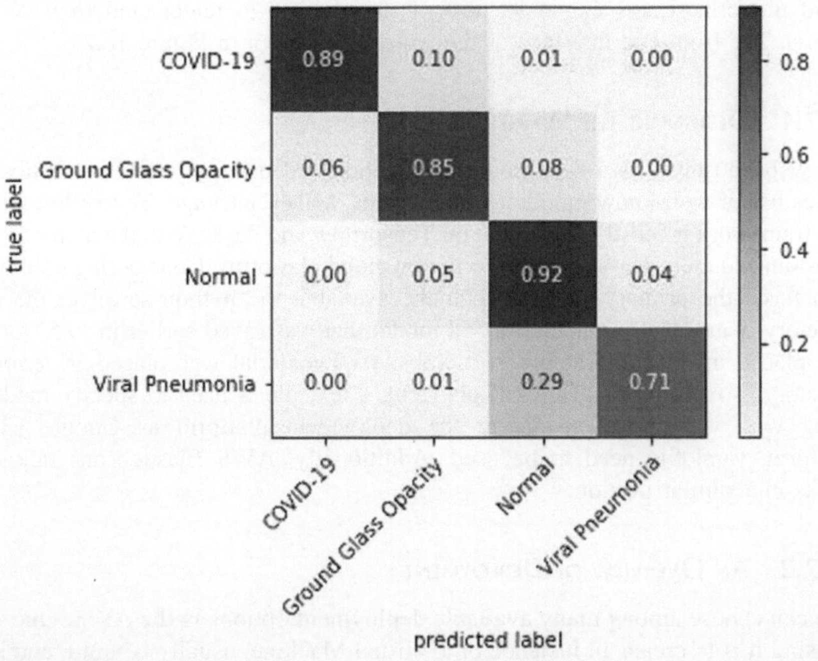

FIGURE 18.18 Confusion matrix of test data of DenseNet201 model.

TABLE 18.1
Evaluation Metrics of All the Four Models on Test Data

Evaluation Metric	Accuracy	Precision	Recall	F1 Score
InceptionResNetV2	0.9416	0.9013	0.9215	0.9314
ResNet152	0.921	0.8806	0.9008	0.9107
Xception	0.909	0.8628	0.8883	0.8903
DenseNet201	0.912	0.8778	0.8909	0.9092

expansion layer follows each block. This gives the network a good performance with a relatively lower computational cost. Figure 18.20 shows the output probabilities of softmax layer for four figures from the testing set each belonging to a different class. It is observed that the model successfully predicts the labels for all of these images. The first value corresponds to COVID-19, second maps to Ground Glass Opacity, third is for Normal and fourth value corresponds to Viral Pneumonia. Clearly, there is a large disparity between the probability of the correct label and other probabilities.

18.7 MODEL DEPLOYMENT

The COVID-19 diagnosis can be made available to public once it gets deployed on cloud platform. Users can make use of the website to understand their X-Ray reports. The front end interface of the website is shown in Figure 18.21.

18.7.1 Designing the Website

The website runs with a background application coded in python. The application makes use of well-known modules like pandas, MIME package, Tensorflow, flask. The framework is mostly dependent on Tensorflow and flask. With the help of flask, a customized hierarchy was made to run on cloud platforms. Considering deploying with flask, the primary focus is to make available the python script in the root directory in any platform. The trained model that was saved earlier in '*.h5*' format was placed in model directory and website UI material was placed in template directory. To deploy on 'Heroku' platform, a text file is used to specify modules along with versions. Considering the deployment platform as Google Cloud Platform, yaml file need to be used. Additionally, AWS Elasticbeans talk also works in a similar fashion.

18.7.2 An Overview of Deployment

One can choose among many available deployment options in the AWS. One way of using it is to create an instance of a Virtual Machine, usually Ubuntu, and host the files from it. This method is difficult when compared to using existing

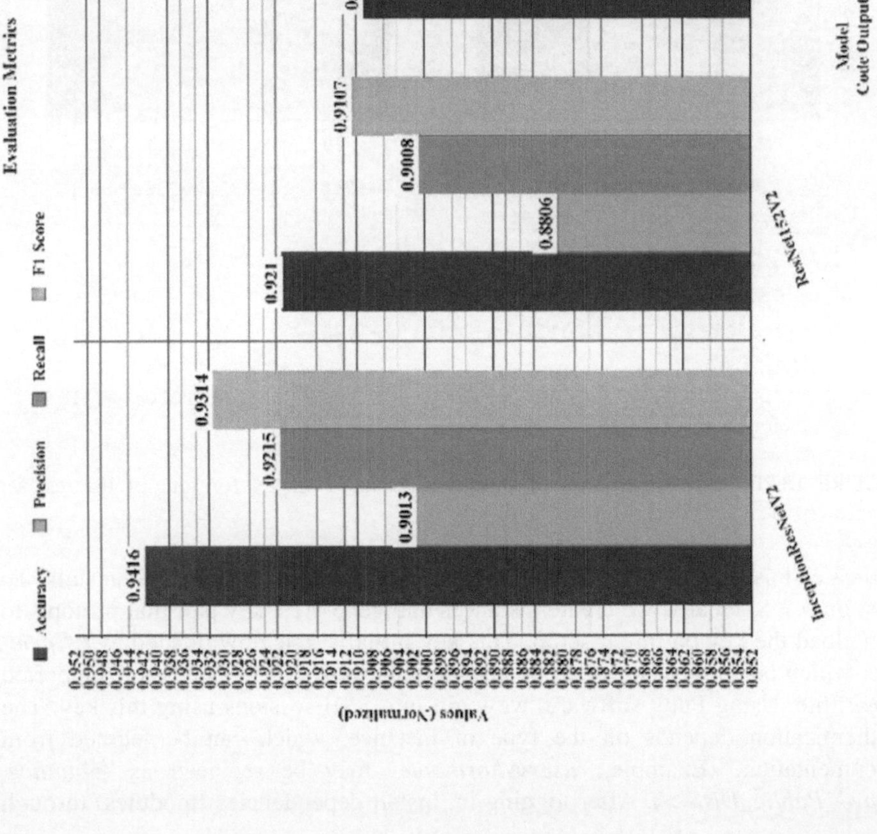

FIGURE 18.19 Bar graph comparing the evaluation metrics of four models.

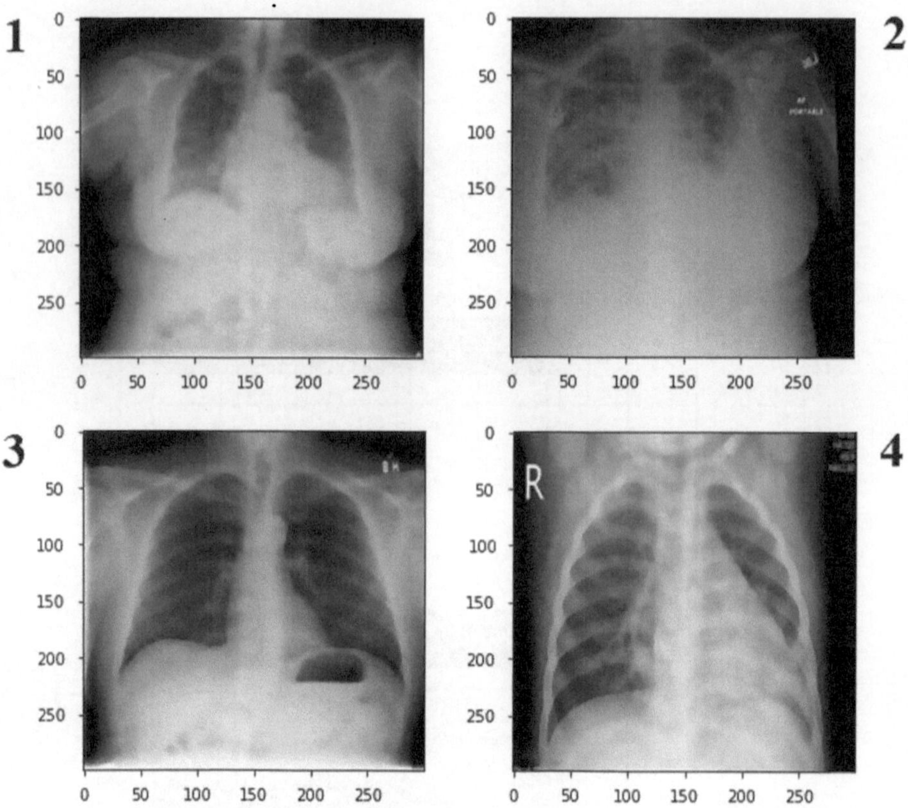

1. `[[1.0000000e+00 6.8145600e-19 2.7904948e-14 0.0000000e+00]]`
   `Diagnosed with COVID-19!`
2. `[[0.000000e+00 1.000000e+00 4.488387e-34 0.000000e+00]]`
   `Diagnosed with Ground Glass Opacity!`
3. `[[1.8685872e-37 7.3012404e-07 9.9999928e-01 0.0000000e+00]]`
   `Healthy`
4. `[[0.0000000e+00 0.0000000e+00 5.6737674e-11 1.0000000e+00]]`
   `Diagnosed with Viral Pneumonia!`

FIGURE 18.20 Output response of InceptionResNetV2 model for four of the test set images.

dedicated hosting models. For example, we can make use of Elastic Beanstalk. To host on AWS, ideally, we create instances and generate a key pair that prompts to download the key on initial setup. This key initially gets downloaded as a *'.pem'* file, which on further steps can be changed and also downloaded as a supported *'.ppk'* file. Using Putty software, we login into SSH sessions using this key. The authentication depends on the type of instance, which can be learned from documentation. (Example, *'user@hostname'* may be replaced as *'ubuntu@ <ipv4_Public_DNS'>*). After logging in, install dependencies (modules) through

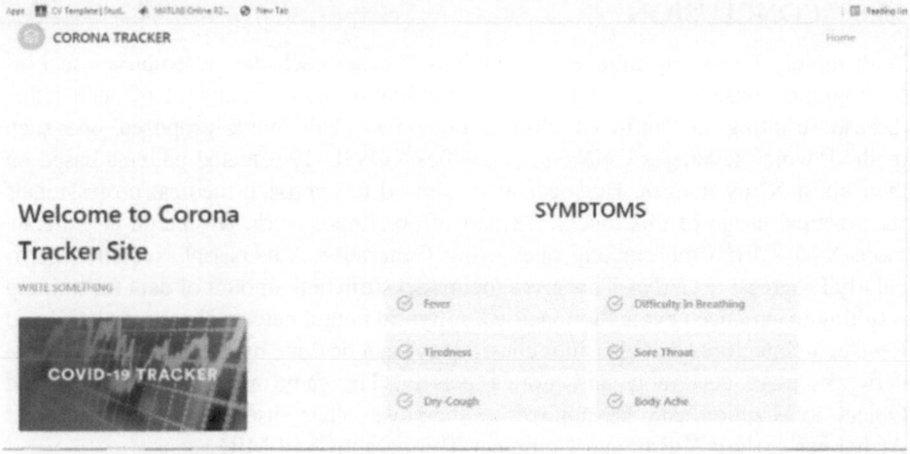

FIGURE 18.21 Website frontend interface.

CLI. Lastly, use applications like FileZilla client or other transferring software to host files. Note that few applications use *'.pem'* keys only, instead of *'ppk'* files to login to servers. The model of output response of diagnosis mail sent to user is shown in Figure 18.22.

18.7.3 Working of Website

The website is open to everyone on the internet and doesn't require any authentication to make use of. Users can simply click on the upload file button on the website and submit their X-Ray image. The file type has to be *'.jpeg'* extension. The image need not have a preset size before uploading. Images uploaded automatically get rescaled. The prediction runs at light speed and the output of severity and likeliness of one being tested positive is also sent to the user's mail ID when provided along with the image during submission.

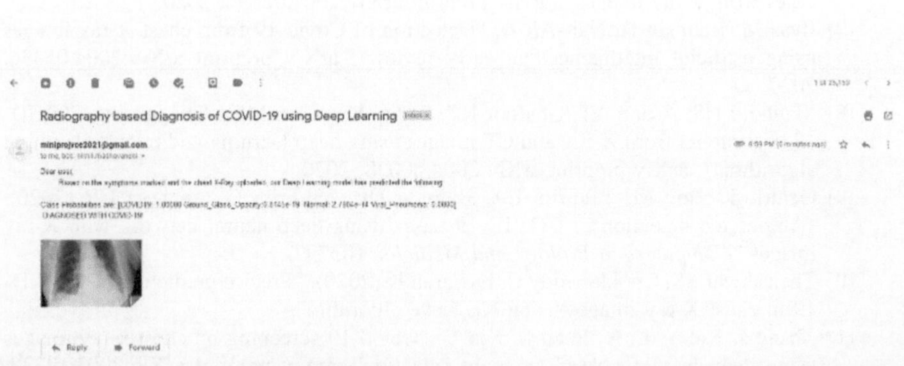

FIGURE 18.22 Diagnosis mail sent to the user.

18.8 CONCLUSION

With rapidly increasing number of COVID-19 cases each day, alternatives such as Radiography based diagnosis can aid in facilitating early treatment of such lethal disease resulting in improved clinical outcomes. This work proposed one such method, which leverages CNNs and classifies COVID-19 affected patients based on their chest X-ray images. However, it is advised to approach medical professionals for practical usage of this model. As part of our future work, we intend to generate more X-rays from the existing ones using Generative Adversarial Networks particularly Progressive GANs. This gives the model sufficient amount of data for training resulting in enhanced evaluation metrics. A hybrid neural network based on VGG and ResNet architectures that classifies chest X-rays can be done by generative adversarial networks more accurately and more precisely. The same approach of CNNs and Object localization can be applied to diagnose other diseases like Cancer and Alzheimer's using X-Ray and Computer Tomography and MRI scans.

REFERENCES

[1] Libster R, Wappner D, Coviello S, Bianchi A, Braem V, Esteban I, Caballero MT (2021), "Early high titer plasma therapy to prevent severe Covid-19 in older adults". *The New England Journal of Medicine*, NEJM.org.

[2] Narin A, Kaya C, Pamuk Z (2020), "Automatic detection of corona virus disease (covid-19) using x-ray images and deep convolutional neural networks". arXiv preprint arXiv:2003.10849.

[3] Apostolopoulos ID, Mpesiana TA (2020), "Covid-19: automatic detection from x-ray images utilising transfer learning with convolutional neural networks". *Physical and Engineering Sciences in Medicine*:1: 635–640.

[4] Afshar P, Heidarian S, Naderkhani F, Oikonomou A, Plataniotis KN, Mohammadi A, "Covid-caps: a capsule network-based framework for identification of covid-19 cases from x-ray images". arXiv preprint arXiv:2004.02696, 2020.

[5] Jain R, Gupta M, Taneja S, Jude Hemanth D (2021), "Deep learning based detection and analysis of COVID-19 on chest X-ray images". *Applied Intelligence*: 1690–1700.

[6] Afshar P, Heidarian S, Naderkhani F, Oikonomou A, Plataniotis KN, Mohammadi A, "Covid-caps: a capsule network-based framework for identification of covid-19 cases from x-ray images". arXiv preprint arXiv:2004.02696, 2020.

[7] Ilyas M, Rehman H, Nait-Ali A, "Detection of Covid-19 from chest X-ray images using artificial intelligence: an early review". arXiv preprint arXiv:2004.05436, 2020.

[8] Maghdid HS, Asaad AT, Ghafoor KZ, Sadiq AS, Khan MK, "Diagnosing COVID-19 pneumonia from X-ray and CT images using deep learning and transfer learning algorithms". arXiv preprint arXiv:2004.00038, 2020.

[9] Ozturk T, Talo M, Yildirim EA, Baloglu UB, Yildirim O, Acharya UR (2020), "Automated detection of COVID-19 cases using deep neural network with X-ray images".*Computers in Biology and Medicine*:103792.

[10] Thejeshwar SS, Chokkareddy C, Eswaran K (2020), "Precise prediction of COVID-19 in chest X-ray images using KE sieve algorithm".

[11] Zhang J, Xie Y, Li Y, Shen C, Xia Y, "Covid-19 screening on chest x-ray images using deep learning based anomaly detection". arXiv preprint arXiv:2003.12338, 2020.

19 Stacked Auto Encoder Deep Neural Network with Principal Components Analysis for Identification of Chronic Kidney Disease

Sanat Kumar Sahu
Department of Computer Science, Govt. K.P.G. College Jagdalpur (C.G.), Chhattisgarh, India

Pratibha Verma
Research Scholar, Department of Computer Science, Dr. C.V. Raman University Bilaspur (C.G.), Chhattisgarh, India

CONTENTS

19.1 Introduction ... 385
19.2 Methodology ... 386
  19.2.1 Stacked Auto-encoder Deep Neural Network ... 386
  19.2.2 Principal Component Analysis (PCA) ... 387
19.3 Result and Discussion ... 388
19.4 Conclusion ... 393
References ... 394

19.1 INTRODUCTION

CKD is a universal public health issue, which concerns around 10% of the people globally. Yet, there is awfully small verification about CKD, due to challenges in identifying efficiently and automatically. CKD or Chronic Renal Disease (CRD) slowly progresses and is difficult to identify and kidney loses its functionality. Normally, it is difficult to detect the disease before 25% loss of kidney's functionality. The beginning of kidney failure of patients cannot be recognized because kidney failure may not give any symptoms initially (Subasi et al. 2017).

DOI: 10.1201/9781003217497-19

There are various types of DL neural networks that are available in computer science used in the healthcare area (Verma et al. 2021). The DL methods help doctors and health care practitioners in accurate diagnosis of diseases. These systems help to detect the disease easily with less time and treatment can be provided at an early stage. This chapter suggests an AE-based structure for CKD identification distinguishing proof, which is foundation of DNN and be developed to acquire best possible solutions for the detection of CKD. The PCA data reduction techniques with a different number of components were used. These DNN are reutilized before and after the application of PCA. The findings depict the performance of post-application of PCA with proposed auto-encoder being much better.

The Deep Learning-based disease diagnosis systems and CKD as a field of research is emerging in the field of computer and health sciences. Zhao et al. (2019) have proposed a DL-based model, namely MHMS. This is AE and its options like Restricted Boltzmann Machines and its categories consist of Deep Boltzmann Machines (DBM), Deep Belief Network (DBN), Recurrent Neural Networks (RNN) and Convolution Neural Networks (CNN). The outcome has shown that the DL-based MHMS doesn't necessitate wide human effort and specialist knowledge. Sri et al. (2018) have proposed a DNN-based AE structure for structural damage detection. The model can be used with DNN and achieve the optimal solution to highly non-linear pattern recognition problems. Kam and Kim (2017) proposed the group choice that adhere to the InSight model. A comparison was made between the findings of DL-based models as compare to InSight model. Xiao et al. (2017) have suggested DL to an ensemble method that incorporated numerous special Machine Learning (ML) approach. In the trial work, they exercise informative gene data elected by discrepancy gene expression investigation to diverse classification models. Finally, a DL model is utilizing to combination the outputs of the five classifiers. They proposed a technique for classification of CKD with the incidence of missing data in the work. Abedalkhader and Abdulrahman (2017) examined the results using K-Nearest Neighbors (KNN), Naive Bayes (NB), Support Vector Machine (SVM) and Decision Trees (DT) using 10-fold cross-validation. Subasi et al. (2017) worked on the ML methods like Artificial Neural Network (ANN), SVM, C4.5, and Random Forest (RF), K-NN. The result was validated with CKD dataset. The outcome showed that the RF classifier performed outstandingly. Manimaran and Muthuraman (2017) used five data mining classification techniques during the study and compared to several factors on a constant set of attributes in MV databases. The experimental outcome shows that C 4.5 and JRIP have the foremost appropriate algorithms for prediction of Kidney Disease (KD) among patients.

19.2 METHODOLOGY

The present work started with the study of background information about classification of CKD by using DNN and SAEDNN.

19.2.1 Stacked Auto-encoder Deep Neural Network

The SAEDNN is a neural organization comprising of several layers of meager AE in which the yields of each layer is wired to the contributions of the progressive layer

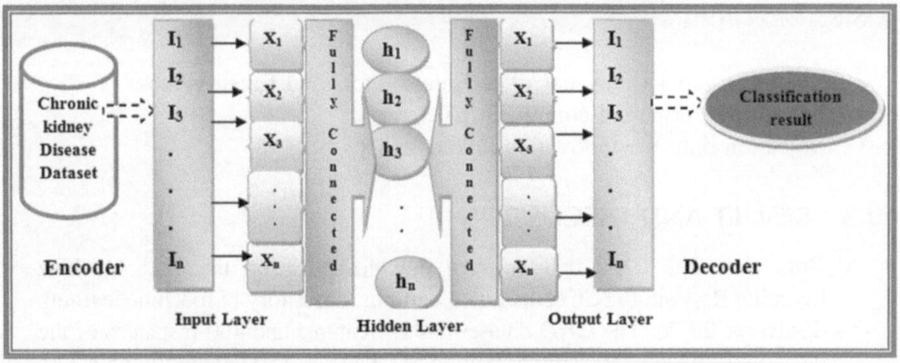

FIGURE 19.1 Stacked auto-encoder deep neural network.

(Tao et al. 2015; Karthikeyan 2017). The features from the stacked AE can be utilized for characterization issues by feeding to a softmax. An AE, auto-associator or Diabolo network is a ANN organization utilized for unsupervised learning of proficient coding. A traditional AE (Kam and Kim 2017; Sri et al. 2018b; Li et al. 2016; Tao et al. 2015) consists of two core segments: a single hidden layer encoder and decoder.

1. **Encoder:** The deterministic mapping $f(x)$, which redesigned a d dimensional info vector $x \in Rd$ into an r-dimensional shrouded representation $h \in Rr$, is called an encoder.
2. **Decoder:** The mapping $g\ h\ ()$, which transforms the hidden representation h (observed in the step described above) back into a reconstructed vector $z \in Rd$ in the input space, is called a decoder (Sri et al. 2018b).

In the Figure 19.1 SAEDNN was developed for helpful identification of CKD using simple DL method. This is the proposed framework for the classification of CKD dataset.

19.2.2 Principal Component Analysis (PCA)

The PCA (Zhang and Wu 2012) is an approach to decrease the dimensionality of a dataset consisting of a huge numeral of consistent variables while keeping up with the edition presented in the dataset (Paul et al. 2013; Yildirim 2015). This is agreed for remodeling to a novel set of variables, the principal components (PCs) and primary ordered Einasto et al. 2011) (Einasto et al. 2011). It is a statistical technique-based approach to discover outline in data and in such a way to show up their relationships and variations. PCA (Miranda et al. 2008) could be useful tool for exploring data. Another major benefit of PCA is that after discovered these patterns in the data, humans may reduce the data by reducing the number of dimensions, allowing for more reasonable dealing without losing information. It provides a road plan and a restriction for reducing a large dataset to a smaller dimension (Verma et al. 2021). It is a mathematical tool that comes from the field of applied algebra. It's a simplified, non-parametric method for extracting relevant data from disconcerting datasets. The PCA basics of statistical measures like variance and covariance (Han et al. 2012; Jolliffe 2002; Sebastian Raschka 2015).

Steps of PCA:

- Eigen decomposition – calculate Eigenvectors and Eigen values.
- Pick out the principal components.
- Projection onto the innovative feature space

19.3 RESULT AND DISCUSSION

A. **Data Set:** The CKD dataset from downloaded from the UCI Machine Learning Repository (UCI Machine Learning Repository of machine learning databases, 2015). The CKD dataset has 24 features and 400 instances of the data, out of which 250 samples belong to CKD and 150 belong to non-CKD.

B. **Performance Measurement:** Performance of classification (Fawcett 2006; Stehman 1997) models can be calculated by using some famous valuation measuring techniques. Classification results are assessed dependent upon information that was utilized for characterization, for example, realized class names. Confusion matrix (Han et al. 2012; Fawcett 2006; Stehman 1997) for binary classes of CKD dataset (ckd, notckd labels) is exposed in Table 19.1.

1. **Accuracy:** In this methodology, accuracy is characterized in the terms of precisely classified instances partitioned by the aggregate number of cases present in the dataset. It can separate CKD and non-CKD cases accurately.

$$\text{Accuracy} = \frac{TP + TN}{TP + TN + FP + FN} \quad \ldots. \qquad (18.1)$$

C. **Discussion:** Calculating the performance of classifier we have used 5 fold cross-validation techniques.

Steps of 5-fold cross-validation

i. Split sample dataset into 5 equal size sample
ii. Used train for 4 datasets sample and test on 1 sample.
iii. Repeat 5 times of steps 2 and obtain a mean accuracy.

The graphical plot is shown in Figure 19.2–19.4 with all features of CKD dataset and selected components of CKD dataset.

TABLE 19.1
Confusion Matrix

Actual Predicted	Positive	Negative
Positive	True Positive (TP)	False Negative (FN)
Negative	False Positive (FP)	True Negative (TN)

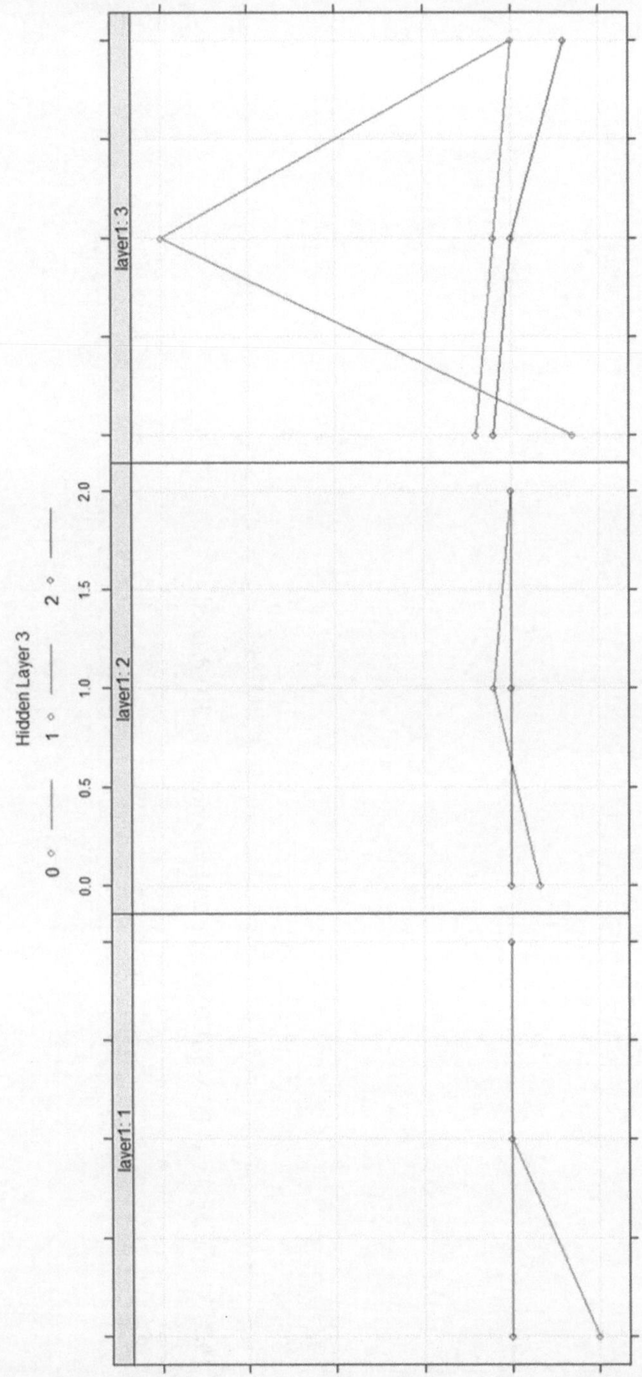

FIGURE 19.2 Graphical plot of SAEDNN with 24 features of CKD dataset.

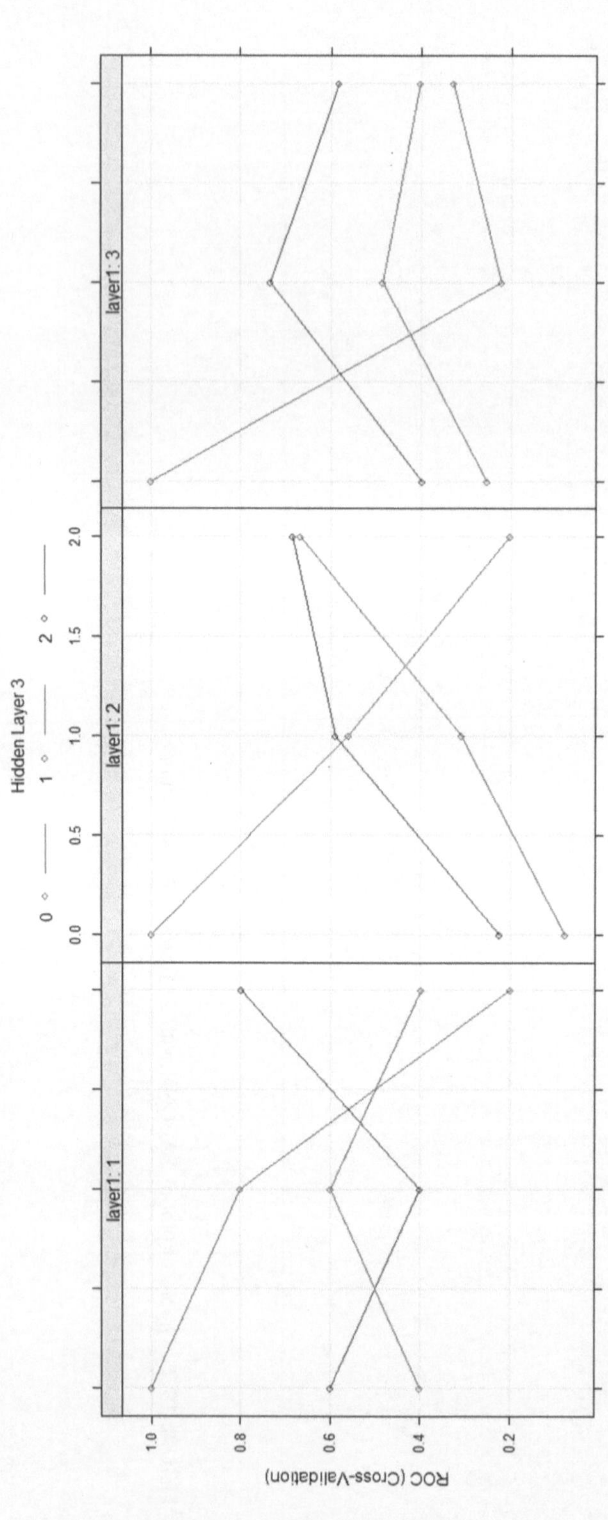

FIGURE 19.3 Graphical plot of PCA-SAEDNN with 20 components of CKD dataset.

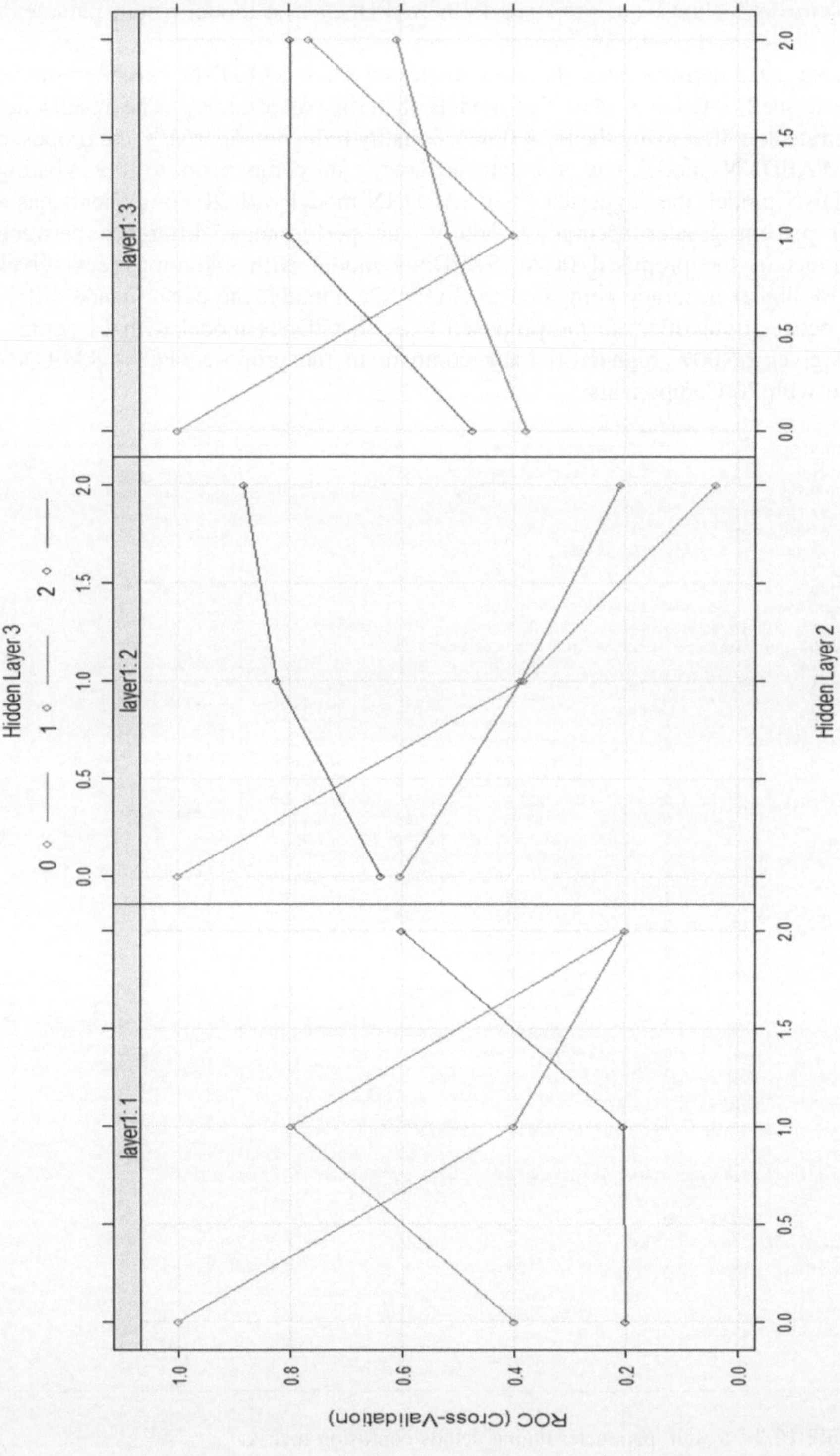

FIGURE 19.4 Graphical plot of PCA-SAEDNN with 14 components of CKD dataset.

Figure 19.5 shows our proposed PCA-SAEDNN best model result, parameter tuning details and confusion matrix.

Table 19.2 demonstrates that the suggested PCA-SAEDNN classifier model outperformed SAEDNN classifier models in terms of accuracy. The results demonstrate that after using the PCA dimensionality reduction approach, the proposed PCA-SAEDNN model has a better accuracy. In comparison to the existing SAEDNN model, the suggested PCA-SAEDNN model with 20 components has a 14.50 percent greater accuracy.Similarly, the performance difference between classifiers in the proposed PCA- SAEDNN model with 14 components gives 20.50% higher accuracy compared to SAEDNN. Finally, the performance difference between classifiers in the proposed PCA- SAEDNN model with 14 components gives 06.00% higher accuracy compare to the proposed PCA- SAEDNN model with 20 Components.

```
> mdeep
Stacked AutoEncoder Deep Neural Network

400 samples
 14 predictor
  2 classes: 'ckd', 'notckd'

No pre-processing
Resampling: Cross-Validated (5 fold)
Summary of sample sizes: 320, 320, 320, 320, 320
Resampling results across tuning parameters:

  layer1  layer2  layer3  ROC         Sens   Spec
  1       0       0       0.99973333  0.968  0.6000000
  1       0       1       0.40026667  1.000  0.0000000
  1       0       2       0.20080000  1.000  0.0000000
  1       1       0       0.40026667  1.000  0.0000000
  1       1       1       0.79813333  1.000  0.0000000
  1       1       2       0.20120000  1.000  0.0000000
  1       2       0       0.20000000  1.000  0.0000000
  1       2       1       0.20053333  1.000  0.0000000
  1       2       2       0.59933333  1.000  0.0000000
  2       0       0       0.99933333  1.000  0.6066667
  2       0       1       0.60186667  1.000  0.0000000
  2       0       2       0.63773333  1.000  0.0000000
  2       1       0       0.38226667  1.000  0.0000000
  2       1       1       0.38826667  1.000  0.0000000
  2       1       2       0.82320000  1.000  0.0000000
  2       2       0       0.03733333  1.000  0.0000000
  2       2       1       0.20826667  1.000  0.0000000
  2       2       2       0.87986667  1.000  0.0000000
  3       0       0       0.99840000  0.992  0.7333333
```

```
> mdeep$finalModel
$input_dim
[1] 14

$output_dim
[1] 2

$hidden
[1] 1

$size
[1] 14  1  2

$activationfun
[1] "sigm"

$learningrate
[1] 0.8

$momentum
[1] 0.5

$learningrate_scale
[1] 1

$hidden_dropout
[1] 0

$visible_dropout
[1] 0

$output
[1] "sigm"
```

```
> confusionMatrix(mdeep)
Cross-Validated (5 fold) Confusion Matrix

(entries are percentual average cell counts across resamples)

          Reference
Prediction  ckd notckd
    ckd     60.5   15.0
    notckd  2.0    22.5

 Accuracy (average) : 0.83
```

FIGURE 19.5 Result, parameter tuning details confusion matrix.

TABLE 19.2
Accuracy of Proposed Model (In %)

Classifiers	Features/ Components	Accuracy
SAEDNN	24 Features	**62.50**
PCA- SAEDNN	20 Components	**77.00**
PCA- SAEDNN	14 Components	**83.00**

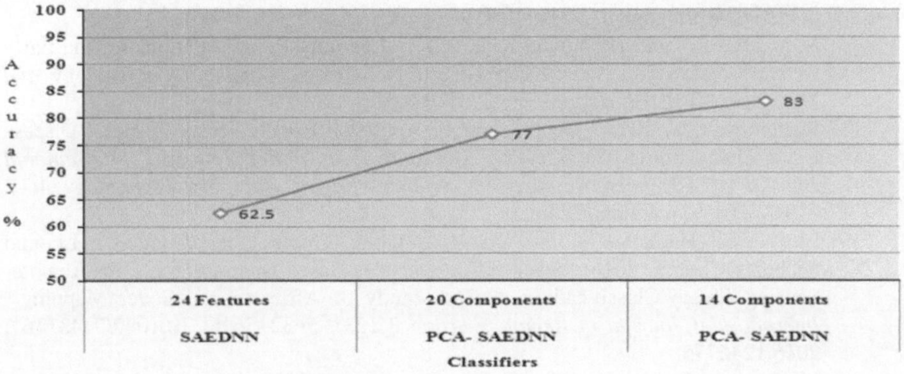

FIGURE 19.6 Comparative graph of all models.

Figure 19.6 clearly showed that the highest accuracy obtained by our proposed PCA-SAEDNN. The fourteen components are sufficient to identify the problem of CKD. Our proposed model performed impressively because of the reduction of the components of the learned perfectly.

19.4 CONCLUSION

In this chapter, SAEDNN and PCA- SAEDNN-based Deep Neural Network-based model were developed using neural network architectures for the identification and classification of CKD. Classification and conditionality reduction techniques participated an imperative role in the rapid and perfect identification of disease. The approach of the system is to use DL techniques like classification and dimensionality reduction. This proposed system can be helpful for doctors and medical professionals for identification of CKD patients. We analyzed the SAEDNN output without using PCA and verification of Auto-Encoder DNNs functionality with selected components. The accuracy of SAEDNN with PCA model was 83.00% higher with few selected components of CKD dataset.

REFERENCES

[1] Abedalkhader, Wala, and Noora Abdulrahman. 2017. "Missing Data Classification of Chronic Kidney Disease." *International Journal of Data Mining & Knowledge Management Process* 7(5/6): 55–61. 10.5121/ijdkp.2017.7604.

[2] "CKD." 2015. https://archive.ics.uci.edu/ml/datasets/Chronic_Kidney_Disease.

[3] Einasto, M., L. J. Liivamagi, E. Saar, J. Einasto, E. Tempel, E. Tago, and Martinez Vicent J. 2011. "SDSS DR7 Superclusters. Principal Component Analysis," 1–13. 10.1051/0004-6361/201117529.

[4] Fawcett, Tom. 2006. "An Introduction to ROC Analysis." *Pattern Recognition Letters* 27:861–874. 10.1016/j.patrec.2005.10.010.

[5] Han, Jiawei, Kamber Micheline, and Pei Jian. 2012. *Data Mining: Concepts and Techniques*. Third Edition. Elsevier.

[6] Jolliffe, Ian T. 2002. *Principal Component Analysis*, Second Edition. Series in Statistics, Springer. 10.1007/b98835.

[7] Kam, Hye Jin, and Ha Young Kim. 2017. "Learning Representations for the Early Detection of Sepsis with Deep Neural Networks." *Computers in Biology and Medicine*. 10.1016/j.compbiomed.2017.08.015.

[8] Karthikeyan, T. 2017. "Deep Learning Approach for Prediction of Heart Disease Using Data Mining Classification Algorithm Deep Belief Network." *International Journal of Advanced Research in Science, Engineering and Technology* 4(1): 3194–3201. www.ijarset.com.

[9] Li, Weijia, Haohuan Fu, Le Yu, Peng Gong, Duole Feng, Congcong Li, and Nicholas Clinton. 2016. "Stacked Autoencoder-Based Deep Learning for Remote-Sensing Image Classification: A Case Study of African Land-Cover Mapping." *International Journal of Remote Sensing* 37(23): 5632–5646. 10.1080/01431161.2016.1246775.

[10] Manimaran, R, and Vanitha Muthuraman. 2017. "Prediction of Diabetes Disease Using Classification Data Mining Techniques." *International Journal of Engineering and Technology* 9 (5): 3610–3614. 10.21817/ijet/2017/v9i5/170905319.

[11] Miranda, Abhilash Alexander, Yann Aël Le Borgne, and Gianluca Bontempi. 2008. "New Routes from Minimal Approximation Error to Principal Components." *Neural Processing Letters* 27 (3): 197–207. 10.1007/s11063-007-9069-2.

[12] Paul, Liton Chandra, Abdulla Al Suman, and Nahid Sultan. 2013. "Methodological Analysis of Principal Component Analysis (PCA) Method." *IJCEM International Journal of Computational Engineering & Management* ISSN 16 (2): 2230–7893. www.IJCEM.org%0Awww.IJCEM.org.

[13] Sebastian Raschka. 2015. "Principal Component Analysis." 2015. https://sebastianraschka.com/Articles/2015_pca_in_3_steps.html.

[14] Sri, Chathurdara, Pathirage Nadith, Li Jun, Li Ling, Hao Hong, Liu Wanquan, and Ni Pinghe. 2018a. "Structural Damage Identification Based on Autoencoder Neural Networks and Deep Learning." *Engineering Structures* 172 (April): 13–28. 10.1016/j.engstruct.2018.05.109.

[15] Stehman, Stephen V. 1997. "Selecting and Interpreting Measures of Thematic Classification Accuracy" 89.

[16] Subasi, Abdulhamit, Alickovic Emina, and Kevric Jasmin. 2017. "Diagnosis of Chronic Kidney Disease by Using Random Forest." *CMBEBIH 2017: Proceedings of the International Conference on Medical and Biological Engineering* (pp.589–594). 10.1007/978-981-10-4166-2_89.

[17] Tao, Chao, Pan Hongbo, Li Yansheng, and Zou Zhengrou. 2015. "Unsupervised Spectral – Spatial Feature Learning With Stacked Sparse Autoencoder for Hyperspectral Imagery Classification." *IEEE Geoscience and Remote Sensing Letters*.

[18] Verma, Pratibha, Awasthi, Vineet Kumar, and Sahu, Sanat Kumar. 2021. Classification of Coronary Artery Disease Using Deep Neural Network with Dimension Reduction Technique. In 2021 2nd International Conference for Emerging Technology (INCET) (pp. 1–5). Belgaum, India: IEEE. 10.1109/incet51464.2021.9456322.

[19] Verma, Pratibha, Vineet Kumar Awasthi, and Sanat Kumar Sahu. 2021. "A Novel Design of Classification of Coronary Artery Disease Using Deep Learning and Data Mining Algorithms." *Revue d' Intelligence Artificielle* 35 (3): 209–215.

[20] Xiao, Yawen, Jun Wu, Zongli Lin, and Xiaodong Zhao. 2017. "A Deep Learning-Based Multi-Model Ensemble Method for Cancer Prediction." *Computer Methods and Programs in Biomedicine*. 10.1016/j.cmpb.2017.09.005.

[21] Yildirim, Pinar. 2015. "Filter Based Feature Selection Methods for Prediction of Risks in Hepatitis Disease." *International Journal of Machine Learning and Computing* 5 (4): 258–263.10.7763/IJMLC.2015.V5.517.

[22] Zhang, Yudong, and Lenan Wu. 2012. "Classification of Fruits Using Computer Vision and a Multiclass Support Vector Machine." *Sensors (Switzerland)* 12 (9): 12489–12505. 10.3390/s120912489.

[23] Zhao, Rui, Ruqiang Yan, Zhenghua Chen, Kezhi Mao, Peng Wang, and Robert X Gao. 2019. "Deep Learning and Its Applications to Machine Health Monitoring." *Mechanical Systems and Signal Processing* 115: 213–237. 10.1016/j.ymssp.2018.05.050.

Index

accuracy 16, 22, 128, 137, 147, 148, 188, 352, 377
actinic keratoses 180
activation function 256
activation functions 10
active learning 197, 290
adam optimizer 255
AOI 31
artificial intelligence 47
artificial neural network 46, 59, 164, 289, 341

balanced multi-class accuracy 188
basal cell carcinoma 180
benign keratosis-like lesions 180
bland-altman analysis 129
block variance 47
blockchain technology 286
blood vessel ratio 114
brain oncology 346
breast cancer 143

carry look-ahead style 28
chemotherapy 266
CIFAR-10 11, 16
cloud computing 126
competitive learning 80
complementary learning fuzzy neural network 48
confusion matrix 56, 377
convolution 5, 6, 7
convolutional neural network 5, 16, 18, 24, 87, 88, 109, 164, 181, 182, 208, 224, 284
covid-19 313
CovXNet 312
cross entropy 372
cup to disk ratio 114

database of mastology research 47
decision tree classifier 216, 338
deep belief networks 284
deep convolutional neural network 2, 16, 18, 24
deep learning 156, 157, 198, 208, 222, 290
deep neural network 124, 126
dermatofibroma 180
diabetic retinopathy 319
dice score 229
discrete wavelet transform 48
drop out 10
drug development 265

efficiency 149
electroencephalography 84
evolutionary learning 198

f1 score 16, 22, 188, 352, 378
false negative 57, 187, 257
false negative prediction 352
false positive 57, 149, 187, 257
false positive prediction 352
feature point image 48
food & drugs administration 46
fully connected layer 10

gastric oncology 351
glaucoma 222
gradient boosting decision tree 110

health care waste management 100
hepatitis b virus 104
hopfield neural network 91, 92
human immunodeficiency virus 104, 106, 107

immunotherapy 267
inceptionresnetv2 371
instance-based learning method 206
intersection over union 229
isic 2019 challenge dataset 178, 180

k-nearest neighbor 145, 213, 288, 341

level set 109
logistic regression 212, 288, 338
lung oncology 349

magnetic resonance imaging 45, 81, 158
mammography 46
matlab 48, 59
mean absolute error 37
mean absolute relative difference 134, 137
melanocytic nevi 180
melanoma 180
MNIST 11, 12
MRI diffusion tensor imaging 158
MRI diffusion weighted imaging 158
MRI fluid-attenuated inversion recovery 158
MRI t1-weighted image 158
MRI t2-weighted image 158

MSE 117
multilayer perceptron -mlp 3, 16, 18, 24, 46
multiplier-accumulator 27

naïve bayes algorithm 144, 288, 340
naïve bayes classifier 215
neuro-retinal rim 114
Neurodegeneration 161
Neuroimaging informatics analysis center 162
nonlinear teager-kaiser filtering technique 111
oncology 346

padding 7
perceptron 84
pneumonia 307
pooling layer 9
precision 16, 22, 188, 352, 377
principal component analysis 48, 125, 343
PSNR 117

q-learning 82
quantum-speck cell automata 29

R^2 regression score 134
radial basis function network 86
random forest 145, 214, 339
raspberry pi 124
rca 28, 29
recall 16, 22, 149, 188, 378
receiver operating characteristics 58
recurrent neural network 89, 90, 284
regression 205
regularization algorithms 206
reinforcement learning 156
reinforcement learning 81, 156, 197, 205, 283, 290
relu activation function 182, 256
resnet152 371
root mean square error 137

semi-supervised learning 156, 197, 205
sensitivity 353
skin oncology 347
softmax 184
sparse code multiple access 284
specificity 188, 353
squamous cell carcinoma 180
striding 7
supervised learning 78, 79, 155, 197, 204, 283
support vector machine 145, 177, 213, 288, 337

transfer learning 185, 291
true negative 57, 187, 257
true negative prediction 352
true positive prediction 352
true-positive 57, 149, 187, 257

unsupervised learning 79, 156, 197, 205, 283, 289

vascular lesions 180
VLSI 27

Xception 185, 372